Critical Thinking in Nursing:
An Interactive Approach

Critical Thinking in Nursing:
An Interactive Approach

M. GAIE RUBENFELD, RN, MS
Assistant Professor
Department of Nursing
Eastern Michigan University
Ypsilanti, Michigan

BARBARA K. SCHEFFER, RN, MS
Assistant Professor
Department of Nursing
Eastern Michigan University
Ypsilanti, Michigan

Illustrations by Mark Steele

J. B. Lippincott Company
Philadelphia

Acquisitions Editor: Donna L. Hilton, RN, BSN
Coordinating Editorial Assistant: Susan M. Keneally
Project Editor: Karen S. Huffman
Indexer: Alberta Morrison
Design Coordinator: Doug Smock
Interior Designer: Joan Jacobus
Cover Designer: Ilene Griff
Production Manager: Helen Ewan
Production Coordinator: Nannette Winski
Compositor: The Composing Room of Michigan, Inc.
Printer/Binder: R.R. Donnelley and Sons Co./Crawfordsville
Cover Printer: Lehigh Press

6 5 4 3 2

Library of Congress Cataloging-in-Publications Data
Rubenfeld, M. Gaie.
    Critical thinking in nursing : an interactive approach / M. Gaie Rubenfeld,
  Barbara K. Scheffer ; illustrations by Mark Steele.
        p.   cm.
    Includes bibliographical references and index.
    ISBN 0-397-55099-5
    1. Nursing—Philosophy.   2. Critical thinking.   3. Nursing—Problems,
  exercises, etc.   I. Scheffer, Barbara K.   II. Title.
    [DNLM: 1. Nursing Process.   2. Thinking.   WY 100 R895c 1995]
  RT84.5.R83 1995
  610.73—dc20
  DNLM/DLC
  for Library of Congress   94-28466
                                                                          CIP

Any procedure or practice described in this book should be applied by the health-care practitioner under appropriate supervision in accordance with professional standards of care used with regard to the unique circumstances that apply in each practice situation. Care has been taken to confirm the accuracy of information presented and to describe generally accepted practices. However, the authors, editors, and publisher cannot accept any responsibility for errors or omissions or for any consequences from application of the information in this book and make no warranty express or implied, with respect to the contents of the book.

Every effort has been made to ensure drug selections and dosages are in accordance with current recommendations and practice. Because of ongoing research, changes in government regulations and the constant flow of information on drug therapy, reactions and interactions, the reader is cautioned to check the package insert for each drug for indications, dosages, warnings and precautions, particularly if the drug is new or infrequently used.

To Rich, for his love, support, and legendary wisdom, and to Jesse and Tyler, for their love and tolerance of my busy schedule.

To Kenn, for his love and encouragement and saying for the last 20 years, "You should write a book," and to Dan and Amanda, whose love and support are always there.

To our students, especially the Eastern Michigan University BSN Class of 1995 for participating in the development of the book and field testing the learning activities. Their thinking has inspired us.

▼ CONTRIBUTOR

Barbara G. Walton, RN, MS, CCRN
President, CEO
Nurse Notes Inc.
Ypsilanti, Michigan

Chapter 11

▼ REVIEWERS

Jean E. Bartels, PhD, RN
Dean, Associate Professor
School of Nursing
Alverno College
Milwaukee, Wisconsin

Margaret W. Bellak, RN, MN
Associate Professor
Indiana University of Pennsylvania
Indiana, Pennsylvania

Bette Case, PhD, RN, C
Independent Consultant
Educational Innovations for Healthcare
Chicago, Illinois

Suzanne Kusserow, RN, CS, EdD
Fulbright Senior Scholar
University of Zimbabwe
Harare, Zimbabwe
Africa

Like two gardeners who planted seeds long ago, we continue to smile with pleasure as we observe the growth and development of ideas about the *nursing process*!

Our work on the *nursing process* began in 1965. We produced the first edition of *The Nursing Process* in 1967, which culminated in four subsequent editions. The framework for the intellectual, interpersonal, and technical skills that are required for its use had been established. Many of the ideas that were presented to the listening professional public 30 years ago have been elaborated by Rubenfeld and Scheffer. With an emphasis on critical thinking, they have taken the framework of the *nursing process* including the three types of skills and have developed all of them explicitly for the nurse and for the consumer of nursing and health care. They have advanced the thinking and doing dimensions of the *nursing process* and have specified the way the consumer can experience "Great Nursing." Since the mid-60s, there have been dialogues, seminars, classes, formal, and informal discussions, as well as oral and written reactions, reports and responses to ideas about the *nursing process*. In the decade of the 70s, more intensive work about *nursing diagnosis* began. The 80s saw the incorporation of the *nursing process*, *nursing diagnosis* and *nursing theory* into daily practice. As the end of the 20th century draws near, it is obvious that the armamentarium of the nurse is more adequate than it was 30 years ago, mainly because the *nursing process* has been clearly identified and accepted as the system that defines and encompasses *nursing*.

As nursing nears the end of the third decade of relying on the *nursing process*, it is with sheer delight that we witness this production by Rubenfeld and Scheffer. They have taken the planted seed of the *nursing process* and have nurtured the growth and development of this significant idea in a way that makes the two original gardeners very proud. The focus on critical thinking places the appropriate emphasis on the *nursing process* and enables the use of intellectual, interpersonal, and technical skills to succeed in nursing.

Rubenfeld and Scheffer have described effectively how nursing has grown and developed over the past three decades. The *nursing process* continues in its traditional form with expansion of its components according to the expertise of the nurse. The use of *nursing diagnosis* has grown and developed, and its application in patient care poses a significant challenge to the nurse who strives for accuracy in defining the patient's needs. Finally, learners are encouraged to select and/or translate theoretical concepts to enable more effective use of the *nursing process* when providing nursing care. Throughout the learning activities of the nurse, the focus of the text is on thinking. Not only will the beginning student benefit from the content and experiences designed in the text, but the experienced nurses who may need to refine their thinking and recapture lost aspects in their practice of the *nursing process* will benefit as well. Most of all, the thinking and doing aspects of the *nursing process* will benefit the consumer of the *nursing process*. The text clearly shows to the consumers and their families and significant others, that great nursing is possible, desirable, and should be demanded.

Having been associated with the *nursing process* in a number of ways, over the years, this production about critical thinking by Rubenfeld and Scheffer provokes a warm, enthusiastic, excited feeling as one reads the presentations. It is a very user-friendly and learner-focused book. In no way does it "speak down" to the reader or to the learner. On the contrary, it seems to hit the level of learner for which it was meant—beginning students. The examples throughout the text are not only interesting but are so well-suited to the context of the *nursing process* and the point the authors wish to achieve that readers will have the "aha" reaction.

The authors have managed to do in this text what all teachers of nursing try to do in planning and implementing learning experiences for nursing students—build on what the student brings to the learning experience, personalize the approach to teaching and learning, enhance the self-esteem of the beginning students, and ease into the diversity of ideas and outcomes when applying the *nursing process* with well and ill consumers of nursing.

A picture is worth a thousand words and so is a good example. Consistent with the sound educational principle of moving from simple to complex learning, less complex situations are used in the early part of the book to illustrate critical thinking. The final situation that is presented as a learning opportunity is a more complex one that employs a greater number of critical thinking skills, more detailed challenges, and requirements for greater depth of knowledge.

Kudos are in order for the authors of this text, for several reasons. They present specific patient situations to illustrate how thinking can enable the use of *nursing process* when providing quality patient care. They include the use of mind-catching terms and phrases such as the Thinking-Learning Checks that make the content a realistic and intimate part of each reader/user's repertoire. The authors encourage using record diaries and logs to enhance thinking and learning. The eye-catching sketches and illustrations designed by Mark Steele make the text more meaningful. The use of selected references completes the picture of the nurse caring for and about patients in any setting through the knowledgable use of the *nursing process*. Throughout the text, students can hear the voice of the built-in mentor urging, supporting, clarifying, and commending them along the way. There are references to a multitude of resources for students that are not overwhelming. There is positive reinforcement at strategic points along the way, and there is a helpful distinction between independent and interdependent nursing practice throughout the text.

Teachers are always seeking learning materials to enable top-notch learning among students. Conscientious and concerned students maintain a vigilance for new publications that will help them improve their understranding of what is essential for their professional knowledge. A happy and joyful declaration is now being sent to teachers and to students: this is IT! This is the text, the new publication that you have been waiting for! This is the book that will make the *nursing process* an even more meaningful part of your professional life. The authors have designed a nursing text that explicates how and why "the *nursing process* is a dynamic entity of multiple processes within a larger process all working in harmony to achieve *great* nursing care." They show with compelling clarity the significance of the intellectual, interpersonal, and technical skills required to become and to be "the *great nurse*."

To those of you who have entertained dreams, ambitions, new ideas and creative ways of approaching the usual, or the well-known—here is the answer! Here is a friendly text that guides, directs, chides, and urges the reader and the learner to reach for new heights and to seek new levels of understanding. Beyond nudging the learner, direction and guidance are provided for which the novice is grateful, and the better-informed student is appreciative. Ultimately, both the novice and the better-informed learner will reap the benefits from using this text.

The legal and ethical bases of practice are inherent in all the presentations. They are portrayed as a natural expectation of critical thinking in following the *nursing process* as nursing care is provided. Lawyers, ethicists, physicians, nutritionists, and the varied health care therapists associated with the nurse and consumer can readily see what it takes to achieve great nursing (in contrast to "okay" nursing or "good enough" nursing).

As old-timers in the business of *nursing process*, we have relied heavily on components of this orderly system of nursing for many years. As users of this text peruse its printed pages, it will become evident that Rubenfeld and Scheffer are comfortable and well-acquainted with the *nursing process*. This book is evidence that they are valuable teachers who have respect and concern for the learner, and have a ready grasp of what the nursing students need in order to provide nursing. Their presentation communicates a respect for learners, as well as a warmth and genuine concern for people—whether student, colleague, or patient. Most of all, they exemplify a true belief in the essential nature of the *nursing process* and an understanding of the merits of the *nursing process* in the care of patients.

Helen Yura-Petro
Mary B. Walsh

▼ PREFACE

This is not a typical textbook. It is an active learning book designed to help beginning students of nursing develop the thinking skills necessary to provide great care. If you, the reader and user of this book, are used to passively reading with no writing implement in your hand, you will find this book to be a change of scene. If you are a margin-scribbler, you will appreciate that there is more than the usual margin space to write as you read.

▶ CONTENT FOCUS OF THE BOOK

This book focuses on critical thinking as it is used with the nursing process. Because critical thinking is often defined in many ways, clarification of this concept is important. Critical thinking is sometimes defined narrowly as inquiry, which is a questioning approach to issues. However, a broader definition, one used by Richard Paul, is advocated here:

"The art of thinking about your thinking while you are thinking in order to make your thinking better: more clear, more accurate, or more defensible" (Paul, 1992, p. 643).

In the spirit of this definition, thinking is conceptualized into five modes which, collectively, represent the broad definition of critical thinking. The five modes, "Total Recall," "Habits," "Inquiry," "New Ideas and Creativity," and "Knowing How You Think," are explored from both a personal and nursing perspective. The readers are helped to build on their existing thinking styles to incorporate the nursing focus.

The nursing process is presented in its traditional four-part format of assessing, planning, implementing, and evaluating as described by Yura and Walsh (1988). Specific discussions of nursing diagnoses as part of the nursing process follow the guidelines of the North American Nursing Diagnosis Association (NANDA, 1992). To keep the content of this book applicable to the majority of potential users, no specific theoretical framework of nursing is advocated. While the classic nursing process and nursing diagnosis approaches are usable with any theoretical framework, some users of this book may want to translate specific terminology to their theoretical language for ease of student learning.

Because this book is intended for use by beginning students, most of the nursing situations in early chapters, while "real," are not overly complex. The nursing knowledge needed to understand the situations is commonly learned early in nursing programs. At the same time, as students progress through the book, their knowledge will be increasing; therefore, in the last section of the book, a more complex case study is used as a learning opportunity.

▶ STRUCTURE OF THE BOOK

This book is divided into four parts and sixteen chapters. Part I provides an overview of thinking, doing, and the nursing process. Part II provides details of the nursing process, with a focus on the thinking that occurs while using the nursing process. Part III focuses on communicating the thinking and the nursing process. Part IV pulls all of the book's content back together and, using a complex patient situation, applies the thinking concepts.

While there is a building of content throughout the book, readers who so desire can feel free to study Part IV, or any part before the others. Each person's brain works in unique ways. Learning occurs best when those natural tendencies are not stifled.

Each chapter begins with *learning outcomes* which provide direction for the reader. The outcomes can be used as a learning check at the end of each chapter. If the reader can meet those outcomes, then the desired learning has occurred.

This book has a combination of information to read and **Action Learning** exercises to complete. The exercises are numbered consecutively throughout the book. Action Learning exercises provide a way for the reader to use several senses as they learn. Multi-sensory learning increases retention of information because more of the brain's capacity is used.

Following each Action Learning exercise is a discussion section. The questions and issues raised can be used for class discussions or as a stimulus for additional thinking.

Because of the unique nature of this book, especially when Action Learning exercises are introduced, there are frequent uses of the word "you." In those places the reader is asked to relate what is being said to a personal perspective.

Another learning enhancer is the use of mnemonics. These are phrases or abbreviations that are easy to remember. Mnemonic devices trigger the brain's memory programs and allow a learner to retain large sets of information more easily. An example of mnemonic devices used throughout the book is the word "T.H.I.N.K.," which represents the five modes of thinking used in nursing.

Each chapter also has periodic **Thinking-Learning Checks**. These are summaries of information presented to that point. Frequent reviews help to check and clarify learning and enhance retention of information. They also give one's brain a chance to sort the new information and plug it into relevant places for future use. They are used more in early chapters where new information is presented. Later chapters that focus on application of previously learned material have fewer Thinking-Learning Checks.

Similar to Thinking-Learning Checks are the **"Thinking Logs"** at the end of each chapter. These logs are designed for learners to keep a diary of thinking. Specific instructions for each thinking log give direction for what should be included. The reader should not feel held back by the directions, however; if something is discovered about personal thinking, each person should feel free to add it to the log. At the end of the book, each learner should be able to go back and see how personal thinking has evolved.

▶ LAST MINUTE REMARKS TO USERS OF THIS BOOK

It is the authors' intent in this book to help you to recognize your existing thinking skills, to build on your current thinking skills, and to enhance your skills so you can apply them to nursing situations. Throughout all the chapters you will be consistently reading, thinking, and doing to achieve this goal. Grab a pen or pencil, find a comfortable place to study and begin this exciting journey into your mind and into great nursing.

REFERENCES

Paul, R. (1992). *Critical thinking: What every person needs to survive in a rapidly changing world* (2nd ed.). Santa Rosa, CA: Foundation for Critical Thinking.

North American Nursing Diagnosis Association (1992). *NANDA nursing diagnoses: Definitions and classification 1992*. Philadelphia: NANDA.

Yura, N. & Walsh, M. B. (1988). *The nursing process: Assessing, planning, implementing, evaluating* (5th ed.). Norwalk, CT: Appleton & Lange.

▼ ACKNOWLEDGMENTS

Many people have been supportive of our efforts on this project. We particularly want to acknowledge our colleagues at Eastern Michigan University who supported our joint sabbatical leave proposals: Dr. Betty Beard, Provost Ron Collins, Dean Elizabeth King, Dr. Regina Williams, Dr. Judy Williston, and Dr. Lorraine Wilson; Dr. Bob Kraft, in addition to supporting our sabbatical leave, provided constant encouragement and outstanding writing workshops and Dr. Georgia Langer gave excellent guidance in effective teaching methodologies. Our gratitude extends beyond EMU to Dr. Marjory Gordon, Dr. Cathy Guzzetta, and Dr. Elizabeth McFarlane, who strongly encouraged our efforts, and to Professor Mary Walsh, whose mentorship planted the seeds for this project over a decade ago. We would also like to express our gratitude to Helen Yura, whose work with Walsh was the original inspiration for this project. We are grateful to Mark Steele for his ability to capture the quintessential meaning of concepts in his illustrations. Conversations with Barbara Morris have provided invaluable learning opportunities. To the "goils," Sue, Sharon, and Chuckie, a big thanks for caring and sharing. We appreciate our dedicated friends, Jane Duerr and Constance Bond, who offered editorial advice and freely assisted with last-minute detail work. We extend a special thanks to the staff at J. B. Lippincott, especially Susan Keneally, Editorial Assistant, for keeping us on track; Karen Huffman, Project Editor, for her attention to details; and, most of all, Donna Hilton, Executive Editor, for her insights and for patiently nurturing us throughout this publishing process. Finally, we offer a huge thanks to our families—Rich, Jesse, Tyler, Kenn, Dan, Amanda, Tosha, Tarzan, Popcorn, and Talon—who have functioned well and supported us in the midst of our preoccupation with this project.

▼ CONTENTS

Part III Communicating Thinking and the Nursing Process

Chapter 10 Written and Verbal Communication of Thinking and Doing

Chapter 11 Consequences of Thinking and Not Thinking When Documenting

Part IV Thinking Through a Complex Patient Situation

Chapter 14   Designing, Doing and Determining Quality of Care for Potential (High Risk) Problems   *311*

Chapter 15   Designing, Doing, and Determining Quality of Care for Wellness Diagnoses, Interdisciplinary Problems, and Problems for Referral   *329*

Chapter 16   Thinking Into the Future: From Linear Equation to a Paradigm of Great Nursing   *345*

Critical Thinking in Nursing:
An Interactive Approach

Overview of Thinking, Doing, and the Nursing Process

Thinking

Here's a new approach to reading a book—start by drawing a picture!

> ▶▶▶▶▶▶ **Action Learning #1: Draw Your Thinking Cap**

Before you read anything, consider how you think right now. Draw a picture of your personal "Thinking Cap." Get something to draw with and be adventurous!

Pretend you have your thinking cap on. Describe in a sentence or two how you *feel* when you are thinking.

Explain your thinking cap drawing to a classmate.

DISCUSSION Now, why do you **think** you were asked to do these three things at the beginning of the book—draw your personal thinking cap, describe your **feelings** when **thinking**, and explain the picture? Here are some reasons. How do they compare with your reasons?

> ▼ Having a picture and written description provides a concrete re-
>   minder of how you think today. Periodically, you can return to your
>   drawing and description to see if or when your thinking has
>   changed.
>
> ▼ Some people process and understand information best when they
>   see it. They are visual learners, and drawing pictures helps them
>   process information visually.
>
> ▼ Some people process and understand information best when they
>   hear it. They are auditory learners, and speaking and listening help
>   them process information.
>
> ▼ Processing and understanding information is a key part of thinking.
>
> ▼ How you feel has a strong influence on how you think.
>
> ▼ Feedback from another person can help clarify your thoughts.

LEARNING OUTCOMES

After reading and doing the exercises in this chapter you will be able to:

Classify ways of thinking.

Explore obstacles to your thinking.

Identify what makes your thinking unique.

Examine the impact of thinking on learning and the practice of
nursing.

Embrace new ways of thinking about your thinking.

▶ WAYS OF THINKING

Based on the above activity with your thinking cap, what conclusion have you
drawn about your style of processing information? Are you auditory? Are you
visual? Are you both? Are you neither? What does this all mean? It means that
people are not alike in the way they process information, nor are they alike in
the way they think about the information; it is not easy to categorize human
processes like thinking into neat boxes.

Thinking is not a static process; it may change daily or even hourly. Because *thinking* is so dynamic (constantly changing) and because all nursing actions require thinking, it is important to understand *thinking* in general. It is
also important to figure out one's own unique styles and patterns and to identify what helps one *think* better.

In the 10 minutes before you began reading this text, you might have
thought, "Should I read now or watch TV?" "Should I lie on the bed or sit in the
chair?" "Should I use a highlighter or just read?" For each of those questions

you thought of an answer. How did you think of that answer? Did you recall a teacher telling you that it improves concentration if you sit at a desk? Are you lying on the bed because you always lie on the bed when you study? Did you consider all of your options and think about their pros and cons before choosing your mode of studying?

Each of these options or their combinations required different modes of thinking. You may have relied on past habits or approached the studying situation as a problem to solve. Perhaps you decided to do something new or different such as reading while you pedalled your exercise bicycle and listened to music. Just about everything you do requires some thinking, but not all thinking is the same. If you are like most people, you have not spent lots of time thinking about the different ways of thinking. You may not even think such delving is important.

▷ Classification of Thinking Modes

Many classifications of thinking can be found in the literature, especially in the field of education. One example is the system used by Costa and colleagues (1985), "The Six Rs"—remembering, repeating, reasoning, reorganizing, relating, and reflecting. Although the six Rs are useful, thinking styles used in nursing are better represented by a slightly different, five-mode classification system. The five modes are TOTAL RECALL, HABITS, INQUIRY, NEW IDEAS AND CREATIVITY, and KNOWING HOW YOU THINK. To help remember the five modes for nursing in this book, each letter of the word *think* is used to represent a mode. T.H.I.N.K., therefore, becomes a mnemonic device, a catchy word or phrase to help remember something important. (Authors' note: mnemonic devices are used several times in this book to enhance the readers' retention of important information. You may recall other mnemonic devices that you have used before, such as the saying that goes with the twelve cranial nerves: "On Old Olympus' Towering Top, A Frog And Groundhog Vaulted A Hedge.")

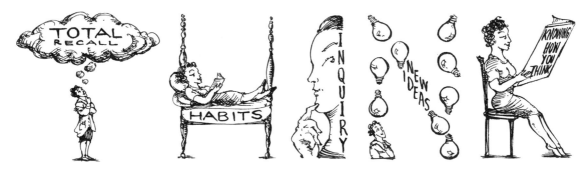

Figure 1-1.   Modes of T.H.I.N.K.

DISPLAY 1-1. Five Modes of Thinking

T = Total Recall
H = Habits
I = Inquiry
N = New Ideas and Creativity
K = Knowing How You Think

The best thinkers, certainly the best nurses, are able to use all of these modes all of the time. The phrase "all of the time" is purposefully used to show that these modes are not used individually so much as in combination with each other. As you will discover, nursing has few aspects that fit into clearly delineated, mutually exclusive categories. T.H.I.N.K. is no exception to that rule. The goal of this book is to help you use all of these modes well. You already use some very well; others probably could use some polish. To start, examine each mode individually, keeping in mind that each one is rarely used alone.

▷ Total Recall (T)

Total recall means remembering facts, such as the date the Crimean War ended, normal values for hematocrit, who Florence Nightingale was, the second disassociation constant of maleic acid, the Krebs cycle, and so on. These are important things. Nurses use TOTAL RECALL by either remembering the facts or remembering where to look for them.

How total one's recall is depends on memory. Memory is a complex process. Some people can remember many seemingly isolated facts effortlessly; others struggle. If you are a struggler, don't despair. There are ways to help you remember. Putting facts into patterns is one way. The T.H.I.N.K. mnemonic is an example—a pattern to help you remember the five modes of thinking. Often, however, patterns are not quite so obvious. You have to make or find the patterns in your brain and use them. Look at this set of numbers: 5555068527. Now, look at the same set written this way: (555) 506-8527. As you can see, it is a telephone number. The numbers are easier to remember because there is a familiar pattern to them. Look at another list. See if you can remember this after reading it: car, train, fork, orange, plate, apple, spoon, airplane, cup, banana, bicycle, watermelon. Now look at the same list arranged in a pattern. There are four items in each of three categories.

car	**fork**	**orange**
train	**plate**	**apple**
airplane	**spoon**	**banana**
bicycle	**cup**	**watermelon**

The way people receive information also affects their ability to recognize patterns. Test this out with a friend. Create a list of items that you know can be categorized, mix up the items, and read them to a friend to see if he or she can remember them. Then show the friend the written words in the order that you originally read them and see if he or she can remember them. Which way was easier? Could the friend recognize the patterns more quickly when hearing or when seeing? Have the friend do the same for you. Learn how your mind processes information to get it into your memory. The experience will also give you some clues on how to study and learn the mountains of "facts" you need to remember in nursing school.

Another process for remembering is the association of a fact with some experience. Most forty-ish people can remember exactly what they were doing the day President John Kennedy was shot. Other associations may be less dramatic. You may remember something you heard in a lecture because the teacher supported the fact with a funny story. You may remember something else because you had to perform some action to or with it. For example, if someone told you how to use jumper cables to start your car, you might remember it. But you would remember it better if you actually got stuck and had to jump start your car with cables.

▶▶▶▶▶▶ **Action Learning #2: Can You Remember?**

Answer the following TOTAL RECALL Questions:

What is your social security number?

What is a normal oral body temperature?

How many days are in September?

What medications would a physician most likely request rapidly during a cardiac arrest?

DISCUSSION Which of the answers do you know instantly? Which are OK to take the time to look up? How do you memorize information? How many facts can you memorize? What patterns do you use to increase your memory ability?

▷ **Habits (H)**

Habits are accepted ways of doing things that work, save time, or are necessary. They are thinking approaches that are repeated so often they become second nature. Habits allow one to do things without having to figure out a new method each time. Riding a bicycle or driving a car are habits for people doing them on a regular basis. Have you ever driven several miles and then realized you could not remember what you saw or what streets you passed? Hopefully, you did not cause any accidents as you got from point A to point B with no recollection of the trip. You could do this "mindless" driving because you had already mastered the basic mechanics of driving and could do it without conscious effort. (This *is not* a recommended way of driving a car, but it does demonstrate how habits work.)

Cardiopulmonary resuscitation (CPR) is a very useful habit in nursing. When someone is lying at your feet looking dead, there is no time to come up with a creative way to bring him or her back to life. A quick solution is needed here. Nursing has many other procedures comparable to CPR—the proper way to give an injection, take a temperature, insert a catheter, and many more such activities. When these actions are first learned, they obviously are not yet habits, but as they are used repeatedly, they become second nature; they become habits. You will appreciate how many of these habits will be formed by the time you graduate.

▶▶▶▶▶▶ **Action Learning #3: Your Personal Habits**

Identify three things in your life that you would call habits.

DISCUSSION   How did these things become habits? Why are these activities useful? What is the best way for *you* to develop habits?

▷ Inquiry (I)

Inquiry means examining issues in depth and questioning that which may seem immediately obvious. It is sometimes called critical thinking, however, this text defines critical thinking as a collective of Inquiry and the other four modes. Inquiry is the primary kind of thinking used to reach conclusions. Conclusions can be reached without using inquiry, but conclusions are better (more accurate) if inquiry is used. For example, one day, while sitting at her desk, Sue glanced up at the window and saw that it was wet. Her immediate conclusion was, "It's raining and I won't be able to go to the beach when I'm done studying." On a closer look, Sue saw that there was no water on the grass; the sun was shining; there were no clouds, and there was a ladder visible on the side of the window. Sue really wanted it to be sunny because she wanted to go to the beach after she finished her studying, so she stopped for a moment to make sure her mind was not playing tricks. She considered that a lawn sprinkler might be spraying the window. She stood up to look at a different angle and there was a window washer on the ladder with a squeegee. Relieved, Sue came to the most accurate conclusion—the windows were being washed.

In this story, Sue used inquiry when she did the following:

▼ saw something (received information)

▼ came to an immediate conclusion

▼ collected additional information to rule in or rule out the first idea (immediate conclusion)

▼ compared new information to what was already known about situations like this by using past experience

▼ questioned any biases

▼ considered one or more alternative conclusions, and

▼ validated the original or the alternative conclusion

This process of collecting and analyzing information to confirm or to make additional conclusions beyond the obvious ones is the essence of inquiry.

In this window-washer situation, the final conclusion is probably quite accurate and fairly simple. Obviously, not all situations in nursing are quite this simple. Most situations in nursing practice require inquiry. Sometimes a single validated conclusion emerges; at other times, several conclusions may seem equally valid. In those cases, the nurse needs to repeat the inquiry until the one conclusion that is *most accurate* is found. This sounds very time consuming, and sometimes it is, but in most cases the process occurs in microseconds, especially for experienced nurses. Many textbooks refer to this process when they describe diagnostic reasoning. In Chapters 5–8 you will see why this thinking is used for diagnostic reasoning.

Examine this example of a fairly simple nursing situation:

It's 3 AM in the hospital and Ms. Avon, the nurse, sees a patient's overhead room light on.

She walks into the room and says, "Hi, Mr. Trent, I noticed your light on. How are you doing?"

The patient smiles and says, "I'm fine."

The nurse observes that there are wads of used tissues on the floor; the sheets are all twisted; Mr. Trent's eyes are puffy and red.

Inquiry is called for here. The nurse must make a preliminary conclusion about something that is not readily apparent. The patient is smiling and saying nothing is wrong. Would Ms. Avon accept his response and conclude he is fine? Not if she was using Inquiry. She would have to put several pieces of information together to make some sense out of the situation. She would recognize that there may be no simple answer, but several possible conclusions.

Using inquiry allows Ms. Avon to consider at least the following four conclusions:

▼ The patient is fine, is normally awake at this hour, and may have been rubbing his eyes because of his allergies.

▼ The patient is fine but can't sleep because he napped all day because of boredom. His eyes are always red and puffy.

▼ The patient is not fine but doesn't want to talk about it or bother anyone.

▼ The patient is not fine but doesn't know how to ask for help.

To say with any degree of certainty that one of these four conclusions is better than the others, the nurse needs to validate her conclusion, to put together as much information as possible, and to ask Mr. Trent directly if he agrees with the final conclusion. (She might say, "Mr. Trent, you said you were fine, but it seems to me you might be upset.") To get the necessary information, the nurse must ask questions and observe reactions and the surroundings. She would need to analyze the information by looking for patterns and determining what was significant. Determining significance is dependent upon the nurse's ability to think about how the information about the patient compares to the nursing content knowledge she has learned.

Note that the content knowledge (Total Recall thinking) is not enough. A nice, neat package or "answer" to many real world situations cannot always be found in a book. Books help nurses see patterns by providing factual information, such as usual behavior patterns or the appearance of eyes, but the nurse has to put that information together with the information found in each unique situation. Books describe the *usual* ways to interpret information and the *usual* rules, but not everyone or every situation fits into these usual patterns (norms). For example, most people are asleep at 3 AM, but not all; most people's eyes are not red and puffy, but some people's eyes are. You have to use inquiry to collect key information and put the pieces together in meaningful patterns. No books can do this for you.

Based on the descriptions of inquiry thus far, how would you judge your present ability to use inquiry on a scale of 0 to 10, with 10 being outstanding? Be sure to write this number down so you can compare it to your inquiry ability at the end of the book.

My ability to use Inquiry on _____
                                (date)

0---1---2---3---4---5---6---7---8---9---10
(poor)   (outstanding)

Compare your answer to that of a classmate. Is there a difference? Talk about the reasons behind each of your decisions and about your inquiry skills.

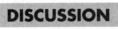 **A**ction Learning #4: Inquiry into Bertha's Body

Answer the following questions about Bertha and then compare your answers to those of a classmate. Bertha is a 31-year-old woman who is 5'2". She recently gained weight and weighs 150 pounds. She is wearing a baggy sweatsuit.

What conclusions are most obvious?

What are your biases about weight? Women? People who wear baggy sweat suits? People named Bertha? Thirty-one-year-old women?

What are some less-obvious possible conclusions?

What information would you need to validate your conclusions?

DISCUSSION Do you think you thought of all the possible answers to these questions? When you compare your answers to those of a classmate, do you find many differences?

(Authors' note: You will be asked to share your work with a classmate many times. The purpose of this sharing is NOT to see if one of you did better than the other, *but* to start a lifelong process of collaboration with peers. Peer *thinking* is a valuable resource that frequently gets ignored in the nursing profession.)

▷ New Ideas and Creativity (N)

New ideas and creativity comprise a thinking mode that is very special to you. This individualized thinking goes beyond the usual to reconfigure the norm. Like inquiry, this mode allows you to go beyond textbook ideas. Creative thinking is at the opposite end of the spectrum from the HABIT mode. Instead of saying, "This is the way things have always been done," the creative thinker says, "Let's try this new way." Creative thinking is not for the faint-hearted; one must be willing to risk looking foolish occasionally and not fitting the mold. A creative thinker appreciates mistakes for their learning value. (This can be uncomfortable if you have been told all your life to avoid mistakes.) Chances are, if you are like most people, you have not been encouraged to be creative to the point of being "different from the rest of the crowd"; however, everybody is creative under certain circumstances.

New ideas and creativity are very important in nursing because they are at the root of individualized care. Many things nurses learn have to be mixed, matched, and reworked to fit each unique patient situation. Nursing has many standard approaches to care that save time and generally work well, but they do not work the same way for everyone. Take for example, Ethel (not her real name), who lived in a nursing home and spent her days wheeling her wheelchair up and down and up and down the same hall. She spoke to no one in spite of repeated verbal prompting by very caring nurses who knew the importance of communication.

When thinking of communication, most people think of talking to somebody; that is the standard way to encourage people to communicate. So that is what most nurses did, except for Maria (her real name). One day Maria knelt down next to Ethel's wheelchair, gave her a big hug, looked Ethel straight in the eye and, with a big smile, said, "Let's sing." Guess what happened? Ethel sang. Not only could she sing, but she had the voice of an Irish folk singer.

Now what is the thinking lesson in this story? Other nurses knew recipes (standards) for therapeutic communication that they learned in the textbooks. They used them with the best intentions. Standard verbal approaches to therapeutic communication work with most patients. Maria, however, expanded the definition of communication to include singing and touching, thus creating an individualized approach for Ethel that was not in any textbook.

From that point on, Ethel always responded to Maria by smiling. She even gave one- or two-word responses to Maria's questions and, on occasion, sang with the other nurses. One small, creative approach that individualizes care often has a way of mushrooming into bigger and better things.

▶▶▶▶▶ **A**ction Learning #5: Your New Ideas and Creativity

Describe a situation in which you were creative or had a new idea. (It doesn't have to be related to nursing.)

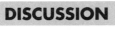

DISCUSSION How did you feel when you were creative or had a new idea? How many times a day are you creative? How many times a week? A month?

▷ **Knowing How You Think (K)**

Knowing how you think, the last, but not the least, of the T.H.I.N.K. modes, means thinking about one's thinking. Thinking about thinking is called "meta-cognition," a word composed of the prefix, "meta," which means "among or in the midst of," and "cognition," which means "the process of knowing." If you get in the midst of your process of knowing, you will get to know how you think.

▶▶▶▶▶ **A**ction Learning #6: How You Think

Write down and explain to someone how you think. Be careful to focus on *how* you think, not what you think.

| **DISCUSSION** | Was this difficult to do? (It is for most people.) Why do you think it is hard to do? One reason why it is difficult is |

that a special vocabulary of analytical terms is needed to describe HOW one thinks. Typically, few people (except for philosophers and some teachers) routinely learn or use such a vocabulary.

Display 1-2 provides a vocabulary useful in describing how one thinks. As you think about your thinking, you may use these words as cues. Ask yourself, for example, what *assumptions* you tend to make, what your *point of view* and *biases* are, and how you *elaborate* on ideas. Think about what *evidence* means to you and how you deal with *contradictions*. Continue in this way until you have considered all the words on the list.

DISPLAY 1-2. Vocabulary for Thinking About Thinking

Ambiguous (ambiguity): unclear, having multiple meanings

Assume (assumption): take for granted

Bias: a neutral, negative, or positive inclination

Conclude (conclusion): make a judgment or decision based on reasoning

Contradict (contradiction): state an opposing view, deny

Credible (credibility): worthy of belief or trust

Distinguish: recognize plainly by the senses; to separate and classify

Elaborate (elaboration): expand on

Evidence: data that support conclusions

Infer (inference): a strong or weak, justified or unjustified conclusion based on information and assumptions

Interpret (interpretation): explain the meaning of, make understandable

Justify (justification): to show to be just, right, or in accord with reason

Point of view: perspective; one's personal way of looking at the world based on background and experiences

Relevance: importance, significant relationship

Validate (validation): to verify; to search for evidence to support a conclusion

---

▶▶▶▶▶ Action Learning #7: Metacognition Check

Look over the vocabulary in Display 1-2 and write down the five terms you use most of the time. Then write out three that you want to use more often. Pay attention over the next week to how much you use the terms. Share this with a classmate.

THINKING VOCABULARY THAT I:

Use Now   Want To Use More Often

DISCUSSION It probably seems artificial at first to use these terms. But, when you talked with your classmate who was using similar words, did the strangeness decrease? Learning the language of a new profession is much like learning a foreign language—pretty soon you are comfortable with new words.

Before reading further, it is time for a quick summary. One of the best ways to learn is to break things into manageable parts and review them periodically before adding more information. Quite a bit of information has been presented in this chapter, so this is a good time for a thinking-learning check.

▼ THINKING-LEARNING CHECK

You should be able to elaborate on these ideas:

- ▼ Classification of modes of thinking as T.H.I.N.K.
- ▼ Why mnemonic devices such as T.H.I.N.K. help you think
- ▼ Details of each part of T.H.I.N.K.: TOTAL RECALL, HABITS, INQUIRY, NEW IDEAS AND CREATIVITY, KNOWING HOW YOU THINK
- ▼ Using the Action Learning exercises to increase understanding and retention of the ideas
- ▼ Using the best words to describe how you think

The reading and activities so far have introduced the five modes of thinking and expanded upon each mode separately. In the real world, all five modes need to be used together. To achieve this unified thinking, it is useful to explore some of the obstacles to thinking as well as factors that make each person's thinking unique.

▶ OBSTACLES TO HIGH-QUALITY THINKING
▷ Habits and Ruts

One of the biggest obstacles to *thinking* is getting into a rut, and the most common way of getting into a rut is to overuse the HABIT mode. Novices do not have many nursing habits, but they develop them quickly. Habits provide security and comfort, so they have definite value. Nurses need habits. Beginning nurses need to follow recipes at first to provide safe, basic nursing care; otherwise they are a menace to patients.

Problems occur, however, when nurses stop *thinking* after they have developed some comfortable, secure, and safe habits of patient care. Habits not only feel good, they discourage the use of inquiry and new ideas. One needs to be a risk-taker to *think* beyond habits. How would you rate yourself in the risk-taking area? (Authors' note: risk-taking here is not the bungee-jumping sort; rather, it is being willing to question what one reads and hears, even if it comes from "authority." Questioning expands one's awareness and solidifies new knowledge. One risk of questioning is that it can be interpreted as defiance. Defiance is focused on the power of authority figures rather than on the information being imparted by those sources. Focusing on the issues instead of the source of information decreases the risk of misinterpretation.)

Nurses care for patients who do not fit the textbook recipe as closely as books say they will. When that happens, it is necessary to use other modes of thinking to find the alternative explanations and creative interventions. This is called individualization. Imagine yourself as the patient. You would not want a nurse who approaches you only with habits and recipes, and presumes you are exactly like everybody else in the book.

▷ Anxiety

The second-largest obstacle to high-quality thinking is anxiety. Increased anxiety turns down the burner on *thinking* and severely limits the I, N, and K modes. When starting a new field of study as you have, one of the strongest feelings you experience is high-level anxiety. Everything is new—new words, new experiences, new language, new books, new pressures. Nursing as a new experience is probably scarier than other new experiences because nurses deal with life and illness situations. Anxiety decreases one's thinking abilities, even about simple things, like talking. Imagine what it does to higher-order thinking, like learning and problem solving. Learning and problem solving comprise 90% of nurse-thinking, so it is worthwhile to find ways to decrease anxiety so that you can think more efficiently.

▶ THINGS THAT MAKE YOUR THINKING UNIQUE

Each of you is unique and special and brings different feelings, backgrounds, and ideas to thinking. Below are just a few key factors that make your thinking special.

▷ Consistency

In the ideal world, nurses would switch on their *thinking* skills, turn up the power to high, and always (consistently) be great thinkers. In the real world, however, many things interfere with consistent thinking. Food, beverages, room temperature, lighting, clothing, energy levels, sleep deprivation, illness, and many other factors create thinking peaks and valleys. Timing also affects consistency. Sometimes thinkers are "sharp as a tack"; other times they are "dense as a fog." It is important to recognize the inconsistencies in your thinking, be aware of what helps and what hinders you, and maximize your best thinking times.

▷ Organization

Would you describe your thinking as neatly ordered or organized chaos? What one person believes to be organized may seem to be disorganized to another person. The important thing is to find the organizational patterns that work best for you. Some people need lists; others need sticky notes pasted everywhere; still others just store things mentally. Identify your style and work to improve it for you.

▷ Memory

How is your memory? Can you remember isolated facts? Do you associate new ideas with things you already know? Do you need some peak experience to remember something? How long do you remember something that you do not use regularly? Do you use memory aids like writing notes on your hand? (You may want to reread the earlier discussion of memory in this chapter.)

▷ Feelings

Feelings, or emotions, are usually identified in one word: mad, sad, glad, happy, frustrated, confused, angry, elated, scared, anxious, and so forth. Feelings are a part of life; they cannot and should not be ignored. But you can learn to recognize them. You can realize how they affect your thinking and develop ways to modify the circumstances that contribute to the feelings.

▷ Intuition

This is your sixth sense, your "gut feeling." It is what occurs when you say to yourself, "I can't put my finger on it, but I know something is wrong." For years, the nursing profession discouraged the notion of intuition, saying it was not scientific and could not be proven. Well, it still cannot be "proven," but it is no longer ignored. Researchers (eg, Benner, 1984; Benner & Tanner, 1987) have found that experts rely on intuition a great deal at times, and frequently are right on target. Beginners also have intuition in varying degrees. Some are very tuned-in to their sixth sense; others need to nurture it for a while. What is important for beginners is to verbalize their thoughts to someone more expert and look for evidence to support their intuition before acting on it.

▷ Experience

How much experience (combination of knowledge, understanding, and active participation) do you have? Your experience in nursing may be minimal, but you have had life experiences in which you interacted with individuals, families, and groups. Life experience is a valuable asset in learning nursing. For each life event, coping skills are developed that can be shared with others. Experience in nursing is a key ingredient in moving from a beginner to an expert. The combination of your unique life experience and nursing experience gives you your individual style as you practice the art of nursing.

▷ Self-Perception of Intelligence

Do you think you are smart or of average intelligence? Do you catch on to things quickly or do you mull them over? When you make statements, do they tend to be sure things or do you leave yourself open for other possible answers? Are you a fast or a more meditative thinker? Do you get personal or outside affirmation when you think, or are you put down for not conforming? Answers to these questions indicate how you feel about your cognitive abilities. In general, with the exception of close-minded egotists, the brighter you think you are, the better you use all your *thinking* modes, and the more willing you are to grow in your thinking. It is very important for you to value your abilities, no matter how different they are from those of someone else.

▶▶▶▶▶▶ **Action Learning #8: What Makes Your Thinking Unique?**

Think back on the last month and recall a situation that required a great deal of thought. Briefly describe how each of the factors discussed above (consistency, organization, memory, feelings, intuition, experience, and self-perception of intelligence) affected the outcome of your thinking. Share your descriptions with a classmate.

DISCUSSION How were your influencing factors different from your classmate's? Were you comfortable with those differences? How were they similar? You can see from this Action Learning that, although the categories of influencing factors are somewhat the same for everyone, they can be defined and experienced very individually.

▶ CLOSING COMMENTS

Hopefully, you now have an appreciation for the complexities and challenges of *thinking*. This chapter has addressed some everyday situations and some nursing situations in which the various modes of thinking were used. The purpose of this was to show you how your existing thinking skills can be further developed and used in nursing. Everything nurses do requires one or a combination of the five modes of thinking.

The exercises in this chapter and throughout the book will help you see how you can use all of T.H.I.N.K., not just the "T" and the "H." To nurture your growing awareness of your thinking styles and abilities, you will be talking and writing about your thinking on a regular basis throughout this book (and, we hope, for the rest of your life.) At the end of each chapter, you will be writing in your personal "Thinking Log," which is a sort of diary about thinking. It is best to get a notebook that you use just for thinking logs.

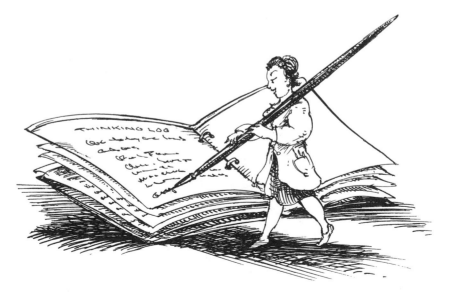

Figure 1-2. Thinking Log.

▶▶▶ *THINKING LOG #1*

This log will be a final Thinking-Learning Check for Chapter 1. Briefly describe what you learned about each of the chapter's Learning Outcomes:

1. Classify ways of thinking.
2. Explore obstacles to your thinking.
3. Identify what makes your thinking unique.
4. Examine the impact of thinking on learning and the practice of nursing.
5. Embrace new ways of thinking about your thinking.

REFERENCES

Benner, P. (1984). *From novice to expert: Power and excellence in nursing practice*. Menlo Park, CA: Addison-Wesley.

Benner, P. & Tanner, C. (1987). Clinical judgement: How expert nurses use intuition. *American Journal of Nursing, 87*, 23–31.

Costa, A. L., Hanson, R., Silver, H. F., & Strong, R. W. (1985). Building a repertoire of strategies. In A. L. Costa (Ed.), *Developing minds: A resource book for teaching thinking* (pp. 141–143). Alexandria, VA: Association for Supervision and Curriculum Development.

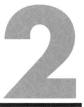

Doing

This chapter and all the rest begin with Learning Outcomes, which provide direction for learning.

LEARNING OUTCOMES

After reading and doing the activities in this chapter you will be able to:

Describe what nurses *do*.

Examine the factors that affect *doing*.

Begin to appreciate how *thinking* and *doing* are intertwined.

▶ DOING IN NURSING

Doing and *thinking* are inseparable in great nursing care, but, for now, some concentration on the *doing* alone is helpful. Knowing what one is supposed to *do* as a nurse will help to clarify *learning how* to *do* it. Learning the *how* before developing an appreciation of the broader perspective of what nurses *do* promotes a reliance on TOTAL RECALL and HABIT modes of thinking. A learner might mimic the steps while learning *how* to *do* nursing, but would not appreciate how each nursing activity fits into the complex picture of great nursing.

If learners know where they are going (what nurses *do*), they will have a better chance of engaging other *thinking* modes (INQUIRY, NEW IDEAS AND CREATIVITY, and KNOWING HOW YOU THINK) along the way. This will lead to better *doing* in the end.

Doing is the outcome of *thinking* in nursing. The last chapter focused on thinking, something that goes on in one's head that cannot be seen. DOING is the part of nursing one can observe, the part that is more easily recognized; people can put labels on it. For example, nurses can be seen giving medication, making a bed, adjusting the intravenous line, teaching the patient how to change a dressing, and so forth. These *doing* activities are seen in real life, on

TV, or in the movies, and are described in books. If the major sources of information were TV, movies, or novels, one might think that all nurses were "attractive" women in high heels and tight, short uniforms flirting with "men of medicine" or gossiping all day. There is no thinking and very little real nursing going on in those depictions of what nurses *do*.

Leaving fantasy behind, it is clear that high-quality DOING in real nursing cannot occur without *thinking*. *Thinking* and *doing* are so interrelated that it is almost impossible to separate them. They will be separated in this chapter, however, so that a strong base of *doing* knowledge can be formed to go along with the *thinking* knowledge. At the end of this chapter, both pieces of the inseparable *thinking–doing* core of professional nursing practice are linked, forming a basis for future chapters on the *how* of *doing* great nursing.

Doing is not as simple as giving a medication or taking a blood pressure. Professional nursing encompasses a gamut of *thinking* and *doing* activities. First, there are many things done that are directly related to patient care. This type of *doing* is called *nursing interventions* or *nursing actions*. Second, there are many other things that provide the background for nursing care; these are called *indirect activities*.

Before studying these basic *doing* categories, it is helpful to consider what you know already. One of the underlying assumptions of this book is that learning occurs best when students can build on what they already know. Triggering one's existing brain patterns gives the learner a place to insert new knowledge. Adding to existing patterns often is more efficient than building entirely new ones for each learning area.

▶▶▶▶▶▶ Action Learning #9: What *Do* Nurses *Do*?

Where have you seen nurses? What have they been *doing*? Write a list of several things you know that nurses DO. Share your list with a classmate and discuss any differences in your perceptions of what nurses do.

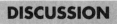 **DISCUSSION**   How many things did you list? Do you see any connections among the things that you listed? Any patterns? How do you feel about your chosen profession's many jobs? How does your list compare with that of your classmate?

DISPLAY 2-1. The Basic Doing List of Nursing

DIRECT PATIENT CARE ACTIVITIES

Caring: Conveying, through verbal and nonverbal behaviors, nurturing, supportive feelings for patients and significant others.

Care-taking: Doing things for patients and their significant others that they cannot do for themselves.

Counseling: Helping patients and significant others to cope more effectively with situations.

Data collecting: Gathering information about the patient.

Teaching: Providing information so that patients and significant others can understand or carry out activities.

Implementing physician orders: Doing activities ordered by the physician as part of the medical plan of care.

Monitoring: Keeping track of relevant information about the patient and the patient's situation.

INDIRECT PATIENT CARE ACTIVITIES

Advocating: Being the patient's "agent," looking out for his or her rights.

Collaborating: Working with other health care professionals and significant others to provide care.

Data collection: Gathering information about the environment around the patient and how he or she is interacting with it and significant others. Sometimes this involves individual patients, at other times groups of patients.

Documenting: Writing down important information about the patient.

Educating self: Being a lifelong learner (even after nursing school).

Managing: Organizing and coordinating the care of several patients at once and supervising other health care workers.

Referring: Connecting patients and significant others with helpful resources.

Research, using and doing: Applying new knowledge developed through systematic study and identifying areas of nursing that need further study, and participating in research studies. (This sounds like heavy-duty stuff, but it can be fun and exciting.)

▷ **The Doing List**

Display 2.1 contains a list of things that nurses *do*. This list is a basic one and is not all-inclusive, but it includes most nursing activities. The list is divided into two categories—"direct care activities" and "indirect activities." Distinguishing between these categories is like distinguishing the categories of things students do. "Direct patient care activities" are analogous to going to class, studying, reading books, taking tests, and writing papers: in other words, the day-to-day student activities. The indirect student activities include registering for classes, getting bookshelves and file drawers organized, and creating a work and living situation compatible with the student role.

This *doing* list of direct and indirect nursing activities may seem overwhelming at first glance. It takes time, practice, and a lot of *thinking* to master the multiple activities that nurses *do*.

Doing, put together with *thinking*, reveals how the activities fit into nursing situations. Learning skills such as how to use a sphygmomanometer to take blood pressure readings, how to prevent a patient from getting bed sores, and how to help patients cope with stress, loss, and grief, provide the content for *doing*. *Thinking* allows the nurse to know when such skills should be implemented and how those activities should be tailored to specific patient situations.

Using the *Doing* List

To discover how this *doing* fits into a real patient situation, read the following situation and the exploration of how nursing care includes all of the *doing* list.

> Mr. Adams cannot dress or bathe himself. He is hospitalized and partially paralyzed after a stroke.

Look at the *doing* list, and think about each item on it. Obviously, **caring** and **care-taking** apply here. It is likely that a nurse would be **teaching** Mr. Adams adaptive ways to bathe himself. His physician would have ordered treatments and medications that the nurse would **implement**. In a hospital setting, nursing assistants often work with the nurse, so **managing** that part of care done by assistants also would be part of the nurse's duties.

Although there is no information on Mr. Adams' emotional state, one could assume that he and his significant others might need some **counseling** to help them cope. This *thinking* assumption would be made based on knowledge about situational crises like strokes and how they cause stress. If the patient is to return to a healthy state, he and his significant others must cope with the stress. The nurse would need to find out how much stress this illness has precipitated. This is a good example of what was mentioned earlier; one cannot avoid *thinking* if one wants to *do* great nursing.

There will be many health care providers involved in Mr. Adams' care with whom the nurse would **collaborate** (eg, other nurses, physicians, physical, occupational and speech therapists, social workers, chaplains, dietitians). Such people might automatically be part of the treatment team or, if Mr. Adams' needs exceeded the nurse's ability to intervene, the nurse might **refer** the patient to other health care providers, such as a home health nurse or counselor.

Often, nurses have the most consistent and frequent contact with patients and their significant others. Nurses are the key people to **monitor** the patient's status and note any changes in that status. The nurse is frequently the **advocate** for the patient and significant others when their needs and the workings of the health care system are not aligned. Because nurses know the patient and the system, they use **management** skills to get everything to flow as smoothly as possible.

All patient situations require **data collection**; that is how nurses know what is going on and when changes occur with the patient. Nurses need to **document** data, plans of care, and results of care. Proper **documentation** is not only good patient care, it is required by laws and institutional policies.

Every patient situation that involves a nurse is a potential **research** situation. Nurses stay abreast of the literature, reading the latest **research** findings and thinking about how those findings could be applied to care. Practicing nurses are also in the best position to identify gaps in the nursing knowledge base and instigate **research** projects.

Related to research is the need to **educate oneself**. Nursing and health care are changing rapidly. The primary ways to keep up on the changes are to read professional literature, go to conferences, and talk to knowledgeable people.

The preceding paragraphs have shown how all the items on the *doing* list could be put into practice. Obviously, some things would be used more than others, depending on the situation. In the example of Mr. Adams, if he had his stroke recently, the nurse might have to provide most of his care for him. If, however, he had his stroke a few days earlier, more time would be spent in teaching than in care-taking because it is important for patients to regain as much independence as possible. The nurse would teach him new ways to bathe himself to compensate for his paralysis, and collect information to see how well he could help himself. If he were at home, the nurse might teach his significant others how to help him or how to help him help himself.

There are lots of factors that need to be taken into account as nurses put the *doing* list into practice. Mr. Adams' case illustrates the importance of considering the situation itself. A nurse needs to pay close attention to the patient in relation to where he is, how sick he is, what he wants done, when things need to be done, and many other factors. That attention means thinking.

▼ THINKING-LEARNING CHECK

Pause here for a thinking-learning check. You should be able to elaborate on these ideas:

- ▼ What nurses *do*
- ▼ Differentiating Direct Care Activities and Indirect Care Activities
- ▼ Tracking *doing* in a patient situation.

▶ FACTORS AFFECTING DOING

What nurses *do* is often dictated by many things other than what nursing books show as "the nursing actions" for "patient problems." Here is where *thinking* makes a big difference. Nurses have to make decisions about how to *do* things by considering all the circumstances of a patient situation. Each patient is an individual with a personal, subjective reality. That reality is shaped by many things, such as cultural norms, values, developmental phase of life, and many other influences. There are no recipes for care that apply to all situations.

Display 2-2 lists factors affecting how nurses *do* nursing. The factors, with examples in parentheses, are not all-inclusive. No one could think of all the possible factors and combinations of factors in any given situation. The items listed are meant to stimulate one's thinking about those issues that could affect *doing*.

The details of the environmental factors and patient factors are studied by students in courses such as psychology, sociology, biology, and the like. The "nurse factors," however, need to be addressed immediately because they are vital to beginning-level *thinking* and *doing*. Find a comfortable place to do some serious *thinking* and reading about the nurse factors.

▷ Values, Beliefs, and Expectations

The first factors affecting *doing* are values, beliefs, and expectations about health and health care. The best appreciation of these factors comes with self-reflection.

DISPLAY 2-2. Factors Affecting Doing

A. Environmental Factors
   1. Setting (hospital, home, clinic, nursing home, school)
   2. Time (Are there 5 minutes available or 2 hours? Will you see the patient again in 20 minutes or in 1 week?)
   3. Resources (supplies, equipment, money, insurance coverage)

B. Patient Factors
   1. Acuity of illness (intensive care, emergency, routine, chronic, health promotion, and so forth)
   2. Values, beliefs, and expectations about health and health care. ("Take care of me totally," "I'd rather do it myself!," "I'm too nervous to do this now," "Leave me alone")
   3. Developmental stage, cultural, ethnic, and socioeconomic factors, and level of education (infant or adult stage; eye contact is inappropriate in some cultures; immunizations are not believed good by some people; level of literacy limits types of teaching tools)

C. Nurse Factors
   1. Values, beliefs, and expectations about health and health care. (Nurses are supposed to do everything for patients. Nurses are supposed to help patients to help themselves.)
   2. Standards, laws, policies, and procedures (what a nurse can or cannot, should or should not do to stay within the law and follow the guidelines of the profession and the agency)
   3. Interdependent and independent role functions (collaborative actions or actions taken solely by nurses)
   4. Level of expertise (how much experience a nurse has had with similar situations)

>>>>>> **A**ction Learning #10: Effect of Values, Beliefs, and Expectations on Nursing Care

Study the following two patient assignments and imagine what, if anything, would be different as you plan care for each of them. Record your perceptions and share them with a classmate.

You are a rehabilitation nurse. Here are two of your assigned patients for the evening.

PATIENT 1

Dolly, a 63-year-old bartender, was in an automobile accident while she was driving intoxicated. She suffered a mangled leg that had to be amputated. She has been very quiet and refuses to wear her prosthetic leg to practice walking. The skin on her back is severely broken down. You have concluded that her impaired skin integrity is related to her immobility.

How do you think you will feel as you plan her care?

PATIENT 2

Monty, a 26-year-old nurse, was in an automobile accident while he was stopped on the side of the road to fix a flat tire. A truck swerved as it came around a corner and hit him and his car. His 3-month-old baby, who was in a car seat, also was injured during the accident and is currently in the hospital. Monty also has an amputated leg because his leg was pinned under the car during the accident. He has tried to use his prosthetic leg, but it has been rubbing on his stump. He has refused to get out of bed for the past 2 days and has two areas of skin breakdown on his back. You have concluded that his impaired skin integrity is related to his immobility.

How do you think you will feel as you plan his care?

DISCUSSION Because these situations are hypothetical, it is possible that what you *think* you would feel would not be exactly what you *would* feel in real life. Hopefully, however, these similar situations have shown you that you might have very different feelings in different patient situations. Notice that the problems of both patients (impaired skin integrity related to immobility) are identical. The surrounding circumstances, however, could make you feel differently. How do your values, beliefs, and expectations influence how you might feel or act with each patient? Would your values, beliefs, and expectations be obvious to the patient because of what you said or did? Or, would your values show only in subtle ways—by what you did not do or say, or even by how you said things?

What you strongly value and believe will not change overnight, but be prepared to have some of your values and beliefs challenged, and perhaps changed, as you continue your nursing career.

▷ Standards, Laws, Policies, and Procedures

Standards of Practice are set by state and national nursing organizations. These standards are nursing's assurance to society that a basic level of safe care will be maintained. Statements about what nurses can or cannot do are included in state Nurse Practice Acts. Those are the laws that govern nursing practice. (Make a note to yourself to get a copy of your state Nurse Practice Act if you don't already have one.) Each institution (agency) also has its own set of policies and procedures that govern what nurses can do while employed at that agency. A full description of such laws, standards, policies, and procedures is beyond the scope of this book. They are taught in several nursing courses. For now, remember that they influence what nurses *do*.

▷ Independent and Interdependent Role Functions

Nursing roles overlap with those of other health care professions, and many nursing activities are done collaboratively with other health care providers. These are called *interdependent nursing actions*. An example of interdependent nursing actions is illustrated by this situation: After finding a patient's blood pressure extremely high, the nurse collaborates with the physician so that the patient's medication may be ordered or adjusted. The physician orders the medication; the nurse gives it and monitors its effects. (Except for some nurses with advanced degrees and certification, such as nurse practitioners and nurse anesthetists, nurses cannot prescribe medications.) A nurse who collaborates with the nutritionist to create an acceptable meal plan for a finicky eater on a new diabetic diet is also performing interdependent nursing actions.

Nurses exercise their *independent* roles when they decide what a patient needs and follow through with nursing interventions. For example, a nurse can decide independently to teach a patient how to use relaxation techniques to counteract anxiety. Or, the nurse can give a back rub to help the patient sleep better. The independent role of the nurse is based on nursing knowledge and nursing judgment, not on medical knowledge or that of another health care specialty.

Nurses use independent and interdependent actions constantly. In any situation, a nurse may move between the two several times and do the two simultaneously. They engage their *thinking* skills to decide which one is appropriate at any given point.

Here is an example of the interplay between independent (I) and interdependent (ITD) nursing actions:

A nurse takes a patient's blood pressure and discovers that it is 160/100. This is a high reading for most people. The nurse might take any or all of the following actions:

Retake the blood pressure (I)

Observe the patient for other physical changes (I)

Ask the patient how he is feeling; note any changes (I)

Ask the patient what he was doing immediately before the blood pressure was taken (I)

Check the patient's record; compare previous readings to these (I)

Check the physician's orders for directions related to blood pressure parameters (ITD)

Report the blood pressure and other findings to the physician (ITD)

Give treatment as ordered by physician (ITD)

Monitor effects of medication (ITD)

Ask the patient what he understands about high blood pressure and how it affects him (I)

Teach the patient relaxation techniques that might help lower blood pressure (I)

Think about how using both independent and interdependent roles helps increase the quality of care. What would be different if the nurse just called the doctor and reported the first blood pressure reading? Would that be wrong? No—but it would be the action of a nurse with low-level thinking. (Incidentally, a non-thinking nurse would simply record the data in the chart and not do anything about it, or worse yet, would not even record it!) The *high-level thinking nurse* (you) uses both independent and interdependent actions, providing great nursing care.

▷ **Level of Expertise**

Level of expertise also influences what nurses *do*. In some situations, nurses are very familiar with patients' problems because they have dealt with similar problems in the past and thus have become more expert. In other situations it is not readily apparent what should be done. Not surprisingly, beginning students of nursing encounter many more of the latter situations than the former. The scale tips in the other direction when experience is gained by nurses who keep their *thinking* caps on.

Much attention has been given lately to how novices (beginners) and experts differ in their *thinking* and *doing* (Perry, 1970; Benner, 1984; Belenky, Clinchy, Goldberger, & Tarule, 1986; Dreyfus & Dreyfus, 1986). Beginners are less likely to "know" quickly what is occurring in most patient situations. Some beginners look at experienced nurses and are amazed at how "easily" they know what to do. Obviously, they were not born as experts; they also started as novices. Table 2-1 outlines some of the differences between beginners and experts. The table does not address the many stages between beginner and expert; one does not just go from one to the other at some point in time. Even this simple set of differences, however, can be helpful. An understanding of the differences can help beginners speed up their transition to the expert level.

Ways of Gaining Knowledge

Beginners sometimes believe that, by finding the right books to read, they will find all the answers to nursing questions and will acquire (gain) all necessary knowledge. This is not true. In the first place, there are not enough books in the universe to answer all the possible questions and give solutions to the problems that occur in nursing situations. Second, the answers are always changing; what was the best answer yesterday may not be acceptable today.

Clearly, books do have useful information in them; they show what is "typical" or "standard" in many or most situations, or what a procedure ought to be like under controlled circumstances. What books cannot provide are all the possible exceptions to the "rules" (and there are lots of exceptions). That is where the *thinking* cap and some study skills help. By reading more than one book on a subject, one gets different points of view. Journal articles usually are more current than books; therefore, it is a good idea to read one or two journals on a regular basis and search in journals for specific topics as they come up. Talking to experts and paying attention to one's own experience and com-

TABLE **2-1 Some Differences Between Beginners and Experts**		
	BEGINNERS	**EXPERTS**
Ways of:		
Gaining Knowledge	Assigned readings and asking authorities	Multiple written and verbal sources, and experience
Thinking	Dualistic	Relativistic
Using Rules	Context free	Situation dependent
Looking at Situations	Narrow	Broad

mon sense also are very helpful. Each of these strategies helps novices move beyond the beginner stage.

>>>>>> **Action Learning #11: Moving Beyond a Beginner's Way of Gaining Knowledge**

Spend a couple of minutes and think about food intake. (If you need a snack at this point, feel free to partake!)

Probably 90% to 100% of this book's readers have been on or heard about dieting and diets for the purpose of weight reduction. How many different diets can you list?

Pretend you are assigned to a patient who really wants to lose weight, and you do not have access to a dietitian. How are you going to find the "right" diet for the patient? Can you just go to your textbook and hand it to the patient and say, "Read this and see me in a month?" Of course not, but how will you proceed? Briefly describe what you would do and share your ideas with a classmate.

DISCUSSION Did you find the "right" diet? What makes you think this will work for this patient? How many sources would you use besides your textbook? What do you think is the role of the patient in planning this new diet?

Ways of Thinking

Dualistic thinking, common for beginners, involves seeing things as only "right" or "wrong," "good" or "bad," "red" or "blue." It does not take into account the real world, where things are usually poor, good, better, or best, or shades of purple. Relativistic thinkers see the wide range of "purple" hues that make up the real world. Here is how this works. The dualistic-thinking nurse who sees a 5-foot, 140-pound woman eating cookies might assume the patient is overweight and should not be eating cookies. The relativistic-thinking nurse might consider that the woman could be pregnant and of normal weight, could be an overweight diabetic who, incidentally, needs to eat something sweet to counteract her hypoglycemic reaction (low blood sugar), or would at least get more information before coming to a conclusion about the merit of this person's cookie-eating behaviors.

Ways of Using Rules

Context-free rules are the "steps in the books." Such steps are methods of acting or doing things without considering the unique circumstances of each patient situation. For example, when first learning how to drive a car, the beginner reads the driving manual, which says, "At a four-way stop, the person to your right gets to go through the stop first." This is a context-free rule. Although this is important to know, a driver has to consider each situation before driving through the intersection. The person to the left might be impatient and start into the intersection even though it is Driver A's right to proceed first.

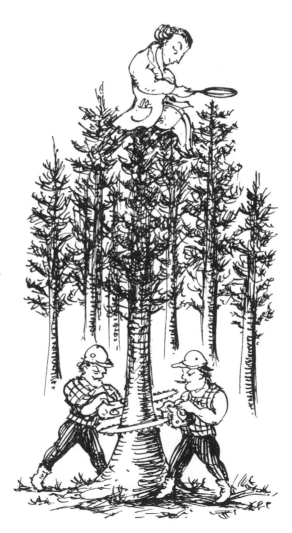

Figure 2-1. Missing the big picture (she can't see the forest for the trees).

Driver A's action needs to be adjusted to put safety first. Therefore, the rules must be interpreted in the context. The same holds true in nursing.

Here is a nursing example. Basic, context-free rules of discharge planning state: "Provide patient with written information on medications and how to take them at home." This is a good idea because written information can be used if a patient forgets what was said verbally. If that patient is illiterate or has a visual impairment, however, the written material is useless. The rule must therefore be adapted to the context of the individual patient situation.

Ways of Looking at Situations

Remember the old expression, "He can't see the forest for the trees?" Beginners often concentrate so hard on the pieces and details of a situation (the trees) that they are unable to see that there is a bigger picture (the forest and maybe even a forest fire coming over the ridge.) Have you ever focused so hard on building a sand castle at the beach that you didn't notice that the tide was coming in and would soon wipe out your hard work? In nursing, missing the big picture is common for beginners because they have to put so much energy into keeping the details straight. For example, students giving their first injection often concentrate so hard on their technique and hitting the right spot that they may not see other serious situations—that the patient's intravenous fluid has run out, the bed is wet, and the untouched breakfast tray is still sitting at the bedside at 3 PM.

Does all of this mean that all beginners are doomed to think dualistically, be slaves to context-free rules or victims of narrowmindedness? To some degree these attributes are unavoidable. Beginners will avoid some of the pitfalls, however, if they engage all *thinking* modes right from the start in their nursing careers. Students of nursing advance their *thinking* and *doing* as they progress through school. At the same time, it also is important to accept that no one is an expert by graduation; nurses may get there only after several years of experience. Nurses move faster along the path to expert *thinking* and *doing* when they pay attention to *how* they think. (Remember, that is *metacognition.*) *Thinking* in all five modes helps compensate for lack of experience. That is what this book is all about.

▼ THINKING-LEARNING CHECK

Pause here for another thinking-learning check. You should be able to elaborate on these ideas:

- ▼ Factors affecting *doing* in the categories of Environmental, Patient, and Nurse Factors
- ▼ Knowledge of environmental and patient factors comes through experience and courses of study
- ▼ Early attention to the nurse factors that affect doing can help beginners avoid pitfalls associated with those factors

To pull all of the ideas in this section together, another case study is presented. With it, you may test your learning about *doing* and factors affecting *doing*.

▶▶▶▶▶ **Action Learning #12: What Is the Nurse *Doing* and What Factors Are Affecting the *Doing*?**

Read the following case study.

First, label the nursing actions according to the items on the "Basic *doing* List of Nursing" in Display 2-1.

Second, for each nursing action, list at least one factor from Display 2-2, "Factors Affecting Doing," that could influence the nursing actions.

Third, share with a classmate your conclusions and how you did this action learning exercise.

CASE STUDY

Julie Wu, RN, has been assigned to Mr. Antler, who is being discharged to his home today. He was hospitalized for 1 week after having a stroke that partially paralyzed his left side. He has had difficulty dressing and bathing himself. He lives with his wife and two teenage sons. Mr. Antler's insurance coverage provides for nursing care at home for 2 weeks. He is having a great deal of difficulty accepting the changes in his body, tries to do things very quickly, and gets easily frustrated. With reminders, he can move more slowly and is able to stand from a sitting position and maintain his balance. His wife also gets impatient and frequently does things for Mr. Antler rather than waiting for him to do things independently.

Ms. Wu has been working with stroke patients for the last 10 years and initiates the following nursing actions while Mr. Antler is still in the hospital:

▼ Explains to Mr. and Mrs. Antler how the stroke has affected Mr. Antler's judgments about his body in space.
DOING:

FACTORS POSSIBLY AFFECTING DOING:

▼ Reminds Mrs. Antler to give her husband verbal cues rather than doing things for him.
DOING:

FACTORS POSSIBLY AFFECTING DOING:

▼ Talks about the importance of decreasing clutter and potential hazards in the home environment.
DOING:

FACTORS POSSIBLY AFFECTING DOING:

▼ Shows Mr. and Mrs. Antler how to simplify bathing and dressing by dividing them into smaller steps.
DOING:

FACTORS POSSIBLY AFFECTING DOING:

▼ Calls the home health nurse and sets up time and date for nurse's visit.
DOING:

FACTORS POSSIBLY AFFECTING DOING:

▼ Checks with physicians on discharge medication orders and makes sure prescriptions are written.
DOING:

FACTORS POSSIBLY AFFECTING DOING:

▼ Asks the patient care assistant to pack Mr. Antler's personal belongings into bags.
DOING:

FACTORS POSSIBLY AFFECTING DOING:

▼ Contacts the office of Mr. Antler's physician after Mrs. Antler could not get through to clarify a medication.
DOING:

FACTORS POSSIBLY AFFECTING DOING:

DISCUSSION   Can you imagine any of the many other things that the nurse was likely to have done in this situation? What kinds of thinking did you use? How was your approach different from or like that of your classmate?

▶ INTERTWINING DOING AND THINKING

Remember, this chapter started with a focus on *doing*; however, it has been impossible to discuss *doing* without discussing *thinking* at the same time. Although Julie's *doing* was influenced by environmental factors, patient factors, and nurse factors, her actions were strongly influenced by her *thinking*. It is practically impossible to *do* nursing without *thinking*! The next chapter will specifically combine *doing* and *thinking* and show how their intertwining results in quality care.

▶▶▶ *THINKING LOG #2*

This time you have an interview assignment. Find a real nurse and ask him or her if you can have 15 minutes of time. Ask the following questions and record the person's response:

1. What are the major things you *do* during a routine day?
2. What are the things you like to *do* best?
3. What are the things you *do* that are most important to good patient care?
4. How much of your day is spent *thinking*?

Make a list of the things the person tells you and compare it to the *doing* list. Share your findings with a classmate. There may be things described by the nurse that are not on the list; be sure to write those things down and discuss them.

REFERENCES

Belenky, M. F., Clinchy, B. M., Goldberger, N. R., & Tarule, J. M. (1986). *Women's ways of knowing: The development of self, voice, and mind.* New York: Basic Books.

Benner, P. (1984). *From novice to expert: Power and excellence in nursing practice.* Menlo Park, CA: Addison-Wesley.

Dreyfus, H. L., & Dreyfus, S. E. (1986). *Mind over machine: The power of human intuition and expertise in the era of the computer.* New York: The Free Press.

Perry, W. G. (1970). *Forms of intellectual and ethical development in the college years.* New York: Holt, Rinehart & Winston.

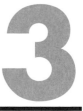

Thinking and Doing and the Nursing Process: The "How" of Great Nursing

LEARNING OUTCOMES

After reading and doing the activities in this chapter you will be able to:

Explain the "how" of great nursing.

Describe the nursing process.

Place the nursing process in its historical context.

Explore possible nursing process sequences.

Define the components of the nursing process, and the thinking and doing related to each component.

The last two chapters have laid a foundation for the examination of great nursing. A basic understanding of the five modes of *thinking* and the many *doing* aspects of nursing provide a beginning for the journey toward great nursing. Keep your thinking caps on as the journey continues.

▶ AN EQUATION FOR GREAT NURSING

A goal of most nurses is to provide high-quality nursing care, or, as some would like to call it, great nursing. How to achieve that goal successfully requires high-quality thinking and high-quality doing. For the beginning nurse, it is helpful to examine a simple equation that briefly illustrates *how* to achieve great nursing.

$$\text{Patient} + \text{You} + \frac{\text{Thinking}}{\text{Skills}} + \frac{\text{Content}}{\text{Knowledge}} + \frac{\text{Nursing}}{\text{Process}} = \text{Great Nursing}$$

This is a simple linear equation. Obviously, there are many other factors that influence great nursing. Also, what appears to be a simple series of additions of one component to another turns out to be much more complex in real life. In reality, the components are intermingled in a variety of ways. But, for now, look just at the components of the equation. As the chapters continue, the relationships among the components of this equation will be explored and examined in much more depth.

▷ Who is The Patient?

The patient may be a person, a family, a group, or a community. The usual description for nursing care with families, groups, and communities is "nursing care for aggregates."

The identical nursing process is used in all cases. The big difference between using the process with individuals and using it with groups is that nurses need different content knowledge to determine what is normal and what is not normal to identify problems accurately, formulate plans, and implement and evaluate care. The following is a list of just a few of the different kinds of content knowledge (information) needed to apply the nursing process to individuals and aggregates:

For *individuals*:
What is normal oral body temperature?
What are typical eating patterns of 2-year-olds?
What are the effects of chronic illness on self-esteem?
For *families*:
How do members react when one person is ill?
What happens to family roles after the first child is born?
What are healthy family developmental stages for single-parent families?
For *groups*:
What are the norms of behavior for this group?
How cohesive is the group?
How do the leaders of the group affect problem solving?
For *communities*:
What community resources are focused on immunization clinics?
What is the frequency of drug and alcohol use among the community's 12- to 18-year-olds?
What health concerns are resulting from high concentrations of lead in the playground soil?

There is a great deal more content knowledge needed to provide effective care of families, groups, and communities. Both required and recommended books in nursing school will help supply some of that information. This text, however, will focus only on the individual. Understanding about the *thinking* and *doing* and the nursing process *with* individual patients is enough for this stage of learning.

▷ Who Are You?

You are a very special, one-of-a-kind person with a desire to be a great nurse. Your personality (feelings, values, and beliefs) as well as your thinking skills will transform the basic skills acquired from textbooks into your own art of great nursing. This will not happen overnight, and it will not even happen by graduation; but it can happen if you accept the challenge to think consistently using all five thinking modes.

▷ What are Thinking Skills?

The five thinking modes and the nurse's ability to use all of them effectively comprise thinking skills. This text is designed to continue to nurture and expand the reader's existing skills. Patients also have thinking skills. A major part of nursing's role is to help patients engage their thinking skills, or, more generally, to help patients to help themselves.

▷ What is Content Knowledge?

Content knowledge is the information learned from written documents (books, journals), through interactions with others, and through nursing practice. All those heavy nursing books provide a great deal of content knowledge. Those texts include many of the facts and concepts required during nursing school **and** during the remainder of one's professional career. The content knowledge from books and articles includes, for example, how illness affects coping skills; what happens to skin if a person is confined to a wheelchair and is incontinent (no bladder control); and all the multiple nursing needs of a teenager or elderly person with diabetes.

The other major sources of content knowledge include clinical experience and nursing research findings. It is impossible to know everything, and it sometimes is barely possible to keep current with the rapidly changing state of knowledge in health care today, but nurses must try to acquire the best content knowledge available.

▷ What Is the Nursing Process?

Before we answer that, first consider the definition of the word "process." Process is a way of *doing* something. That something could be organic gardening, fly fishing, cutting hair, practicing medicine, repairing cars, or nursing. The word "process" means moving from one point to another and changing things (hopefully, for the better) along the way. Many processes involve problem solving.

The nursing process which includes problem solving, is how nursing is done. It is presented in its totality in this chapter; subsequent chapters explore the components and the whole process in greater detail.

▷ What is Great Nursing?

Great nursing is a concept that is hard to capture in a simple definition. It's the point at which the nurse goes beyond good, safe nursing skills. Great nursing practice focuses on patients as human beings with unique strengths and unique health needs. Great nursing is creative and individualized; it is an art as well as a science.

Great nursing is not some elusive ideal that can only be aspired to and achieved in scholarly dissertations. Great nursing is practiced daily by nurses around the world. The key to practicing great nursing is the effective use of all the components of the equation **and** the nurse's belief that every patient is unique.

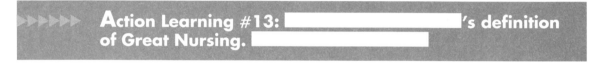

▶▶▶▶▶▶ **A**ction Learning #13: _____'s definition
of Great Nursing. _____

(insert your name and today's date above)
Think about how you would describe great nursing. Write out a brief description. Share it with a classmate.

DISCUSSION   Having a description of great nursing is one of the first steps in becoming a great nurse; it provides direction and a personal goal. Save your ideas and look back to them occasionally. You may find that your ideas change as your *thinking* and learning evolve.

With this preliminary understanding of the basic components of great nursing, it is time to focus on some details of the equation's components, specifically the nursing process. Understanding and effectively applying the nursing process requires constant use of thinking caps.

▶ THE NURSING PROCESS

The intertwining of *thinking* and *doing* in nursing is the nursing process. This process is the essence of professional nursing practice. The nursing process is the means by which nurses identify patients' strengths and responses to health and illness situations, design ways to assist patients in dealing with those situations, implement the needed nursing care, and determine the effectiveness of that care by looking for changes in patient behavior. Again, the nursing process is frequently a problem-solving process.

Translated into everyday language, the nursing process would look like this: A nurse meets a patient and *thinks*, "What does this patient need from me, if anything?" To answer that question, the nurse thinks about and collects some information. The nurse thinks about what the information means, draws some conclusions about what the patient needs, and makes sure the patient agrees with those conclusions. Then the nurse thinks about and works with the patient to identify the best ways to meet the needs. The nurse performs whatever nursing care is required. After the nurse has helped the patient, the nurse and patient determine if the patient's needs have been met.

The process that the nurse goes through is similar to that used by car mechanics who must find out what is wrong with a car in order to fix it. It also is similar to the process that many others, such as hairdressers, telephone repair people, social workers, and physicians use. Although the processes are similar for these and other groups of workers, the "focus" of each process varies. For mechanics it is car repair; for physicians it is disease care. For nurses it is nursing care.

This process of determining what is needed and taking care of the needs may seem like common sense because it is practiced in everyday problem solving. Nursing, however, like other disciplines, has refined the basic process specifically for itsclf.

For many years, nurses have used specific terms to identify parts of the nursing process: *assessing*; *planning*; *implementing*; and *evaluating*. Some authors insert *nursing diagnosis* between assessing and planning for the purpose of highlighting the problem identification portion of the process. This appears to lengthen the overall process and is not really necessary, because diagnosing is an integral part of assessing.

It is time to talk about how all this works with real patients. Remember, this text concentrates on *thinking* and *doing* and on the nursing process with individuals, but in reality, families, groups, and communities (aggregates) also are recipients of nursing care. Also, whether it is with aggregates or with individuals, the focus of care is **with** the patient.

▷ The Role of the Patient

In the preceding paragraph, the word "with" was highlighted. Although at times, nurses do things "for" patients who cannot participate in their care, most of the time nurses work with patients collaboratively. Patients' active participation in the nursing process is a key factor in success because it indicates that patients have active roles in care. Active participation in care nurtures the patient's self-esteem and problem-solving skills. When patients are merely the passive recipients of care (when care is provided "for" or "to" them), they become overly dependent on the nurse and cannot achieve their optimum level of functioning.

Working "with" patients implies teamwork. The nurse asks questions, the patient responds. The patient asks questions, the nurse responds. The nurse uses *thinking* skills and professional judgment and comes to conclusions about the patient's strengths and health concerns. The conclusions are shared with the patient, who agrees or disagrees. If the patient agrees, the nurse and the patient plan care with specific outcomes in mind. The nurse does the nurse *doing* activities (teaching, bathing, changing dressings) and the patient does the patient activities (relaxing, exercising, washing, eating). Both evaluate the results—togetherness is the watchword.

▷ Applying the Nursing Process, Thinking, and Doing

What does this nursing process look like when applied to an individual patient? Read the following example, and try to identify the components of the nursing process as well as the *thinking* and *doing* of the student nurse, Ms. Calli Mooradian.

Ms. Calli Mooradian, SN, is assigned to care for Mr. Steinberg. Mr. Steinberg is confined to bed with no weight-bearing on his legs. Both legs were broken when he was hit by a car 1 week ago. While Ms. Mooradian is helping with his bed bath she observes (**assesses**) a pinkish-red area on his lower back. She **thinks**, "This is not normal. The skin over the lower back should be the same color as the rest of the patient's skin." She next **thinks**, "When skin is pink it could mean: 1) sunburn, 2) a normal color for this patient even though it is not normal for most patients, or 3) the beginning of a pressure sore (decubitus ulcer).

After asking some questions (**assessing**), she comes to the conclusion that this is the beginning of a pressure sore and makes the nursing diagnosis of:

> Impaired Skin Integrity, related to decreased circulation to the lower back secondary to immobility

The evidence to support her nursing diagnosis (a conclusion of assessment) is:

> The skin on Mr. Steinberg's lower back is pinkish-red.
>
> This is not normal skin color for this patient's lower back.
>
> This patient has been lying on his back without turning for extended periods of time because he is confined to bed (immobility).
>
> Immobility leads to increased pressure and decreased circulation to areas of the body.
>
> Pressure and decreased circulation promote the development of pressure sores (decubitus ulcers).
>
> Decubitus ulcers are not good.

Ms. Mooradian develops a **plan** of nursing care to increase circulation and mobility, which should allow the skin to return to its usual color. She immediately **implements** (*does*) the plan, which includes explaining to the patient the importance of turning off his back at regular intervals. She writes the plan in the patient's chart so all nurses can follow it.

At the end of her shift, she checks (**evaluates**) to see if there is any change in the skin color on Mr. Steinberg's back and if Mr. Steinberg is turning off his back every 2 hours. When asked, Mr. Steinberg says he has been faithfully turning, and there is less pinkish-red color to the skin of his lower back. She **thinks** there is good evidence to validate that she accurately identified a nursing problem and selected an appropriate intervention. She will continue to monitor Mr. Steinberg's skin for several more days.

▶▶▶▶▶▶ **A**ction Learning #14: Find the Nursing Care with **M**r. **S**teinberg

Think about what the nurse did that specifically involved the patient as an active participant in his care. Write your ideas down.

DISCUSSION It is important, as a beginner, to see how the active participation of the patient moves you closer to great patient care. The two episodes that clearly demonstrate patient involvement are explaining to the patient the need to turn, and asking if he is turning. What else could Ms. Mooradian have done to increase care **with** Mr. Steinberg?

Do you think all nurses would have applied the nursing process the same way Ms. Mooradian did in this situation? Today, the answer is probably "yes" because such use of the nursing process in caring for patients and their skin has become a standard practice. A brief look at nursing's history shows how and why nursing has come to the point at which patients can expect a consistent approach to care from all nurses.

▶ A BIT OF BACKGROUND: TRACKING THE ROOTS OF NURSING PROCESS

For many, the idea of looking back at history conjures up unpleasant recollections of memorizing meaningless dates and events. Others appreciate that there are past patterns and events that have significance for the present; such is the case in nursing history.

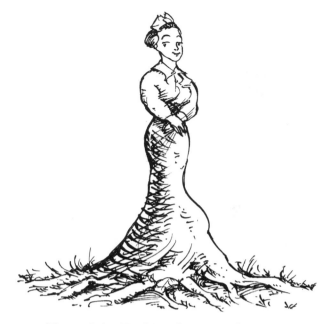

Figure 3-1. Tracking the roots of nursing.

There were several historical events significant to the development and understanding of the nursing process. Since the time of Florence Nightingale, nurses have attempted to define and describe what nursing is and what nurses do. This text's discussion, however, goes back only to 1967, when a group of nurses in Washington, DC, met and formally described what nurses do and how they do it. They called this the nursing process.

The two leaders of this group, Helen Yura and Mary Walsh, compiled the proceedings of the first efforts of the group (Yura & Walsh, 1967) and went on to write four more editions of a book called *The Nursing Process: Assessing, Planning, Implementing, Evaluating* (Yura & Walsh, 1988). Their work on the nursing process has become the standard for nursing for the last 25 years.

Discussion of or references to the nursing process can be found in all current nursing textbooks. The nursing process has become the underlying approach for nursing's Standards of Practice. (Standards of Practice were introduced in the last chapter under "Factors Affecting *doing*.")

The terms assessing, planning, implementing, and evaluating describe the traditional parts or components of the nursing process. Assessing is the process used by nurses to draw conclusions about patients' strengths and health concerns. Planning is the development of approaches to meet patient needs. Implementing is the actual care. Evaluating is a determination of the patient outcomes and the quality of the care.

▷ Nursing Diagnoses and the Nursing Process

An important addition to the original nursing process work was the development of nursing diagnoses. Until recently, there was no universal set of labels for most of the conclusions reached through assessment. In the early 1970s, work was started by a group of nurses in St. Louis, Missouri, to define more clearly the problems for which nurses provide care (Gebbie & Lavin, 1975). The set of labels identified by the St. Louis group are collectively called "Nursing Diagnoses." In 1976, the St. Louis group expanded into an international nursing organization called The North American Nursing Diagnosis Association (NANDA). Although the nursing process is firmly established, the work of standardizing the terminology for nursing diagnosis work is still in progress, and revisions are made every 2 years. The profession currently has a working document called the "NANDA Approved Nursing Diagnoses" (NANDA, 1992; see Appendix A).

▷ The American Nurses' Association Definition of Nursing and the Nursing Process

Another significant development in nursing that affected the nursing process was the publication in 1980 of a "standard" definition of nursing by the American Nurses' Association (ANA). The ANA is one of the major professional organizations for nurses. Its definition of nursing is as follows:

> Nursing is the diagnosis and treatment of human responses
> to actual or potential health problems (ANA, 1980, p. 9).

The term "human responses" was selected to clarify the difference between caring for the actual illness (typically a disease or medical condition—eg, diabetes), which is usually in the domain of medicine, **and** caring for patients as they deal with those health concerns or illnesses (eg, lack of knowledge about giving insulin). Human responses generally include a patient's physical or emotional *reaction* to a disease, change in health status, or potential for reaching a higher level of health (eg, fear of dying, inability to bathe self, or effective coping. Human responses, therefore, are the situations or conditions that nurses diagnose and for which they plan, implement, and evaluate care.

▷ Nursing Interventions and the Nursing Process

In 1992, a group of nurses in Iowa developed a set of terminology to describe what nurses do, called the "Taxonomy of Nursing Interventions" (McCloskey & Bulechek, 1992). This work, like that of the NANDA group, is an attempt to define, with standard language, the realm of nursing care. The "Taxonomy of Nursing Interventions" does for implementing what the NANDA Taxonomy does for assessing.

▷ Nursing Theories and the Nursing Process

One final historical development that is important to align *thinking* and *doing* with the nursing process is the development of nursing theories. The nursing process is just what it says it is—a process; it is the *how* of nursing. But this process cannot stand alone. It needs to be combined with some framework (theory) of *what* nursing is all about. Nursing theories provide direction as to what information needs to be assessed and what to do with the information. The *how* (assessing, planning, implementing, and evaluating) is always the same, no matter what theory (framework) is used, but theories may vary in their conceptualizations of the *what* of nursing.

To appreciate the difference between a theory (framework) and a process, think about gardening.

Gardening theory A says the best way to grow plants is to:

1. Rub the seeds six times before planting them
2. Water the seeds every 10 days
3. Check for insect damage to leaves

Gardening theory B says the best way to grow plants is to:

1. Be careful not to rub the seeds before planting
2. Water the seeds with fertilizer every other day
3. Play music for the plants to get greener leaves

No matter which theory (framework for growing good plants) the gardener uses, the process of planting is the same: you put a seed in the soil, give it water (and maybe fertilizer), and take care of the plant when it comes up. This is basically how nursing theories and the nursing process work together. With all nursing theories, the nursing process of assessing, planning, implementing, and evaluating remains constant, even if different terms are used to describe what nurses do.

Because the nursing process can be used with just about any nursing theory, this book does not try to link the process specifically with one theory or another. Rather, it focuses on the process and shows how **thinking** and **doing** are inseparably intertwined throughout the process. This provides a sound beginning for the practice of great nursing. The preferred nursing theory or theories to support practice can be selected at a later time.

These brief historical highlights provide the basis for a beginning appreciation of the events and time frames of activities that have contributed to the development of the nursing process and the nursing profession. Although the formal terminology, "nursing process," is fairly recent, the problem-solving methodology used by nurses is much older. Ongoing nursing research and clinical practice continue to make giant strides in clarifying and refining the use of the nursing process in the achievement of great nursing.

Pause here for a thinking-learning check. You should be able to elaborate on these ideas:

▼ The *how* of great nursing includes the patient, you, thinking skills, content knowledge, and the nursing process.

▼ The patient, whether an individual or an aggregate (family, group, or community), has unique strengths and health concerns.

▼ Content knowledge comes from books, clinical practice, and nursing research findings.

▼ The nursing process components, assessing, planning, implementing, and evaluating, are constantly intermingling, but some assessment is done first.

▼ The roots of the nursing process include:

Identification of the components of the nursing process and how they work

Development and refinement of nursing theories

Development and refinement of Nursing Diagnoses

Definition of nursing by ANA

Development of an initial "Taxonomy of Nursing Interventions."

▶ CAUTIONS ABOUT USING LABELS AND STANDARDIZED CARE

Part of the ongoing task of a socially responsible profession is to continue to define and describe clearly what it does for the protection and safety of the public. This movement continually to refine, clarify, label, and develop standards of care, although necessary, is a double-edged sword. Although definitions, descriptions, and standards are professional mandates, they also carry with them the danger of making nursing appear to have cookbook-type recipes for care.

Some nurses strongly criticize the use of any labels or standardized approaches. The major criticisms are based on two beliefs. First, attempts to label and standardize care are too simplistic for the uniqueness of individuals and their needs. Second, the dynamic nature of people, their environment, and nursing care is too complex to infer any direct cause-and-effect relationship between nursing care and the results of care.

In most cases, however, it is not the standardized approaches that are at fault, but rather what is done with those approaches when they are used as cookbook recipes, devoid of much thought. Unfortunately, the *thinking* and the necessity for focusing attention on the individual can be lost along the road to defining and standardizing terminology and approaches.

A standardized approach, like the nursing process, is similar to a cake recipe. The recipe works fine if the cook has all the correct ingredients in all the right amounts, the right-sized pan, and the correct oven temperature. But what happens if one ingredient is missing? Can some other ingredient be substituted? What happens if the oven doesn't get as hot as the recipe calls for? Can a lower temperature be used, or is it better just to bake the cake longer? Without the ability to think and make adjustments in the recipe, the result will be something much different from the desired cake. The *thinking* cook, however, can modify the recipe and still end up with a great cake.

The same principle applies in nursing. Standards and labels are only guides; the nurse must think and adjust standards and labels to fit each patient's unique needs. Thinking provides the nurse and the patient with multiple avenues to achieve the same goal. It is continually necessary for both beginning nurses and experienced nurses to keep those *thinking caps* on and avoid the rut of cookbook nursing.

Some say that there has always been a focus on thinking in nursing; others say it has been lost. Regardless of the view taken, a brief review of the original work on the nursing process reveals a strong focus on thinking as integral to the components of the process. In their second edition of *The Nursing Process*, Yura and Walsh stated, "The skills the nurse must have to use the nursing process are: intellectual, interpersonal, and technical. Intellectual skills entail problem-solving, critical thinking, and making nursing judgements" (Yura & Walsh, 1973, p. 69).

Nursing has come a long way in 30 years, but there is still much to do. Some may find that prospect overwhelming; others get excited by the challenge. Part of what is exciting is that the nursing leaders, who will guide thinking and doing and the nursing process into the 21st century, are the beginning nurses of today. Keep those thinking caps on and take good care of the profession and the patients.

▶ SEQUENCING THE COMPONENTS OF THE NURSING PROCESS

With the recognition that the nursing process and *thinking* and *doing* are the foundation of successful practice, comes the question, "Where does the process start?"

▷▷▷▷▷▷ **Action Learning #15: Where to Start**

Take a minute now and imagine yourself as the student nurse in the situation below. Remember that nursing is a process of *thinking* and *doing*. What is the *first thing* you, as a student nurse, are thinking about in the following nursing situation?

You are assigned to care for Mrs. Svensen for the morning. She is 85, very independent, and does not like to bother people. Today she is confined to bed after her hip surgery yesterday. You walk into her room and find her struggling to complete her bed bath even though she can't reach the lower part of her legs. The first thing I think about is

_____

DISCUSSION Those of you who wrote, "I need to help the patient finish her bath" are thinking about *implementing* first. Others of you may say, "I need to get some information about the patient first." You are thinking about *assessing*. Still a third group of you might say, "I need to sit down and decide what is the best way to help this patient. Should I do it myself, or find another way to help her finish the task so she doesn't have to give up her independence?" Your group is approaching this from the point of *planning*.

▷ Right or Wrong Sequences

As with most of nursing, it all depends . . . . Basically, there is no absolute right or wrong place to start. Although thinking may focus on any component of the nursing process first, the most logical DOING starts with assessment. Logically, if the nurse has never seen the patient before, some information (assessment) is needed before doing anything if safe nursing care is to be achieved. All encounters begin with some degree of assessment. How much information is needed depends on other circumstances, such as how immediate the patient's need is (severe bleeding, not breathing), how much experience the nurse has (beginner or expert), and how much time is available to spend with the patient (10 minutes during an office visit or many months in a nursing home).

Similar circumstances will influence how much time and energy nurses put into planning care. Sometimes planning is instantaneous, on the spot. Other times the nurse can sit for an hour or two and write out a lengthy, long-term plan of care. Likewise, implementation may vary depending on the situation.

Evaluation always occurs *after* something is done. It does not make much sense to try to evaluate changes in patient behaviors before any care is provided.

▷ Traditional Assumptions About Sequencing the Components of the Nursing Process

Most traditional nursing books describe the nursing process as a sequence of steps with simple feedback loops. This method provides a basic explanation of the components of the process and the importance of feedback. Unfortunately, this method has several problems. First, it promotes the idea that the nursing process can be effectively used like a "cookbook." The second problem is that the components become a series of concepts to memorize without any appreciation of their dynamic relationship to each other beyond feedback.

▷ Actual Sequencing of the Nursing Process Components

In reading about the nursing process as it was described above, do not be lulled into believing that the nursing process is a simple 1-2-3-4, lock-step procedure. In any given patient encounter, the nurse may assess, plan, implement, and evaluate several times as well as use all the components at the same time. The nurse also may spend varying amounts of time and energy on each component of the process. Consider this example; the nurse may *assess* for a new problem (eg, diaper rash) while *evaluating* care outcomes for an old problem (eg, how well Mom learned to diaper the baby). Likewise, as the nurse *implements* care for a patient's problem (eg, turning a patient on his side to relieve pain), the nurse may *assess* for other concerns (eg, skin condition, mobility) and even *evaluate* the results of care for another problem (eg, how well the patient has learned to use the trapeze to help with moving in bed), while *planning* care for yet another problem (eg, the best toileting schedule). And, believe it or not, this may be accomplished in several seconds by more experienced nurses. Although it may take a little longer for beginning nurses, the same events in thinking and doing will occur if the nursing process is used effectively.

The "bottom line" here is that there are four key components to the nursing process. All four are critical to high-quality nursing care, and all four are used repeatedly for each nursing concern. Where to start and how much emphasis to place on each component at a certain point in care depend on many factors, including the patient situation, the nurse's expertise, and the amount of time available. Some degree of assessment, even if it takes only microseconds, is usually the starting point.

▶ DEFINITIONS OF THE NURSING PROCESS COMPONENTS

Each of the components of the nursing process serves a special role. To understand those roles better, it is useful to examine the definitions of the components first.

▷ Assessing

Thinking about what information to collect, collecting information, *thinking* about the significance of that information, and drawing conclusions about how the patient is responding to his or her health or illness condition. The conclusions of assessment include two basic categories: strengths and health concerns. Health concerns focus on: 1) issues the nurse can deal with independently (nursing diagnoses), 2) issues that a nurse and another health care provider work on interdependently (interdisciplinary problems), and 3) issues that need to be referred to another health care provider (eg, medical or nutrition problems).

▷ Planning

Thinking about (and usually writing down) how to help with the patient's response to his or her health or illness condition. Working with the patient in deciding which problems have priority, in developing patient goals and objectives, and in determining what the nurse and the patient need to do to meet those goals.

▷ Implementing

Doing specific activities to help the patient meet the goals in the plan, while continuing to *think* about what is being done, how it is being done, when, where, and why it is being done.

▷ Evaluating

Thinking and collecting information about the patient's responses after some nursing care is provided. Working with the patient to determine if the patient's goals and objectives have been met and how well.

Anyone can memorize the above or any other definitions. However, understanding and recognizing the concepts that are defined requires more than TOTAL RECALL. The following learning activity was designed to illustrate how all the components of the nursing process are used with thinking and doing, and to move the reader's thinking beyond the TOTAL RECALL mode.

▶▶▶▶▶▶ **Action Learning #16: Identifying Components as the Nursing Process is Used**

Reread the definitions carefully, then read the following case study. Find the components of the nursing process as used by Ms. Louise Lamay, Student Nurse. Circle the sentence(s) that demonstrate one or more of the components of the nursing process, and write the appropriate label or labels (assessing, planning, implementing, or evaluating) next to your circles.

CASE STUDY

Louise Lamay, Student Nurse, just started her rotation in a Pediatric Nursing Clinic. Preparing for her clinical day, she reviewed information on growth and development, pediatric dosages of medications, immunization schedules, and family processes.

In the morning before the patients arrived, Louise reviewed 4-year-old Jesse's clinic record and learned the following:

Date of birth: 3/4/89

Last visit to clinic 1 year ago

Normal labor and delivery, successfully breast fed for 9 months

Immunizations up to date (needs fourth DPT booster and oral polio vaccination)

Ht. = 38 inches (50th percentile for 3-year-old boys)

Wt. = 33 lbs. (50th percentile for 3-year-old boys)

History of two to three ear infections each winter, effectively treated with amoxicillin

Parents' concern about fussy eater after the age of 18 months

No known allergies

Louise greeted Jesse, who was accompanied by his father, Mr. Frazier. She introduced herself and escorted both to the examining room where she asked, "How are things?" Jesse smiled and said, "Fine, you want to see my drawing?"

While Louise examined the multicolored crayon drawing of teddy bears, Mr. F. stated, "Jesse seems OK, but we are really concerned that he is not eating enough to keep a bird alive. His diet consists solely of american cheese, french fries, peanut butter, white bread, bananas, and milk. He also doesn't want to take naps anymore and gets up three to four times before finally falling asleep at night. He generally sleeps from 10 or 11 PM until 8 AM. He hates breakfast! We also see that he gets a rash when he is outside on windy days in the summer."

Louise summarized for Mr. F., "It sounds like you have several concerns about Jesse—his eating, his sleeping, and his periodic rashes. We will examine them all, but which one is the biggest problem from your perspective?" Mr. F. replied, "Well, the eating is really our biggest headache."

Louise asked Jesse to get on the scale. She found the following:

Ht. = 40 inches (25th percentile for 4-year-old boys)

Wt. = 35 lbs. (25th percentile for 4-year-old boys)

In response to Louise's questions about his eating, Jesse replied, "I don't like other stuff. They feel funny when they crunch and they make my belly hurt. I like fries best, but Mom and Dad won't let me eat them all the time."

At this point, Louise looked at the available data and compared them to the norms for 4-year-old boys (height/weight norms, dietary requirement norms, and behavioral norms). She suspected that nutrition was a problem because Jesse's diet was deficient in fruits and vegetables. She also realized she needed more information, specifically, the amounts of each of the foods he ate over a period of days. She needed a 3-day, 24-hour diet record.

After obtaining a diet record through Mr. F.'s recall, she verified her initial hunch that the diet needed more fruits and vegetables. The question then was, what was causing this eating problem? She considered that he might have food intolerance; he might be trying to control his environment; he might just not like the taste of things; or he might be hesitant to try new things. She asked questions to rule in or rule out these possible causes, and discovered that he was hesitant to try new tastes and textures because they were different. He often interrupted their food discussion with excited remarks about his drawings and new computer painting program.

At first Louise thought this was going to be tough. He didn't seem interested in food at all. Then it occurred to her that her mother used to get her to eat new foods by shaping them with cookie cutters. She smiled to herself at the memory of eating stars and hearts.

Louise considered what she knew about children's learning styles and, realizing that she must keep things simple, came up with a plan involving rewards and short-term goals that would entice Jesse to eat a larger variety of foods. The goal was to get him to eat one new vegetable or fruit each week. The plan included having him create pictures with selected foods, cutting food into bear shapes, and increasing computer time for every new food tried.

Louise told Mr. F. and Jesse that she would call them in a week to see how things were going. She said to Jesse, "When I call, I'd like you to tell me about the food pictures you've eaten and which ones tasted best."

After they left, Louise took a minute to review her encounter with Jesse and his dad. She realized she forgot to ask about the rest of the family's eating style. She made a note to ask about this during her follow-up phone call. She also realized that she came up with a very clever plan and hoped it would work. She recorded the plan in Jesse's chart and made a note on the calendar to call next week when she returned to the clinic.

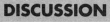 **DISCUSSION** How easily could you see the components of the nursing process? Could you see the intertwining of the components? Was it sometimes difficult to separate the components?

In Action Learning #16 you focused on what the nurse was *doing*. Now, the focus is on finding the *thinking* in the same case study. Refer back to Chapter 1 to review the five modes of thinking in more detail if needed, but the modes are listed below.

▶▶▶▶▶▶ Action Learning #17: Thinking and the Nursing Process

Reexamine the case study about Jesse, his father, and Ms. Lamay, this time looking for evidence of the thinking. For now, just focus on Louise's *thinking*, not Jesse's and his father's thinking. Use a different colored pen than the one you used in Action Learning #16 and label the thinking according to the *think* mnemonic.

> T = Total Recall
> H = Habits
> I = Inquiry
> N = New Ideas and Creativity
> K = Knowing How You Think

Remember, the *thinking* may be very evident in the descriptions of *doing* in the case study, or the *thinking* may be implied. Identify the type of thinking that is occurring. Again, a combination of modes may be in operation all at once.

DISCUSSION   What kinds of thinking did you see happening? Do some types of thinking occur more frequently with some components of the nursing process than with others?

▶ SUMMARY OF LOUISE'S THINKING AND USE OF THE NURSING PROCESS

Louise's **assessing** involved pre-encounter, encounter, and postencounter **thinking and doing**. **Assessing** started before Louise met Jesse and his dad (pre-encounter). She engaged TOTAL RECALL when she looked up some facts that she thought she should know. She was anticipating her needs and checking things that could help her with **assessing** and **planning** care. As a nurse's expertise grows, more facts are stored in memory for retrieval, but do not ever expect to know it all. Nurses, even very experienced ones, continue to look up facts to help them provide care. Sometimes nurses look up information they anticipate needing; sometimes they find gaps in their knowledge and seek reference material during the patient encounter.

As Louise started **data collection** as part of **assessing**, she reviewed records, which are important sources of pre-encounter data. When she encountered Jesse and his dad, she **collected data** from them. She was **thinking** about the data and **forming conclusions** during the encounter when she verified her hunches about Mr. F.'s concerns.

Louise was also starting to **think** about **planning** care when she asked which problem was a priority. Then she went back to **data collection** to get more information about Jesse's nutritional status. Louise used INQUIRY **thinking** when she **analyzed** the data and considered various **conclusions** about Jesse's problems with eating and the factors that could be contributing to those problems. She didn't jump in with easy solutions as she **planned** what to offer as possible solutions. She used INQUIRY to consider various options, and used her NEW IDEAS AND CREATIVITY when she recruited Jesse's strengths (his interest in art and computers) to improve his eating.

Louise **implemented** the first part of her plan by telling Jesse and his dad her suggestions for how to entice Jesse to eat new foods. She anticipated **evaluation** by letting her patients know she would call to see how things were going. KNOWING HOW YOU THINK was used when Louise reflected on her thinking after Jesse and his dad left; she could see what she needed to do to compensate for her forgetting something.

The review of the thinking and doing in this case study illustrates how the components of the **nursing process** and various kinds of **thinking** are used. All of the *think* modes, except HABITS, were evident. Louise probably used HABITS when she checked Jesse's height and weight. Those measurements are associated so commonly with nutrition that almost anyone would check them automatically.

In the next chapter, the details of using the nursing process are addressed. It is helpful, however, periodically to *think* back to Louise and Jesse for a full picture of the process. Learning about and using the nursing process along with *thinking* and *doing* is not something that happens with one reading. Rereading, practice, and asking questions will help you continue on your journey toward great nursing.

▶▶▶ THINKING LOG #3

Put yourself in Louise's shoes and identify all the things you would do differently or in addition to what she did. Write out your thoughts below and compare your thoughts with those of a classmate.

REFERENCES

American Nurses' Association (1980). *Nursing: A social policy statement*. Kansas City: Author.

Gebbie, K. M. & Lavin, M. A. (1975). *Classification of nursing diagnoses: Proceedings of the First Conference*. St. Louis: CV Mosby.

McCloskey, J. C. & Bulechek, G. M. (Eds.). (1992). *Nursing interventions classification (NIC)*. St. Louis: CV Mosby.

North American Nursing Diagnosis Association. (1992). *NANDA nursing diagnoses: Definitions and classification 1992*. Philadelphia: Author.

Yura, H. & Walsh, M. B. (Eds.). (1967). *The nursing process: Assessing, planning, implementing, evaluating*. Washington, DC: The Catholic University of America Press.

Yura, H. & Walsh, M. B. (1973). *The nursing process: Assessing, planning, implementing, evaluating* (2nd ed.) New York: Appleton-Century-Crofts.

Yura, H. & Walsh, M. B. (1988). *The nursing process: Assessing, planning, implementing, evaluating*. (5th ed.). Norwalk, CT: Appleton & Lange.

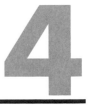

Application of Thinking and Doing in the Nursing Process

LEARNING OUTCOMES

After reading and doing the activities in this chapter you will be able to:

Apply your personal thinking approaches to using the nursing process.

Track the thinking path of a student nurse using the nursing process in a patient care situation.

Appreciate the variety of thinking styles used with the nursing process.

The last chapter showed how the components of the nursing process and thinking were used by one student nurse, Louise Lamay. Although many details are needed to understand the nursing process completely, this chapter continues to focus on the whole of the process. Seeing the whole several times helps to make more sense out of the details, which are addressed in later chapters.

This chapter also nurtures beginning students' growing appreciation for their existing thinking skills. Beginning students do not come into nursing with blank slates in their heads, they come with many existing thinking skills. Students bring a whole repertoire of thinking skills that they have developed over the last two to six decades of life. These skills can and should be built on, and not ignored by pretending to start learning at "ground zero." To enhance all thinking modes, especially INQUIRY and NEW IDEAS AND CREATIVITY, students must focus on KNOWING HOW YOU THINK. KNOWING HOW YOU THINK is the key to nurturing all thinking modes.

► APPLYING PERSONAL THINKING APPROACHES

To accomplish the task of incorporating personal thinking into the nursing process, the first part of this chapter is one big Action Learning (#18). Several questions are posed to stimulate multiple modes of thinking. The second part of this chapter presents another nursing situation accompanied by a report of one style of thinking as the nursing process was applied. Please do not read the second half of the chapter before doing Action Learning #18. This will make it easier for you to appreciate your existing skills and build on them.

In the following nursing situation you will be asked to *think* through the whole process, even though many questions may remain at this beginning stage. Keep in mind there are no right or wrong answers here, so be adventurous in your thinking. *Thinking caps on?*

▶▶▶▶▶▶ **Action Learning #18: The Big Think**

Read the following case study and answer the questions. Then find at least two classmates with whom to compare your answers. Remember, the purpose of comparing is not to see whose ideas are better, but to see how differently people approach thinking. Peer collaboration is a great way to learn about a variety of thinking skills.

CASE STUDY

Dan Christopher is a 20-year-old college sophomore in a Physical Therapy program. He has come to the student health service, where you are a student nurse completing an experience in Ambulatory Care. Dan is hoping to get a prescription for sleeping pills. He complains of not sleeping well for the last month; midterm exams are coming up soon and he needs some rest. He is 6'1" tall, 170 pounds, neatly dressed, alert and oriented. He has dark circles under his eyes and yawns several times during the interview. Dan says he is really stressed out this year with his studies, his part-time job, and his roommate who plays hard rock until 3 AM every night. A classmate suggested he get some sleeping pills. He's a little afraid of them because he's never taken anything stronger than aspirin before, but he's willing to try anything.

Questions to Stimulate *Think* Modes

1. How would you feel if you were Dan? Why?

_____

_____

_____

_____

2. What are your first impressions of Dan? Why do you think those were your first impressions?

_____

_____

_____

_____

3. What initial hunches would you make about this situation and why would you make them?

_____

_____

_____

_____

4. What questions do you have and why do you have them?

_____

_____

_____

_____

5. What do you think Dan wants to see happen in this situation? Why do you think that?

_____

_____

_____

_____

6. What would you like to see Dan achieve? Why?

_____

_____

_____

_____

7. What would you do *with* Dan? Why?

_____

_____

_____

_____

_____

8. After you did what you thought should be done, how would you determine if it was the best thing to do? Why is it important to determine that?

_____

_____

_____

_____

_____

9. What would you write in Dan's record? How would you write it down and why?

_____

_____

_____

_____

_____

10. What do you think is unique about your approach to Dan? Why do you think it is unique?

_____

_____

_____

_____

_____

11. How and why did you use these thinking modes in this situation?

T:

H:

I:

N:

K:

12. Which thinking mode(s) was (were) easiest? Hardest? Why?

_____

_____

_____

_____

DISCUSSION How different or alike were your answers and those of your classmates? Are you beginning to appreciate what is unique about your thinking and theirs? Isn't it interesting how three people can look at the same thing and see some things so differently and some things exactly the same? How did you feel about the differences?

The questions for Action Learning #18 are somewhat broad to allow individual thinking styles to emerge. The questions also are arranged in a typical sequence that many nurses use to begin and follow through on their thinking during patient care. The questions, however, could be arranged differently to fit personal thinking styles. Action Learning #18 also encourages awareness of the feelings associated with thinking, how they might be unique, and how they might be different from other nurses' feelings.

▷ Feelings About Personal Thinking Abilities

Students may have several reactions when they compare their work to that of others. Some feel anxious; others don't. Some feel insecure when they see their work is different from someone else's. Others feel superior when they think they have the best approach or answer. Still others feel all of the above. Although all of these responses are normal, it is important to recognize that they can significantly influence thinking in positive and negative ways.

Think back to how you felt while doing this exercise; on a scale of 1 to 10, with 10 being the highest, what was your anxiety level? Remember, anxiety tends to shut down higher-level thinking skills and shunt thinking energy into survival mode. Therefore, the best thinking occurs when anxiety is not too high. If your anxiety was high while doing Action Learning #18, think about ways to decrease that anxiety. For example, remember that these exercises are for learning, not for grading or even evaluating your ability to do nursing. It is okay to recognize areas for further development, areas you would like to enhance. Acknowledging these areas for development is a great way to learn and to expand thinking, especially in the NEW IDEAS AND CREATIVITY and the KNOWING HOW YOU THINK modes. Recognizing and accepting that there is always room for growth is a true sign of a thinking nurse.

For those who felt insecure after seeing how others had responded, consider how this affects your thinking. If feeling insecure hinders thinking, it will hinder nursing care. If feeling insecure is a common response, seriously consider ways to increase self-esteem. Unfortunately, low self-esteem is a common feeling among college students. The good news is that low self-esteem is a learned behavior; people are not born with low self-esteem. It can, therefore, be unlearned if there is a desire to do so. Many helpful techniques are available besides spending years in psychoanalysis.

Because this text does not allow time for a crash course in improving self-esteem, one simple but effective way is offered. Write a list of 10 of your positive attributes. If you cannot instantly think of 10, list as many as possible. Post the list on your bathroom mirror and read it *aloud* every morning until it is firmly etched in your brain. Add a new item to your list every day and continue to read it aloud. You will be impressed with how much more you can appreciate and respect yourself.

At the other extreme are people who feel they have all the "right answers." This attitude can be a serious threat to patient safety. Students who feel superior are less apt to question their judgments or use INQUIRY in planning nursing care. No nurse has all the answers, not even those who have worked for many years. Even experts have questions and doubts. If nurses do not ask questions and challenge their own thinking, their patients' health may be in serious jeopardy.

Have all the options for feelings been removed? Don't feel superior; don't feel insecure; don't feel anxious. What's left for those who are human? Well, as with most things in life, balance is needed. Strive for a healthy self-esteem with openness to all five modes of thinking. With that combination, the great nurse in every student can emerge.

▶ TRACKING THINKING THROUGH THE NURSING PROCESS

Now it is time to demonstrate the thinking of a nurse using the nursing process. Thinking is not always easy to track, but it is important to try to visualize this very abstract process. Many textbooks describe what to do and why, but most do not discuss the thinking that occurs. Only recently have educators recognized the importance of describing the thinking process.

Part of the reason that thinking has not been discussed may be that expert nurses and nursing instructors, who have practiced nursing for a long time, find it difficult to explain their thinking, which has become automatic. Think about something you have been doing for years, such as riding a bicycle. How easy is it to describe verbally the balance and coordination acquired so many years ago? Most of the process has become second nature for the long-time bike rider. Thinking about how to describe the fine-tuned skills of bike riding is a big challenge.

But challenge or not, describing thinking is one of the best ways to nurture better thinking in beginning students, and examining a case study role model is the next-best thing to real life. The student nurse in this case study is Ken Tanaka. His clinical course focuses on gerontology and rehabilitation care.

Examine Ken's thinking carefully and compare it to yours with an open mind. Draw on the things that make sense and add them into your thinking skills repertoire. Set aside the things that do not make sense, but do not discard them immediately. Read several more chapters on thinking skills, then decide if some of these thinking approaches are worth keeping after all.

CASE STUDY

Ken is doing a clinical rotation in a nursing home. This morning, part of his assignment is to care for Mrs. Poski, a newly admitted, 82-year-old patient.

Mrs. Poski came to the skilled nursing home facility after a short hospitalization for malnutrition. She is a retired piano teacher who has been living independently since her husband's death 10 years ago. Three months ago, after her bout with the "flu," her appetite and strength diminished. She lost 20 pounds, which led to her hospitalization.

Mrs. Poski has three sons who visit regularly and are supportive of her returning to her home when her strength improves and her nutritional intake is stable. She is a pleasant woman who is cooperative and agreeable with the current plan for her recovery. Her sons describe her as extremely sociable, enjoying numerous activities and interactions with others. The nurses, however, have observed her interacting very little with other residents and spending much time in her room alone. When asked about this apparent change in her socialization pattern, Mrs. Poski says she just doesn't want to bother people by asking them to repeat things she can't hear. She is very hard of hearing. She admits that her hearing has gotten worse since the flu and that she should have it checked. However, she assumed she would have to wait until she got home for an appointment with an ear specialist.

Mrs. Poski is alert and oriented. Her medical diagnoses are osteoarthritis and malnutrition. Her current medications are ibuprofen 200 mg qid and multivitamins, 1 qd. She wears glasses for reading and has her own teeth. Her vital signs this morning were: BP = 106/78, pulse = 76, respiration = 18, temp. = 98.6°F. She has no edema or shortness of breath, no smoking or history of alcohol abuse. Her present weight is 95 lbs. With a height of 5'4", her ideal body weight is 120 lbs ± 10%. Before the flu, her weight was 112 lbs. Although she gained 3 lbs. since arriving at the nursing home, her appetite is still poor to fair. She consumes 50% to 75% of meals. She is continent of bowel and bladder and denies problems with constipation. She had lots of diarrhea during the "flu" and for 1 week thereafter. Mrs. Poski continues to experience decreased strength and stamina since the flu, but is improving with physical therapy five times per week and increased food intake. Her gait is unsteady and her balance is poor during transfers from wheelchair to bed. She is able to bathe and dress herself with moderate assistance. Her skin is intact, but fragile.

▷ Assessment

The process of assessment includes data collection and data analysis. Both of these concepts will be explored more fully in Chapters 7 and 8, but for now think about data collection as the gathering of information and data analysis as making sense out of the information. Data analysis includes recognizing important pieces of data, seeing relationships among pieces of data and groups of data, and making conclusions.

Data Collection

Ken began care for Mrs. Poski by listening to the morning report and reading Mrs. Poski's medical and nursing record. This is described as pre-encounter data. He continued his data collection when he talked to (interviewed) Mrs. Poski, observed her during the interview, and took measurements (eg, blood pressure, pulse, respirations, and temperature.) The thinking that is required before collecting data is not addressed here, but is dealt with in Chapter 7 ("Health Detectives"). Ken's thinking for analyzing the data will be studied first.

Data Analysis

First Impressions

For starters, Ken acknowledged his overall first impression. Mrs. Poski reminded him of his Aunt Millie. He thought, if this were Aunt Millie, I know she'd want really good nursing care and I'd want it for her. Ken thought about what was going through his mind; he knew that when he could positively identify with a patient, he thought more clearly and efficiently. When he didn't like the patient as much, he spent more time making sure he was being nice because he was afraid his feelings about the person would be seen as negative. (Ken was demonstrating the KNOWING HOW YOU THINK mode.)

Overall, he thought, Mrs. Poski is getting better and has good family support. She is likeable, but keeps to herself. Her isolation, her nutrition, and her difficulty in transferring are areas of concern that require more thinking. These thoughts all were preliminary hunches that were used to guide his data collection further and refine his conclusions later.

Comparing Data to Norms

Next, Ken thought about the information he had. What was normal? He used his recall (TOTAL RECALL) of knowledge from his course work to decide what was standard (normal) for most people, but remembered to check if these things were normal for Mrs. Poski. He decided the following data were not normal, or at least questionable, and therefore considered "relevant data."

20-lb. weight loss during "flu"	Hard of Hearing
Ht. 5'4" with Wt. of 95 lbs.	Appetite poor to fair
Consumes 50%–75% of meals	Decreased strength
Unsteady gait	Decreased stamina
Poor balance	Interacting little
Spending much time alone	Not wanting to bother people
Hearing getting worse	Unable to bathe and dress alone

Initial Hunches

With this list in mind, Ken developed some more formalized hunches that focused on problems with hearing, socialization, nutrition, and mobility. He also suspected that Mrs. Poski had some risk factors for other problems, but he could not be sure just what those were yet. Again, using his recall (TOTAL RECALL) of lectures on aging, he knew that some normal risks accompanied aging. He knew he wouldn't feel sure of his preliminary conclusions until he reviewed some information on aging and on mobility problems for patients with osteoarthritis (again, exhibiting the KNOWING HOW YOU THINK MODE when he was looking for ways to feel more comfortable with his conclusions).

Finding Clusters

At this point, Ken had lots of ideas in his head, but he had to organize them to come to some final conclusions that could be supported with relevant data. He also thought about what else he needed to know. He decided to jot down the data in clusters (groups) to see what patterns emerged and to see if there where gaps in information (data gaps). He used INQUIRY to question what else he should consider. He used his RECALL of information about usual patterns of human responses to organize his clusters. Here are five clusters of data he initially developed:

▼ CLUSTERS

Ht. 5′4″ Wt. 95 lbs.
Appetite poor to fair
Lost 20 lbs. during "flu"
Gained 3 lbs. in nursing home
Consumes 50%–75% of meals

_____

Decreased strength and stamina
Gait unsteady
Balance poor
Unable to dress and bathe alone

_____

Interacting little
Spending much time alone
Not wanting to bother people
Hard of hearing
Previous pattern of being very sociable

_____

Assuming she would have to wait for appointment with ear
   specialist
Hard of hearing

_____

Supportive family
Independent lifestyle
Music interests
Stable vital signs
Communicates effectively
Mentally alert and oriented
Recent weight gain of 3 lbs.

Ken thought about these clusters. The data were so interrelated, he wasn't sure that these clusters were the best, but he could see that there were definite factors that "painted a picture" of her strengths as well as health concerns. He also realized that some of the problem areas were primary problems, whereas others seemed to be contributing to the primary problems. For example, Ht. 5′4″, Wt. 95 lbs., 20-lb. weight loss during "flu," consuming 50% to 75% of meals, showed a picture of nutrition that was less than adequate. Poor appetite was contributing to that problem. The data and the data clusters were interrelated to some extent. He decided he could draw some conclusions that had a good probability of being accurate because he had enough supporting data. More data on the hearing and specific data on the types of food Mrs. Poski liked or did not like would have allowed him to draw conclusions with even higher probabilities of accuracy, so he made a mental note to get more information as soon as possible. This analysis of the relationships among the data exemplified the use of TOTAL RECALL and INQUIRY.

Thinking About Conclusions

Ken concluded that Mrs. Poski had many strengths that could be used in planning her care. He also recognized there was a definite problem with nutrition, but it was getting somewhat better. If Mrs. Poski's appetite could be increased, she would eat better, which would increase her strength and speed up her recuperation. He'd have to talk to the dietitian before finalizing plans for nutrition.

His second conclusion concerned the hearing problem; this was a mystery. He decided the doctor should evaluate that, and perhaps a referral to a specialist would be advisable. He knew Mrs. Poski was getting physical therapy (PT), so he would coordinate plans with PT to help with the mobility issues (a third conclusion). He thought that something should be done to help her interact more with people because she seemed socially isolated (a fourth conclusion). He deduced that the hearing problem was a strong contributor to the social isolation. This fifth conclusion about the related factor required him to use his knowledge of human behavior and the effects of physical impairment, and then to see a relationship between those two sets of information. Again, TOTAL RECALL and INQUIRY were the major thinking modes used here.

There also were risk factors to consider. The data cluster about decreased mobility led him to think about a potential for falls and injuries (a sixth conclusion). If the nutrition and mobility problems didn't continue to improve, Mrs. Poski's skin would be at risk (seventh conclusion). He recalled from lectures and textbooks that skin, especially that of older people, could break down easily when people didn't move around sufficiently and they were undernourished. This thinking about relationships between pieces of data required the use of TOTAL RECALL and INQUIRY.

Conclusions

As Ken prepared to write his conclusions in the patient's record, he thought about the best wording to use. He wanted his conclusions to be clear enough that others could understand them. He got out his nursing diagnosis books to look for labels whose definitions fit with his conclusions. When he found similar wording and definitions, he compared his clusters of relevant data to the defining characteristics listed for the textbook diagnostic labels. Because his clusters fit with the clusters in the book, he used the standard NANDA terminology. (The discussion of NANDA diagnoses is in Chapter 3, and the Taxonomy list is in Appendix A.)

As well as recording the data clusters that supported his conclusions, he charted the following conclusions:

Strengths: Past history of socialization, participation in PT, increased food intake, supportive family, vital signs stable, skin intact, continent, artistic interests, effective communication skills, mentally alert and oriented.

(Ken was aware that many of Mrs. Poski's strengths might be considered for inclusion in a Wellness Diagnosis, but he decided to talk to his instructor before developing one.)

Health Concerns:

Problems for Referral: Progressive hearing loss (refer to MD).

Interdisciplinary Problems:

Decreased strength and stamina (PT)

Altered Nutrition: Less than Body Requirements, related to decreased appetite 2° "flu" (dietitian)

Nursing Diagnoses (problems and related factors):

Self-Care Deficit for Bathing and Dressing related to generalized weakness secondary to decreased nutrition and prolonged diarrhea post "flu."

Social Isolation related to increasing hearing loss, not wanting to bother people.

High Risk for Injury related to generalized weakness, poor balance, and unstable transfers from bed to wheelchair.

High Risk for Impaired Skin Integrity related to immobility, frail skin, and inadequate nutrition.

Sharing Conclusions With Patient and Setting Priorities

This is the point in the nursing process where assessment and planning start blending together. Sharing conclusions with the patient for validation of those conclusions is part of assessment. Setting priorities is part of planning. For the sake of time, however, both activities are usually done together.

The above conclusions were shared with Mrs. Poski. Ken thought about how important it was for the patient to be actively involved in all aspects of care. He also knew that validating conclusions (making sure the patient agreed with the conclusion) was vital before anything else was done. Mrs. Poski agreed that the conclusions matched her perceptions of her needs. She was most interested in the social isolation diagnosis because she was feeling very alone. She helped to set the priority because no conclusion represented an immediately life-threatening problem or a major safety issue. Involving the patient in validating conclusions and setting priorities is another example of using INQUIRY.

Pause here for a thinking-learning check. You should be able to elaborate on these ideas:

▼ Beginning nursing students have a wealth of life experience and thinking skills to draw on and nurture.

▼ Feelings about personal thinking abilities can help or hinder thinking skills.

▼ Ken's thinking can be tracked in all five modes as he collected data and analyzed data (noting first impressions, comparing data to norms, developing initial hunches, finding clusters, thinking about his conclusions, validating his conclusions, and setting priorities with Mrs. Poski).

▶ CONTINUED TRACKING OF KEN'S THINKING THROUGH THE NURSING PROCESS

▷ Planning Care

In collaboration with Mrs. Poski, Ken developed a plan of care to address *all* the conclusions and build on her existing strengths. For the sake of time, however, only a portion of the complete care plan is presented here.

Patient Goals

Examine the care plan. Study it and then continue to read about Ken's thinking as he prepared his plan. First, consider the "Patient Goal":

> By the end of 1 week, Mrs. Poski will have diminished social isolation

The goal is the first thing Ken thought about after the conclusion (nursing diagnosis), "Social Isolation related to increased hearing loss and not wanting to bother people," was validated with the patient and by the data. While developing the goal for socialization, Ken thought about socialization and how personal an issue it was. He knew it was important to have Mrs. Poski develop the plan with him. They agreed that a decrease in social isolation was a reasonable goal to achieve in a week's time.

Patient Objectives (Expected Outcomes)

It wasn't enough just to have the broad goal of decreasing the social isolation problem. The factors contributing to the problem had to be addressed as well.

▼ **Sample Care Plan 4-1**

Student Ken Tanaka   **Date** 9/3/93   **Patient** Mrs. Poski

Nursing Dx. # 2

Social Isolation related to (R/T) increased hearing loss and not wanting to bother people

Defining characteristics: Interacting little, previous pattern of being very social, spending much time alone, not wanting to bother people, hearing loss.

Patient Goal Statement:

By the end of 1 week, Mrs. Poski will have diminished social isolation as evidenced by (A.E.B.):

PATIENT OBJECTIVES (EXPECTED OUTCOMES)	NURSING ACTIONS (ORDERS)	RATIONALE
1. Sharing her thoughts and feelings about her isolation and hearing loss and their affect on her health (9/3/93).	1. Ask her to share her thoughts and feelings about: Her recent social isolation How the isolation affects her emotional health, physical health, and recovery. How her hearing loss affects her isolation.	1.a. Identification of pt's feelings is helpful in planning effective behavior change. Assessing pt's insight into relationship between life situations determines where to start interventions.
2. Discussing ways to obtain information without feeling like a bother (9/3/93).	2.a. Assess her feelings about bothering people b. Explore with her appropriate ways to get info. without feeling like a bother: Tell people at beginning of a conversation that she needs them to speak slowly, clearly, and in normal tone. Ask if other person would mind if she occasionally reminds them to speak up. Carry pad and pen to offer others as needed. c. Role play an interaction with pt.	2.a. Identification of pt's feelings is helpful in planning effective behavior change. b. Mutual problem solving reinforces pt role as partner in care as well as promoting independence. Providing several suggestions allows pt to expand own thinking of solutions and select ideas best suited to individual needs. c. Role play allows pt opportunity to try new behaviors before using with others.
3. Describing changes in her hearing and things that help and hinder her hearing (9/3/93).	3.a. Assessing hearing loss in depth re: Onset, quality, and quantity of change, Chronology of change, aggravating and alleviating factors, associated problems. b. Ask her to explain what she understands about hearing and hearing problems.	3.a. Accurate and complete data collection increases probability of accurate conclusions and effective care plan. b. Assessing what pt knows saves time in teaching and acknowledges pt as a care partner.

Continued

▼ **Sample Care Plan 4-1** *continued*

PATIENT OBJECTIVES (EXPECTED OUTCOMES)	NURSING ACTIONS (ORDERS)	RATIONALE
4. Agreeing to participate in hearing exam (4/3/93).	4.a. Assess her willingness to have hearing exam. b. Obtain M.D. order for exam and schedule exam. c. Arrange transportation and be sure results are addressed.	4.a. Determining level of pt cooperation avoids waste of time and inappropriate referrals. b. M.D. needs to order all exams. Nurse needs to schedule exam. c. Facilitating pt attendance at exam and follow-up on recommendations increases chances of behavior change.
5. Participating in two activities/day that require interaction with other residents (9/5/93).	5.a. Identify with pt which activities she would be most comfortable with: music group, ceramics, bingo, exercise groups, needle crafts. b. Plan daily care to allow adequate time for activities. c. Monitor pt participation in activities and talk with her afterward to assess what worked and what didn't, and how to modify plans.	5.a. Mutual problem solving reinforces pt's role as a partner in care as well as promoting independence. b. Providing opportunity for behavior change increases probability of change. c. Evaluating pt behavior and adjusting plan as needed increases chance of successful behavior change and resolution of problem

EVALUATION:	RELEVANT INFORMATION RE: PARTIALLY MET OR UNMET OBJECTIVES	
Obj. # 1 Met/Partially Met/Unmet Date 9/3/93	Actions effective.	
Obj. # 2 Met/Partially Met/Unmet Date 9/3/93	Stated hearing loss hard to cope with. Agreed to all except reminding people.	Was receptive to new ideas. Successful role play.
Obj. # 3 Met/Partially Met/Unmet Date 9/3/93	Helps: Facing patient while speaking, speaking slowly and distinctly in a moderate voice tone. Hinders: High-pitched voice, environmental noise, and lots of people talking in the same room.	
Obj. # 4 Met/Partially Met/Unmet Date 9/5/93	Hearing exam scheduled with Dr. Otology for 9/10/93, 10 AM. Son will provide tlransportation.	

Continued

▼ **Sample Care Plan 4-1** *continued*

Obj. # 5 Met/Partially Met/Unmet Date 9/6/93	Prefers one activity/day for now. Enjoyed the music group. Bingo was too noisy. Will try ceramics and exercise next week.
Obj. # _____ Met/Partially Met/Unmet Date _____	
Obj. # _____ Met/Partially Met/Unmet Date _____	

Looking at those factors, Ken thought about smaller increments of change in Mrs. Poski's behavior that would ultimately reduce her social isolation by eliminating or diminishing the contributing factors. If Mrs. Poski could meet these small increments (patient objectives or expected outcomes), Ken, other nurses, and Mrs. Poski would have tangible evidence that progress toward the goal was being made. For the first objective, it was important for Mrs. Poski to talk about her feelings. Then, she needed to figure out how to interact without feeling as if she were bothering others. Three other objectives were developed (see objectives 3, 4, and 5 on plan). Ken studied the set of objectives and, using INQUIRY, asked himself, "Are these objectives reasonable? Are they measurable, are they client-centered, do they address all of the etiologies of the diagnostic statement? If they are achieved, will the goal be met?"

Nursing Actions (Orders)

Once the objectives were developed, Ken designed the nursing actions or interventions (the middle column in the sample care plan) that would help Mrs. Poski achieve the objectives to meet the goal. The nursing actions specifically identify what Ken and other nurses needed to do to increase the probability of Mrs. Poski achieving the objectives to meet the goal and resolve the problem.

The plan so far may look like a neat package, but not all nurses think or work in this sequence. Sometimes, for some problems, nurses think about the nursing actions before they think about patient objectives. This will not seem backwards if one remembers that the nursing process is not a linear set of steps. The best way to achieve open thinking with the nursing process is to remember that all the pieces are interrelated, intertwined, and inseparable. The order in which they are written down on paper is rarely an exact replication of the patterns of thinking that produced the plan. In this case, it made more sense to Ken to decide first where Mrs. Poski should be going than to figure out how to get there. Therefore, he developed the goal and objectives before the nursing actions. He could have figured out what the nurses needed to do and then related that to what the patient should be achieving. Some books (eg, Smeltzer & Bare, 1992) present care plans with the nursing actions or interventions column preceding the expected outcomes column. Others (eg, McFarland & McFarlane, 1993) put objectives first, as Ken did. As long as the final plan is consistent in its relationships of goals to objectives and nursing actions, the order in which the parts are constructed in the nurse's mind or on paper is unimportant. KNOWING HOW YOU THINK is a mode to use when making decisions about *your* "logical" way to approach planning.

Supporting Rationale for Actions

As a student nurse, Ken couldn't just pull the nursing actions out of a hat (or his head). He used his textbooks to help him find actions based on sound rationales (reasons). Also, because he was a student who needed to show his thinking to his instructor, he wrote the rationale down next to each nursing action (see the right-hand column on the care plan example). *Note*—Many instructors also require students to write down the reference they used for each rationale. For example, for the nursing action, "use mild soap," the documented rationale with a reference could read: "these contain no detergents, dyes or hardening agents" (Smeltzer & Bare, 1992, p. 1456).

Developing the nursing actions required Ken to use TOTAL RECALL, INQUIRY, and NEW IDEAS AND CREATIVITY modes of thinking. If Ken were an experienced nurse, some actions would have been HABITS in his mind. Because he was a student, he had not developed nursing action HABITS yet. TOTAL RECALL was used when he remembered which books to use, which lectures notes to check, and which nursing care references to locate. He used INQUIRY to make decisions about which nursing actions were appropriate for Mrs. Poski's care and which were not. He used NEW IDEAS AND CREATIVITY to adapt the standard nursing actions found in a textbook to Mrs. Poski's unique situation.

Ken repeated the process of planning for the remaining three nursing diagnoses, Self-Care Deficit for Bathing and Dressing related to generalized weakness secondary to decreased nutrition and prolonged diarrhea post flu; High Risk for Injury related to generalized weakness, poor balance, and unstable transfers from bed to wheelchair; and High Risk for Impaired Skin Integrity related to immobility, frail skin and inadequate nutrition. Those parts of the plan are not included here but, as a review, see what you can do with one of these diagnoses.

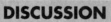 **Action Learning #19: Developing a Goal and Objectives**

Look at the diagnosis "Self-Care Deficit . . . ." What do you think would be an appropriate goal for Ken and Mrs. Poski to be working toward in trying to resolve this problem?

Goal:

What do you think would be one of the objectives that would show Mrs. Poski was moving toward the goal?

Objective/expected outcome:

What resources would you use to decide what is appropriate nursing care for this problem?

DISCUSSION   What was the hardest part about doing this Action Learning? Often, students say it was coming up with concise wording that really said what they wanted it to say. Many students find the wording a challenge at first. Do not despair; you will find that after you have written goals and objectives for a while, you learn there are patterns to the wording. The goal is usually a restatement of the words in the problem indicating that the problem is "fixed." (By the end of 1 week Mrs. Poski will have increased her self-care ability.) The objectives are usually restatements of the words in the related factors, indicating that they are not related factors any more. (Demonstrate ability to bathe and dress self without assistance in 1 hour and not feel worn out.) Note the word "usually" in these sentences. There are no hard and fast rules, only general guides. Developing goals and objectives is addressed more fully in Chapter 9.

▷ More Planning

Planning for Other Conclusions in Addition to Nursing Diagnoses

Back to Ken and Mrs. Poski. In addition to planning the care for all the nursing diagnoses (Social Isolation, Self-Care Deficit, High Risk for Injury, and High Risk for Impaired Skin Integrity), Ken reviewed his other conclusions. For the hearing problem, he left a note for Mrs. Poski's physician, recommending that her hearing be evaluated. For the nutrition problem, Ken talked to the dietitian and, together, they developed an interdisciplinary plan. Likewise, he talked to the physical therapist and learned about realistic mobility goals. The recommendations from the physical therapist were added to the part of the nursing plan that focused on the risks for injury and the self-care deficits. Some agencies call these collaborative, interdisciplinary or master treatment plans.

Ken thought about the best way to communicate these parts of the plan to other nurses. He could have developed a specific nursing plan for the mobility and balance problems, but the nursing actions would have overlapped those on the plan for self-care and preventing injury. To avoid duplication of effort, he picked what he saw as the most logical part of the plan into which to incorporate the recommendations for increasing mobility and balance. INQUIRY was used to make these decisions about where to write what. Chapter 8 ("Making More Sense Out of the Clues: Cluster Analysis") provides details on the thinking required to consolidate care planning.

Streamlining Care Plans

Decisions about where to write on a plan are sometimes very individual. Nurses do not have time to duplicate efforts, yet they want to make sure that others understand what they and the patient are trying to achieve. Sometimes

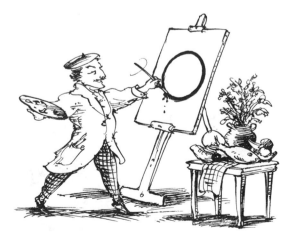

Figure 4-1. Streamlining.

it is necessary to refer to another part of the plan, for example, "See plan for safety." One thing that will soon become obvious, if it hasn't already, is the interconnectedness of human responses. Few things fit into tidy boxes. The actions to alleviate one problem usually affect another problem.

Nurses streamline plans to communicate complexities simply. Experienced nurses can shorten plans because they can assume that other experienced nurses have the knowledge necessary to fill in the details. Although it is necessary, streamlining should be approached cautiously. Too little streamlining can cause redundancies and use up much time; too much streamlining can leave out something important. Students are expected to err on the side of too little streamlining, because they must show what they are learning. As experience is gained, so will skill in streamlining. Below is what a streamlined part of the plan might look like for the problem, "High Risk for Injury related to generalized weakness, poor balance, and unstable transfers from bed to wheelchair." Notice that although there is a reference to physical therapy exercises, the specifics are not duplicated. The rationale for each action is not written on the plan; it is assumed that experienced nurses know the rationale for their actions. There are fewer details in the actions, and the specific actions are not linked directly to specific objectives. They are addressed collectively.

▼ Streamlined Sample Care Plan 4-2

Patient: Mrs. Poski

Nursing Diagnosis: #3 High Risk for Injury related to generalized weakness, poor balance, and unstable transfers from bed to wheelchair.

GOALS/EXPECTED OUTCOMES	NURSING ACTIONS
9/3/93 **Goal:** Pt will have no injuries during stay in N.H. **Outcomes:** 1. Exhibit enough strength to hold herself up during transfers by 9/9//93 2. Maintain balance during transfers by 9/9/93 3. Demonstrate safe pivot transfers by 9/9/93	1. Reinforce exercises recommended by physical therapist, especially on weekends. 2. Encourage ball squeezing for 10 min tid 3. Remind pt to do body lifting while in chair q 1 hr. 4. Teach pt about keeping feet apart to maintain balance during transfers. Remind pt not to over-lean. 5. Show pt how to transfer by sliding bottom forward on chair, leaning forward, pushing down on arms of chair, and moving hips to new position. 6. Stand-by assist during transfers. Remind pt to call for help before getting up.

▷ Implementing Care

Ken began implementing the plan of care as soon as he and Mrs. Poski agreed it was appropriate. During implementation he continued to assess and also think about how well the plan was working (evaluation). This is another example of how phases of the nursing process overlap. Checking for effec-- tiveness of the plan as the plan is being implemented is a sign of a thinking nurse.

▷ Evaluating Care

The evaluation process actually began when Ken and Mrs. Poski developed ob- jectives during the planning phase. It is these objectives that become the crite- ria for judging changes in patient behaviors after care is provided. Because they are outcome-oriented, objectives are often called "Expected Outcomes."

Here is Ken's thinking when he evaluated the implemented plan. First, he thought about the time and compared it to the planned time for the goals and objectives. When the expected dates for the objectives on the plan arrived, he reviewed each objective for that date and asked himself, "Has that objective been met by Mrs. Poski?" He compared the data he had about Mrs. Poski with what he and Mrs. Poski planned as objectives. They decided if each objective was met, partially met, or not met, and he recorded this information on the patient record.

Look at the evaluation section at the end of the sample plan for Mrs. Pos- ki's social isolation problem. In the left column, notice the circled conclusions about each objective. In the right column are Ken's comments supporting his conclusions.

Ken's written comments for each objective serve two functions of evalua- tion. First, they address the specific patient behaviors that indicate whether or not the objective was met. Second, the comments address how effective the nursing actions were. The first is called outcome evaluation; the second is called process evaluation.

Ken used INQUIRY to do the evaluation. He questioned what he saw, made decisions about the quality of care, and thought about what should and could be done to improve the care. He did this not only for the diagnosis of Social Isolation, but for the whole plan with all conclusions.

In some ways, evaluation is similar to the initial data collection. Evalua- tion makes the nursing process a cycle as the nurse moves back to collecting data and, from that data, draws conclusions. These conclusions become the basis for new or changed plans for care. This process continues until all the problems are resolved or the patient is discharged from service.

THINKING-LEARNING CHECK

Pause here for a thinking-learning check. You should be able to elaborate on these ideas:

▼ Planning includes working with the patient to set priorities, establish goals and objectives (expected outcomes), develop nursing actions, support nursing actions with rationales, and write out a care plan.

▼ Streamlined care plans are used by experienced nurses to save time and energy while maintaining high-quality planning.

▼ During implementation of care the nurse is also assessing and evaluating the results of care.

▼ Evaluation of care begins with developing objectives, and includes outcome evaluation (comparing patient behaviors to the objectives) and process evaluation (judging the effectiveness of nursing actions).

▶ REEXAMINING YOUR THINKING

This chapter, long though it may have seemed, is only the beginning of tracking thinking and using the nursing process. It was designed to show the whole of the nursing process, not *all* the details. Think about what you have added to your *thinking* repertoire as you complete Action Learning #20.

▶▶▶▶▶▶ Action Learning #20: Re-Thinking Action Learning #18

Review your answers for Action Learning #18. After seeing how your classmates answered the questions and after reading about Ken's thinking process with Mrs. Poski, indicate any changes you would make in your original answers. The numbers below correspond to the original questions in Action Learning #18.

1.

2.

3.

4.

5.

6.

7.

8.

9.

10.

11.

12.

DISCUSSION   What were the most significant changes? Did most of your answers stay the same, or did most change? Why? What mode(s) of thinking did you use the most?

▶▶▶ *THINKING LOG #4*

Given the large amount of information in this chapter, the complexity of the nursing process, and the thinking that goes into using the nursing process, it is likely that you have identified areas about which you are still fuzzy. List five questions that you now have about *thinking* and the *nursing process*.

REFERENCES

McFarland, G. K., & McFarlane, E.A. (1993). *Nursing diagnosis and intervention* (2nd ed.). St. Louis: CV Mosby.
Smeltzer, S. C., & Bare, B. G. (1992). *Brunner and Suddarth's textbook of medical-surgical nursing* (7th ed.). Philadelphia: JB Lippincott.

Nursing Conclusions

After reading and doing the activities in this chapter you will be able to:

Describe the purpose and characteristics of nursing conclusions.

Examine existing conclusion-making skills.

Explain the relationships among hunches, directed data collection, and ruling in and ruling out hunches.

Appreciate the thinking required to develop nursing conclusions with the highest probability of accuracy.

The last four chapters have focused on the big picture of thinking and doing and the nursing process. Now it is time to start looking at the specifics. Nursing conclusions will be discussed first. Conclusions are judgments made after thinking. This chapter examines the purpose of nursing conclusions, the importance of addressing conclusions at the beginning of a study of thinking and the nursing process, several characteristics of nursing conclusions, and the thinking required to develop conclusions.

▶ THE PURPOSE OF NURSING CONCLUSIONS

The overriding purpose of nursing conclusions is to guide effective and efficient nursing care, that is, great nursing. Achieving such nursing care can be challenging because there are so many pieces of information about patients and their situations that the nurse has to address. The nurse needs to make sense out of all the information instead of just remembering the individual pieces. The "sense" the nurse makes results in conclusions, which lead to even more conclusions.

Conclusions are part of all phases of the nursing process. Some of those conclusions are major ones; others are smaller steps along the way. With assessment, for example, the major conclusions provide direction for planning

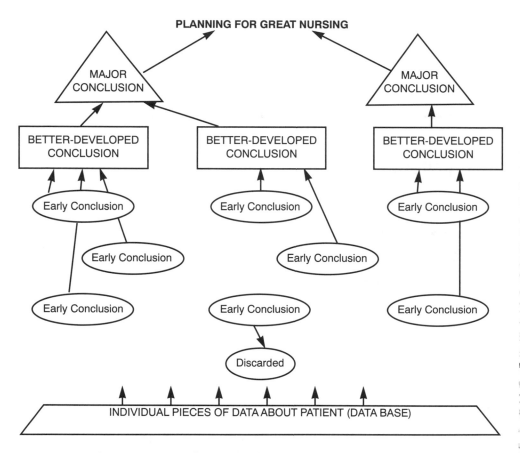

Figure 5-1.   Conclusion development during assessment.

great nursing care, but there are many conclusions leading to the major ones. Figure 5-1 illustrates this progressive series of conclusions.

▶ WHY LEARN ABOUT CONCLUSIONS AT THE BEGINNING?

It may seem that discussing the details of conclusions before describing the earlier parts of the nursing process, such as data collection, is illogical. By studying conclusions first, however, one can see where one is going. If that destination is known, it is easier to figure out how to get there.

Where one is going is not actually an end point. Most conclusions in nursing are more like rest stops on a journey; they provide guidance for travel along the nursing process path. Consider a driving trip from New York to California. A decision is needed for the first day's end point; otherwise, one might be stuck with no hotel room. If Pittsburgh is selected as the first stop, it allows for some detail planning for the best way to get there at the end of the journey's first day. Likewise, in the nursing process, interim "end points" allow the nurse to move on a well-designed path from data to nursing care.

The conclusions made during the assessment phase of the nursing process are stop-overs that feed into planning. Conclusions made during planning feed into implementation. The conclusions reached during implementation result in evaluation; conclusions from evaluation feed back into planning, and, often, back to assessment. At each of these points, and at other such points in the nursing process, the conclusions represent the nurse's thinking about the information at hand.

▶ PERSONAL CONCLUSION-MAKING STYLE

Because everybody thinks, everybody makes conclusions all the time. Many scholarly dissertations have been written on conclusion making, but what is important here is to get a sense of your personal conclusion-making style. Think about the conclusions you made today—conclusions about what to wear, what to have for breakfast, what to think of the class you are attending, and so forth. And this barely begins to enumerate the numerous conclusions you make on a daily basis. But, have you ever thought about how you come to those conclusions? It is time to use the KNOWING HOW YOU THINK mode.

▶▶▶▶▶▶ **Action Learning #21: Tracking Your Thinking Through a Conclusion**

Think of an *important* conclusion that you made recently. Write out the process you went through to arrive at the conclusion, paying special attention to what you were thinking *and* how you were thinking. Consider how your conclusion making might have been tailored to the importance of the conclusion. In other words, do you think differently about important conclusions than you do about less important ones? (Reminder: the *how* of thinking can be described with the vocabulary listed in Display 1-2, "Vocabulary for Thinking About Thinking"—assume, infer, interpret, distinguish, perspective, point of view, and so forth.)

| **DISCUSSION** | What did you learn about the process you use for developing conclusions? Does the process vary depending on |

the situation or the importance of the conclusion? How easy was it to track the *how* of your thinking? As you recall the discussions of nursing in the previous chapters, can you project what parts of your present conclusion-making thinking you will bring to nursing?

▶ NURSING CONCLUSIONS

Nursing conclusions are made the same way conclusions are made in other areas of life. It is important to see these similarities to build on existing skills, and not assume this is a whole new process to learn. After reading about the characteristics of nursing conclusions, the process used to develop nursing conclusions, and the thinking required, compare them to your existing process of making nonnursing conclusions. Some of you may decide they match very closely; some may discover it is time to enhance and modify approaches.

▷ Characteristics of Nursing Conclusions

Judgments

Nursing conclusions are judgments formed after thinking about patient data. Those judgments form the basis of care. They are part of all phases of the nursing process—assessing, planning, implementing, and evaluating. Nurses make conclusions about patients' needs before they intervene; they make conclusions about patients' strengths and health concerns, how the patient is progressing, and what changes are needed in the care.

Evidence of Thinking

Nursing conclusions, written or verbal, demonstrate evidence of thinking. The necessity of designing care based on conclusions "forces" thinking. The thinking that is required to develop conclusions is discussed in much more detail later in the chapter. For now, suffice to say that conclusions reflect the nurse's thinking ability in collecting adequate data, logically analyzing the data, appropriately identifying a label to describe the patient's concerns or state of health, effectively planning, implementing, evaluating care, and evaluating patient outcomes.

Conclusions are made by analyzing pieces of data and clusters of data. It would be impractical to act on individual bits of information. Think about that for a minute: If a child were crying, one would not act on the crying without getting more information. One would find out the source of anguish—stubbed toe, lost toy, or lost child. Acting on individual pieces of information would be a waste of time and potentially harmful because one might be acting prematurely or misinterpreting the problem.

Probability Statements

Nursing conclusions are probability statements. Probability refers to the chances of something occurring. There are many familiar examples of conclusions that are probability statements. The weather forecast is one example. Meteorologists can conclude that an area of the country will get rain by nightfall by using such information as the weather in other parts of the country, temperature patterns, wind velocity and patterns, and past experience with similar weather conditions. Ultimately, they put all of that together and arrive at a conclusion—"70% chance of rain in the next 24 hours." The percentage is an indication of the probability for accuracy. The higher the percentage, the higher the probability of accuracy.

There are few conclusions, especially those made about human behavior, that have 100% probability of accuracy. However, it is important, sometimes vital, that nurses make conclusions with the highest possible probability. The patient's health and well-being are at stake. High-probability conclusions depend on high-level thinking. Methods to increase the probability of accuracy are discussed later in this chapter.

▷ The Process of Making Conclusions

Some beginning students believe that the process of making nursing conclusions consists of finding the "right" label in a book, writing it down, copying the corresponding care plan, and putting it into action. Unfortunately, the standard conclusions presented in textbooks do not correspond exactly to all patients. Textbooks provide lists of labels for existing nursing diagnoses and lists of the typical signs and symptoms that a patient may demonstrate to qualify for a particular label. But what about all the early- and intermediate-level conclusions the nurse needs to make to get to the point of selecting one label or another? And what about all the conclusions that need to be made after that label is selected? Don't bother looking; these early- and intermediate-level conclusions are not in the books.

To make conclusions at all levels accurately and efficiently, the nurse must learn an effective conclusion-making process. Again, a nursing conclusion-making process is best learned by enhancing the existing conclusion-making process used in everyday life. A simple example of developing a conclusion is as follows:

> Mei Song, age 10, has not been feeling well for the last 24 hours.
>
> Her eyes are red, her nose is running, and she is sneezing.
>
> Her mother suspects (has 2 hunches) that she may be getting a cold or her allergies may be acting up.
>
> To determine which is more likely (higher probability), her mother checks things out (collects more data).

Mei Song doesn't have a temperature, so her mother assumes it probably is not a cold (rules out an infectious process).

Her mother remembers that it is the time of year that the ragweed is worst, and Mei is allergic to ragweed.

Her mother gives her the prescribed allergy medicine.

Mei Song feels much better by dinner time (the accuracy of her mother's conclusion was very high because the intervention worked).

Hunches

In this example, the term "hunch" is used. A hunch is an early-level conclusion or a "possible" conclusion . Hunches are stimulated in many ways. Sometimes a critical piece of information (the allergy history) points to an obvious conclusion because "that's always found with this problem." At other times it is the volume of related pieces of data that points to an "obvious" conclusion. For example, if a patient has pain and difficulty with bowel movements 4 days in a row, when he normally has no problems moving his bowels daily, it is fairly easy to see that "constipation" is a good hunch in the path toward a final conclusion.

Sometimes it is not the significance or the amount of data as much as it is a "gut feeling" or a "sixth sense" that leads to hunches. These gut feelings or sixth senses comprise intuition, and should not be ignored. Intuition is being studied with more interest lately. Expert nurses often confide that they do things intuitively. Their thinking skills are so fine-tuned that various levels of thinking occur beyond conscious awareness. It is difficult to explain this thinking by breaking it into steps. Their intuition allows these nurses to make accurate conclusions quickly and seemingly effortlessly; it almost looks like magic. Remember, however, as you admire these "expert" intuitive nurses, that they started at the same point you did.

Hunches are very important pieces of thinking that lead to accurate final conclusions. Because expert nurses make hunches so automatically, their hunches rarely get discussed, let alone written down anywhere. Thus, hunches rarely get the credit they deserve as significant parts of the thinking process.

Although having and acknowledging hunches is very important, they also must be approached cautiously. "Gut-level" hunches can be triggered by nurse biases or prejudices about certain groups of people. Therefore, a hunch that is not obviously data related should be questioned. If, for example, a nurse has a hunch that a patient would not understand something, that nurse should mentally ask, "Am I thinking that because the patient is young (old), of a certain ethnic group (or not)," and so forth. Everyone has biases; they become problematic if they are not recognized and challenged.

It is especially important for beginning nurses to acknowledge hunches and nurture their development. Nurturing hunch development can be achieved by writing them as "possible" conclusions. "Possible social isolation," "Possible activity intolerance," "Possible vision problems," and "Possibly delayed development" are examples of how to write hunches (early conclusions).

►►►►►► Action Learning #22: Hunch Development

Read the following situation and write down at least three hunches you have about why this man is not taking his medication.

Mr. Hernandez, a 48-year-old widower and insurance salesperson who travels quite a bit, has been coming to the clinic to have his blood pressure checked every 3 to 4 weeks because he was diagnosed with high blood pressure 6 months ago. At the last visit, Allie Bahe, Student Nurse, found Mr. Hernandez's blood pressure to be quite a bit higher than usual. She asked Mr. Hernandez if he had been taking his medication as directed, and got this reply, "Well, I know I should, but I didn't take it every day last week; I guess I shouldn't do that." He quickly changed the subject and told Allie about his fiancée, Maria, and about all the social events they had attended lately because of Maria's move to a new modeling agency. He said, with a huge smile, "I feel like a new man these days; I may even be a father again soon."

Hunch #1: Possible . . .

Hunch #2: Possible . . .

Hunch #3: Possible . . .

DISCUSSION Did some things "jump out" at you? Or, did you really have to dig to come up with hunches? How strong were your "gut feelings?" If they were strong, why do you think they were? Do you know anyone like Mr. Hernandez?

Consider and compare these hunches about the factors that might be related to Mr. Hernandez's apparent nonadherence to his medication regimen. Think about why a nurse might have these hunches.

Possibly:

▼ When not feeling bad, he doesn't take the medicine, thinking he would feel bad if his blood pressure were high.

▼ He thinks high blood pressure is an old man's problem and he feels too young for it.

▼ He is very busy and forgets to take the medicine.

▼ When he is traveling, his schedule is unusual and he forgets to take it.

▼ He is experiencing the side effect of impotence and may be reluctant to talk about it.

▼ The label on the medicine says not to take it with alcohol and he drinks during social occasions.

Ruling In and Ruling Out

When there are several hunches about one issue, the nurse must differentiate among them to determine which one(s) is/are the most accurate conclusion(s) about that one situation. This process of differentiation is called "validating hunches" or "ruling in and ruling out." Collectively, the process of identifying two or more possible conclusions about one situation, distinguishing among them, and arriving at the most accurate conclusion is called "differential diagnosing." This makes sense when one considers that diagnoses are conclusions, and "differential" means "distinguishing among possibilities." A nurse's ability to make differential diagnoses (multiple hunches about one situation) and rule

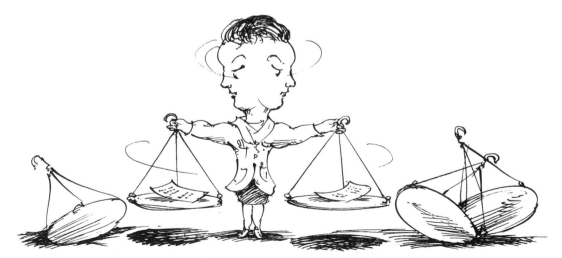

Figure 5-2.   Ruling in and ruling out.

hunches "in" or "out" is directly connected to that nurse's ability to make accurate conclusions. Without accurate conclusions, the rest of the care plan is a waste of time and money for the patient, the nurse, and the health care delivery system.

One of the classic methods to determine which hunches are best to keep and which are best to drop (process of validating hunches) is called *directed data collection*. Gaps in the data picture are identified and the gaps are filled in to give a more complete picture of the patient situation. The additional data collected are "directed" toward supporting or not supporting the hunch(es).

An example: It is the end of the shift and a new patient is transferred to the unit. The assigned nurse starts to collect data and finds that the patient is breathing very hard after moving from wheelchair to bed. The nurse suspects the patient has Activity Intolerance, but there is not enough information yet to say that for certain. In this case, the nurse might write on the chart, "possible Activity Intolerance" with a note, "data gap regarding patient's vital signs during exertion."

To know what additional data are needed, beginners usually go to books that have lists of defining characteristics (signs and symptoms or objective and subjective data) for each nursing conclusion (in this case, "Activity Intolerance"). The patient needs to be observed and questioned to determine if he or she has any of the classic defining characteristics of "activity intolerance" that match what is listed in the book. If the patient's data do not fit well, an alternative hunch must be made about an alternative nursing diagnosis.

▶▶▶▶▶▶ **Action Learning #23: Ruling In and Ruling Out Hunches**

Look at the hunches you made in Action Learning #22. What additional data (identifying data gaps) would you need to collect from Mr. Hernandez to rule in or rule out those hunches?

Hunch #1 Data Gaps:

Hunch #2 Data Gaps:

Hunch #3 Data Gaps:

DISCUSSION How did you figure out what additional data were needed? How would you obtain that additional data? How does your experience and knowledge about hypertension, hypertensive medication and its side effects, and middle-aged Hispanic men affect your ability to make hunches and identify data gaps? Could you make any decisions on "ruling in" or "ruling out" at this point? This process of directed data collection to rule in or rule out is discussed further in Chapter 8.

Accuracy and Conclusions

Achieving accuracy in your conclusions *does not mean finding the "one" right answer.* Accuracy means selecting a conclusion that has the highest probability of matching and making sense out of the raw data. It is very important to aim for the highest accuracy because it will save time and will allow care planning to focus on the "best" strengths and health concerns. If the focus of care is blurry, the nurse's and patient's time and energy are wasted. Meanwhile, an unidentified problem may be getting worse.

It is important to remember that conclusions are rarely 100% accurate because they are probability statements. There is a certain probability that this or that is the most accurate conclusion to make. In some cases, nurses can be 99.99% sure, but, in other cases, they have to live with lower odds. The odds of accuracy are usually increased with more data, but not always. Nurses cannot collect data forever; eventually they have to start making conclusions.

Because collecting volumes of data is not always possible or realistic, nurses can increase accuracy by looking for critical data. Critical data (also called critical indicators) are clearly more significant than others. Here is an example: The nurse sees a patient wringing his hands, sweating, and pacing, and has a hunch that the patient is anxious. The probability of that hunch being accurate is perhaps somewhere around 50%. Now, when the patient says, "I'm really anxious," the probability jumps much higher. The statement by the patient is a critical indicator because it is clearly significant for the anxiety conclusion. All the other signs (wringing hands, sweating, pacing) have some probability of pointing to something other than anxiety. Without that critical indicator, the probability for accuracy is much lower.

High probability for accuracy is directly related to one's skill with the INQUIRY mode of thinking and one's ability to tolerate ambiguity. Remember, from the vocabulary in Chapter 1, "ambiguous" means "having multiple meanings or possible interpretations." INQUIRY skill is necessary to ask the best questions: Do the data support this hunch? What data would make this a stronger hunch? What data do not support this hunch?

The issue of probability forces one to acknowledge ambiguity in conclusion making. Ambiguity and tolerance for ambiguity can be challenging for many, especially for those who prefer to see the world as having only "right" or "wrong" answers to questions. It is not uncommon for beginning college students, nursing students included, to demonstrate this style of thinking, which is called "dualistic." A "right" or "wrong" perspective for finding answers is, however, extremely unusual for the expert nurse. Expert nurses use more relativistic thinking, which allows for gradations in perspective (awful, poor, good, better, best) and seeing the many shades of green instead of just "yellow" and "blue." The expert not only has learned to deal with ambiguity, but has fine-tuned his or her data collection skill to achieve conclusions with high probabilities of accuracy.

▶▶▶▶▶ **Action Learning #24: KNOWING HOW YOU THINK About Ambiguity**

Awareness of your tolerance for ambiguity will add to your self-understanding. Think about how you feel in situations in which you cannot fit things into neat "boxes." On a scale of 1 to 10, with 10 being the most relativistic (able to accept the gradations), mark where you think you are comfortable now.

Dualistic   Relativistic
(only "right" or "wrong")   (accepts gradations)
1----2----3----4----5----6----7----8----9----10

DISCUSSION Do you think you are in a good place? Does your dualistic or relativistic perspective vary depending on the situation? Do you think you need to learn to think more relativistically? You will likely find nursing most "comfortable" if you are tolerant of ambiguity and practice relativistic thinking.

Validating Conclusions

When one considers the importance of the patient's verbal report in the earlier anxiety example, it is clear that asking patients about their perceptions is critical to increasing accuracy. Therefore, one way to increase accuracy of conclusions is to validate conclusions with patients (or their significant others, if it cannot be done directly with the patient). Validation also can be done by involving the patient directly in formulating the conclusion. The nurse might say something like this to the patient: "It seems to me that these are your strengths and your problems [name the strengths and problems], and these are the things contributing to the problems. What do you think?" It is surprising how different and how similar patients' and nurses' conclusions can be sometimes. As you validate conclusions with patients, you soon see the value of this process.

Another major value of validation is that patients have more control over their care, and nurses are not spinning their wheels on problems that patients do not think exist. This seems so logical; however, it is surprising how little validation goes on in health care.

Pause here for a thinking-learning check. You should be able to elaborate on these ideas:

   ▼ The purpose of conclusions: to guide effective and efficient nursing care (ie, great nursing).

   ▼ The value of studying conclusions at the beginning of a study of the nursing process.

   ▼ Transferring conclusion-making skills from everyday life to making nursing conclusions.

   ▼ Nursing conclusions as judgments based on thinking, evidence of thinking, and probability statements.

   ▼ The process of making conclusions: having hunches, ruling in and ruling out hunches, and validating for accuracy.

   ▼ Differential diagnoses: identifying all possible conclusions about one situation.

   ▼ Directed data collection: identifying and filling data gaps for all conclusions.

   ▼ Ruling in and ruling out: making decisions about which conclusions are the most accurate.

▶ TYPES OF THINKING REQUIRED TO DEVELOP NURSING CONCLUSIONS

Many people say "critical thinking" is the key ingredient in making the best nursing conclusions. If critical thinking is defined broadly enough to incorporate all modes of thinking, then that is true. Often, however, as discussed in the introduction to this book, critical thinking is seen only as inquiry-type thinking. In reality, all five thinking modes are necessary to develop accurate conclusions and act on them. Each mode adds an important piece to the process of conclusion making and clinical judgments. Some studies have shown that subjects who demonstrate good critical thinking do not necessarily have good clinical judgment (Kintgen-Andrews, 1991; Miller & Malcolm, 1990). It is a bit like having a lot of "book smarts" but no "common sense." The five modes of thinking must work together to produce skillful clinical judgments.

▷ Total Recall

Think about the *thinking* involved in the conclusion-making process. TOTAL RECALL is used to remember factors that usually go together—cold weather and sweaters, for example, or frail skin, immobility, and incontinence as risk factors for decubitus ulcers. Other information recalled from textbooks may relate to usual clusters of data or critical indicators of certain problems. All of this RECALL knowledge is vital to making accurate conclusions.

▷ Habits

Certain conclusions can easily become HABITS—when nurses see a confused person, they almost always conclude that safety must be addressed. One or two factors just automatically lead to certain conclusions. HABIT-type conclusions can save time and generally reflect conclusions that nurses have made many times with similar sets of information. Although HABITS save time, they also have limitations; they can lead too easily to prejudicial conclusions if the nurse is not careful. Not all old patients are senile, but some people might quickly jump to the conclusion of senility based only on a knowledge of the patient's age.

▷ Inquiry

INQUIRY is the "guts" of conclusion making; it is what is required to make complicated conclusions and important ones. Mentally, nurses put together pieces of information, make early conclusions (hunches), question the validity or completeness of the early conclusions, add more information, revise, and make final conclusions. (For a review, refer again to Figure 5-1.) INQUIRY helps nurses keep an open mind to many possible interpretations of data, and keeps them collecting relevant data. But, remember, it is not the amount of data, but the quality of the data that is most important. Thinking about which data provide the best picture helps a nurse to achieve accuracy. Knowing what is needed is not easily figured out. It depends largely on one's knowledge, or TOTAL RECALL, about nursing care, biology, psychology, sociology, physiology, and all those other "-ologies" that nurses are required to study.

Knowledge helps nurses avoid a pitfall associated with INQUIRY. INQUIRY, like HABITS, can be a double-edged sword; nurses, especially novices, can get in a rut of endless data collection in the hope of developing the most accurate conclusions, so that they never get to the actual conclusion. At some point, data collection has to be interrupted so something can be done for the patient. The key is to know when there are enough data. Inquiry, combined with knowledge and experience, provides the ability to zero in on critical data. Recognizing and collecting critical data increase efficiency and accuracy. Efficiency is almost as important as accuracy. The next chapter focuses on how to collect the best data to make the most accurate conclusions efficiently.

▷ New Ideas and Creativity

Some of the best and most innovative conclusions are developed by people with a well developed thinking mode of NEW IDEAS AND CREATIVITY. The NEW IDEAS AND CREATIVITY mode allows a nurse to see different relationships among pieces of data and to consider options not in the books. Thinking in this mode leads to conclusions that are most closely suited to individual patient needs. Individualized care, care that is uniquely suited to the patient rather than copied out of the book, can be provided only when NEW IDEAS AND CREATIVITY are used in developing conclusions. For example, the "standard" approach for colostomy care is to have the patient irrigate and empty the colostomy in the bathroom. If the patient lives in an area with no indoor plumbing, however, it takes NEW IDEAS AND CREATIVITY to modify the plan to suit the patient's environmental constraints.

▷ Knowing How You Think

Because accurate conclusions are a result of high-quality thinking, the better you understand your thinking, the better the conclusions you will develop. Understanding your thinking requires you to KNOW HOW YOU THINK. It's time for some Action Learning to gain more insight into how much you know about your individual thinking while developing conclusions.

▶▶▶▶▶▶ **Action Learning #25: KNOWING HOW YOU THINK and Developing Conclusions**

Think about and write a response to the following questions about your knowledge of your thinking. Share your answers with a classmate.

Do you question your assumptions? Why, why not?

Have you identified your biases? Why, why not?

Are your conclusions usually supported with data? Why, why not?

Can you usually see more than one "answer" to a problem? Why, why not?

Do you ever make premature conclusions? Why, why not?

How does your point of view generally fit with the views of other nurses, other student nurses, and patients? Why does it fit or not fit?

What is the best way for you to analyze data and then see relationships among data and data clusters? Why?

DISCUSSION   Did you notice the similarities between this Action Learning and Action Learning #21 ("Tracking Your Thinking Through a Conclusion")? It is important to do many Action Learning exercises focused on the KNOWING HOW YOU THINK mode because self-analysis is a slow, building-up process. Each time you study yourself, you discover aspects of your thinking that you may not have thought about before. Each new discovery then needs to be addressed in relation to other discoveries.

▶ "CONCLUDING" COMMENTS

The first purpose of this chapter was to emphasize the importance of developing conclusions and to begin to examine the process of making conclusions. Without accurate conclusions, the rest of nursing care is on very shaky ground. The second purpose of this chapter was to develop an awareness of existing conclusion-making skills and build on them. If conclusion making in nursing is viewed as a totally new process to be learned "from scratch," learning the nursing process will be significantly delayed. The Thinking Log for this chapter was designed to nurture this growing awareness of your current skills.

As is probably obvious by this point, thinking and conclusion making take time and energy. At first, the pay-off for the time and energy spent may not seem worthwhile. The value is enormous, however. High-level thinking resulting in accurate conclusions provides a basis for nursing care that is individualized to each patient, focused on the highest priorities, time saving, money saving, and safe. Beginners will find that the thinking is long and arduous, but, as with any skill, practice makes it easier and quicker. Accepting the challenge in the beginning pays off down the road to great nursing.

▶▶▶ **THINKING LOG #5**

Look back to the conclusion-making example you used for Action Learning #21. Go through it with your new perspective on conclusion making and identify if and how you did the following:
   ▼ Made early conclusions (hunches): Yes_____, No_____, Partially_____
      If "Yes," give an example.
      If "No," what could they have been?
      If "Partially," explain.
   ▼ Used directed data collection: Yes_____, No_____, Partially_____
      If "Yes," give an example.
      If "No," what could have been done?
      If "Partially," explain.
   ▼ Ruled in and ruled out hunches: Yes_____, No_____, Partially_____
      If "Yes," give an example.
      If "No," could you have done so?
      If "Partially," explain.
Briefly summarize the skills you currently use that will be beneficial to your conclusion making in nursing. Share this with a classmate.
(Note: This activity is designed to focus on the positive. Everyone has areas for improvement and it usually is easier to find those, but we frequently forget to take credit for our strengths. It is just as important for beginning nursing students to build on their strengths as it is to help patients build on their strengths.)

REFERENCES

Kintgen-Andrews, J. (1991). Critical thinking and nursing education: Perplexities and insights. *Journal of Nursing Education*, *30*(4), 152–156.
Miller, M. A., & Malcolm, N. S. (1990). Critical thinking in the nursing curriculum. *Nursing and Health Care*, *11*(2), 57–73.

Major Nursing Conclusions of Assessment

After reading and doing the activities in this chapter you will be able to:

Describe the major nursing conclusions of assessment—strengths and health concerns—and the thinking required to develop these conclusions.

Explain the differences between the three categories of health concerns: nursing diagnoses, interdisciplinary problems, and problems for referral.

Explain the differences between diagnosing actual problems, wellness responses, and potential problems.

Diagram the process of making the major nursing conclusions of assessment.

As described earlier, conclusions are made in every phase of the nursing process. Many levels of conclusions, from minor to major, are made throughout the process. This chapter focuses on the major conclusions that are made during assessment. Conclusions made with the other phases of the nursing process are addressed in later chapters.

The major conclusions made during assessment are nursing judgments, based on analysis of data, about patients' strengths and health concerns. Health concerns fall into three categories—nursing diagnoses, interdisciplinary problems, and problems for referral. The nurse's ability to formulate these major conclusions of assessment efficiently and effectively depends on using all five thinking modes. If minimal thinking occurs, inappropriate assessment conclusions may be made, and nursing care ranges from useless to dangerous.

▶ STRENGTHS

Strengths are factors or characteristics of the patient that are positive, are resources, and are important in planning care. It is easy to forget to make conclusions about strengths for at least three reasons. First, because many nurses work with patients who are sick, they often focus on identifying problems they can "fix." (Nurses who work with well populations are less apt to do this.) Second, human nature often seems to direct people toward the negative more than the positive. Third, nurses often see strengths as issues that take care of themselves and therefore do not need to be identified. It takes some extra effort, including a shift in perspective, to *think* about and make conclusions with regard to patients' strengths.

Strengths are unique to each patient and must be determined based on the patient's values, not the nurse's values. For example, Demitri, 23 years old, has a very concerned, attentive mother who wants to participate actively in his rehabilitation after his motor vehicle accident. Is his mother's helpfulness a strength in the form of "good family support?" A nurse might come to that conclusion; but, if Demitri perceives his mother as domineering, pushy, and always meddling in his affairs, then the mother's actions are not a strength from his perspective.

Nurses need to identify patients' strengths so they can use those strengths to help overcome the problems. It is not only good practice to help patients recognize all the strengths that can work for them, it is very cost effective to draw on patients' existing resources. Moreover, it is demeaning to patients not to recognize their abilities. For example, Ms. Tohatchi has a medical diagnosis of diabetes mellitus; she needs to learn how to deal with new ways of eating, caring for her skin, and performing routine activities. If Ms. Tohatchi has a college degree in biochemistry, her knowledge about how living organisms work is an educational strength. By building on this strength when designing teaching strategies, the nurse will need less time to teach her self-care.

Strengths usually are identified during the initial assessment but, because assessment continues throughout care, nurses can identify strengths at any point in the care process. Nurses make a note of them mentally and write them down so they can be incorporated into the nursing care plan.

▶▶▶▶▶ Action Learning #26: Finding Patient Strengths

Read this scenario about Priscilla Domphopper. Answer the questions on making conclusions about strengths. Share your responses with a classmate.

Priscilla F. Domphopper is a 46-year-old professor of art history. She describes herself as a basically happy person who enjoys her life and her job. Recently, however, she has "developed sleep problems." This started about 6 months ago, about the same time her husband's snoring "escalated to the freight-train-through-the-house decibel level." The sleeping problem is aggravated because Priscilla is a light sleeper. She usually gets about 6 hours of sleep each night, waking several times. Because it relaxes her, Priscilla usually drinks a glass of milk or a cup of hot tea right before bedtime.

Priscilla's typical day includes rising at 5:30 AM. She takes a brisk 2-mile walk, showers, and eats a light breakfast of granola cereal, plain yogurt, and 6 oz. of orange juice. Her teaching schedule prevents her from eating lunch most days. After school she picks up her kids, starts dinner, helps the kids with homework, grades papers, and prepares for the next day's work. Because she doesn't have enough time for housework, the house is a bit of a mess. This bothers her husband, but she has gotten used to it. She relaxes by watching one or two of her favorite weekly TV programs.

1. Identify Priscilla's strengths.

2. Describe the process you used to determine Priscilla's strengths.

3. Discuss how you felt about looking for her strengths.

4. Describe the challenges you encountered while identifying her strengths.

DISCUSSION   Think about how identifying Priscilla's strengths might help as you plan care for her sleep problem. If you were not doing this exercise, but were Priscilla's nurse, would you have focused on her strengths as much as you did when you were specifically asked to do so? Do you see that it would make sense to ask her what her strengths were?

It might be helpful to think of reminders for focusing on conclusions about strengths in the future. As you shared your responses with your classmate, did you notice that what some people think is a strength may be seen as a problem by others? The housework issue, for example, can be interpreted several ways. It would be imperative to validate your ideas about her strengths with Priscilla to arrive at the most accurate conclusions about her strengths.

▶ HEALTH CONCERNS

Health concerns are the conclusions many students typically think of as the real nursing issues. These are the illness and wellness issues that usually bring patients to the health care system. There are three categories of health concern conclusions—those that nurses can care for independently (nursing diagnoses), those that nurses work with others to care for (interdisciplinary problems), and those that nurses refer to other health care providers (problems for referral). Figure 6-1, "Overview of Health Concern Conclusions," illustrates the many levels of conclusions. The next several pages will explain the concepts in the diagram, but the diagram may help you to visualize the overview before the details are examined. Continue to refer to the diagram during reading.

▷ Nursing Diagnosis

The number of books and articles written on the topic of nursing diagnosis is mind-boggling. Refer to those sources for the details regarding label definitions, defining characteristics, and related factors (eg, Alfaro, 1994; Carpenito,

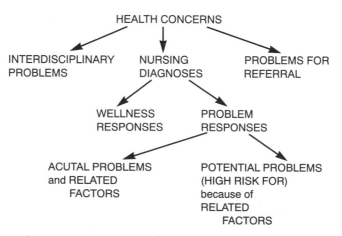

Figure 6-1. Overview of health concern conclusions.

1993; McFarland & McFarlane, 1993; North American Nursing Diagnosis Association [NANDA], 1992.) This text, rather than duplicating those other sources, focuses on a few key issues that are critical to the thinking processes involved in making nursing diagnosis conclusions.

To use nursing diagnosis references most effectively, it is important to understand these terms:

Label Definitions: descriptions of the conclusions that are listed as nursing diagnoses

Defining Characteristics: (also called "indicators" or "criteria") the data typically found to support the conclusion as labeled

Related Factors: (also called "contributing factors" or "etiologies") possible patient issues or concerns that are "causing" the concern

Later discussion in this chapter elaborates on these definitions.

Nursing diagnoses are conclusions about those patient phenomena in the domain of independent nursing practice. (Refer to Chapter 2 for the differences between independent and interdependent nursing practice.) These conclusions are health concerns that nurses can and must independently diagnose and treat fully within the legal parameters of their profession. Refer to Appendix A for a review of the current nursing diagnostic labels identified by NANDA.

Nursing diagnoses are labels accepted by the profession to describe patient responses. A response represents the combined signs and symptoms (objective and subjective data) exhibited by the patient that can be grouped together and given a label that means the same thing to most nurses around the world. For example, one of the accepted labels is, "Impaired Skin Integrity." This label is defined as "a state in which the individual's skin is adversely altered." The defining characteristics (patient data) are "disruption of skin surface, destruction of skin layers and/or invasion of body structures" (NANDA, 1992, pp. 34–35). These labels and corresponding criteria (signs and symptoms or defining characteristics) can be found in nursing diagnosis books and most nursing textbooks.

Determining the Nature of Patient Responses

A series of conclusions is required to determine the nature of patient responses and the factors related to the responses. First the nurse must determine if the response is a problem or a wellness response. If it is a problem, the nurse must determine if it is an actual problem or one for which the patient is at high risk. The nurse must then make conclusions about the factors that are contributing to the specific problem. Conclusions at each of these points lead eventually to the final conclusion, to which an appropriate diagnostic label can be given. Refer again to Figure 6-1 to see this illustrated.

Conclusions About Problem Responses Versus Conclusions About Wellness Responses

The process of making conclusions is the same whether nurses make diagnoses about problem or wellness responses. In both cases the thinking and the conclusions are based on analysis of groups of data. Whether nurses make more conclusions about problems or more about wellness responses depends largely on the focus of their practice. Nurses who work with well populations, such as healthy babies, family health promotion, sports health, and so forth, are more likely to make conclusions about wellness responses and intervene to support that healthy behavior. Nurses who work with ill populations are apt to make more conclusions about problem responses and base their practice on restoring healthy responses. Not all responses, however, clearly fit into problem or wellness categories. For example, many problem responses of patients with chronic or terminal illnesses do not lend themselves to restoration of health. Patients with these problem responses need care designed to maintain a current level of functioning or to promote comfort and dignity as the patient approaches death.

If the distinction between wellness and problem responses seems fuzzy, it is because human responses seldom fit into neat boxes (remember the discussion of ambiguity in Chapter 5?). It helps to keep in mind that, ultimately, what the patient validates is the most accurate conclusion. If, for example, a nurse identifies a patient response as a "problem," but the patient says "I'm managing all right with this," then the conclusion could be a wellness diagnosis rather than a problem diagnosis.

Consider the case of Amanda Gale, the new school nurse. While talking to the parents of Tyler Graham, a kindergarten student, Amanda said, "Mrs. Graham, I think Tyler has a problem with his motor development. His walking is very stiff and he has trouble running." Mrs. Graham smiled and said, "He's doing great. He was born with severely clubbed feet and has had surgery. He wore casts for a long time. A physical therapist and nurse have been working with him and he has made great strides." Amanda then knew that what she thought was a problem was actually a wellness response. She rephrased the conclusion as "Potential for Enhanced Mobility." (NANDA recommends the format of "Potential for Enhanced . . . " as wording for wellness diagnoses) (Carroll-Johnson, 1991). The patient and his family were adapting well, and Tyler would likely improve his mobility. Amanda's care would focus on supporting the family's continued wellness response.

Wellness diagnoses are similar to conclusions about strengths, but they do differ. Wellness diagnoses are focused on transitions in responses, whereas strengths may not be in transition. NANDA has defined a wellness diagnosis as a conclusion about a patient " . . . in transition from a specific level of wellness to a higher level of wellness" (Carroll-Johnson, 1991, p. 375). Nurses making wellness diagnoses develop plans to support the patient's move to higher level wellness. All nurses, regardless of their practice areas, should make conclusions about patient strengths, but, in most cases, specific care plans to do something about those strengths are not developed. The strengths are used to help patients overcome problems. Wellness diagnoses, on the other hand, are often the focus of care plans for nurses who work with well populations.

▶▶▶▶▶▶ **A**ction Learning #27: Identifying Wellness Diagnoses

Examine the diagnostic labels in Appendix A. Write down all the diagnoses you believe would qualify as wellness diagnoses.

DISCUSSION   How many did you find? What do you think this means? Remember, the NANDA work started only in the 1970s. Early in NANDA's development, there were debates over the necessity of including wellness diagnoses in the taxonomy; it is only in recent years that they have been added. The nursing profession has a long way to go before it has a complete taxonomy of nursing diagnoses. Many more wellness diagnoses need to be developed and added to the taxonomy. Later in this chapter, some suggestions will be offered for naming conclusions for which no diagnostic label is developed as yet.

Conclusions About Actual Problems Versus Potential Problems for Patients Who Are at "High Risk"

Conclusions about actual problems and those about problems for which patients are at high risk (potential problems) differ in two ways. First, the conclusions for actual problems are based on data that "paint a picture" of an *existing* problem—hence the use of the word "actual." Conclusions about potential problems are based on data that indicate a strong likelihood, or high risk that a problem will occur in the near future if something doesn't change. Nurses make many conclusions about risk factors because a large part of nursing is focused on preventing problems.

Conclusions about risks are conclusions about related factors. If factors are present that usually contribute to a problem, but the problem has not occurred, the nurse would conclude that a patient is at "high risk for" that problem.

The second difference in the conclusions about actual or potential problems is the diagnostic statement. Diagnostic statements for actual problems start with the problem label, for example, "Anxiety," "Ineffective Airway Clearance," or "Constipation." The diagnostic conclusion statement for potential problems begins with "High Risk for," for example, "High Risk for Impaired Skin Integrity" or "High Risk for Infection."

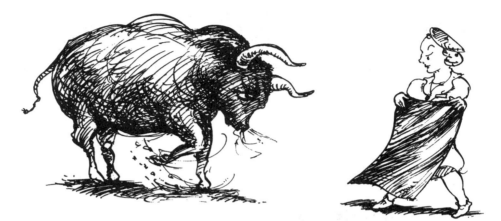

Figure 6-2a.   Potential problems.

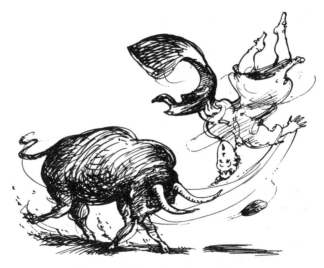

Figure 6-2b.   Actual problems.

▶▶▶▶▶▶ **A**ction Learning #28: Differentiating Actual
From High-Risk Problems

Read the following three situations and determine if the patient has an actual
problem or is at high risk for having the identified problem. Use textbooks
with nursing diagnoses to help with this exercise. Explain your reasoning to a
classmate.

Situation	*Type of problem and reasoning*
#1 Sue, a marathon runner, is confined to a wheelchair for 3 weeks to rest the ligaments damaged in both legs. (Impaired Physical Mobility)	
#2 Bob is 5′10″ and weighs 160 lbs. He wants to increase his muscle mass and plans to eat only steak and eggs for the next month. (Altered Nutrition)	
#3 David has attempted suicide three times in the past. His female companion has just left him. (Self-Directed Violence)	

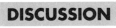 **DISCUSSION**   How did you come to your conclusions? How did the
textbooks help? How did your reasoning compare to that
of your classmate's?

Conclusions About Related Factors

The last conclusions made in the larger nursing diagnosis conclusion-making
process are those focused on the related factors. Once a nurse concludes that a
patient has a problem response, then the factors that are "causing" that problem must be determined. The term "cause" is not used because nurses, dealing
with human behavior, know how difficult it is to pin down behaviors in terms
of a direct cause-and-effect relationship. Human beings are so complex, with a
multitude of individual coping mechanisms, that the nurse can only say, "there
is a high probability" that some factors contribute to problems or influence the
problems. Therefore, when nurses write nursing diagnostic statements, they
link the problem and related factors together with the words, "related to" rather than "due to" or "caused by."

Although related factors are listed along with the label for problem nursing diagnoses, they are used less often with wellness diagnoses. NANDA rec-

ommends that wellness diagnoses be written as one-part statements without the related factors, but many nurses add the related factors just as they do with problem diagnoses.

Related factors are also called "contributing factors" or "etiologies." These terms generally mean the same thing in nursing. "Etiology" is used more often in medicine when referring to causes of diseases. Most books that include information on nursing diagnoses also provide lists of related factors that could go along with the nursing diagnosis label. Related factors, however, are unique to each individual, which means that the lists in the books are used only to trigger thinking. For example, one of the related factors listed for the diagnosis "Diversional Activity Deficit" is "problematic time management." That related factor would be individualized to a patient and might be written as, "Diversional Activity Deficit related to excessive amount of time spent with AM care to the point of missing morning craft class."

As demonstrated in the example above, nursing diagnostic statements, as they are used to describe conclusions in the independent nursing realm, are written in terms of actual problems or high risk for problems, and accompanied by related factors (etiologies). The two components of the statement are linked by the words, "related to." Wellness diagnoses usually are not accompanied by related factors, but some nurses write them in the same format as that used for problem responses. Display 6-1 illustrates three written examples of diagnostic statements that represent the culminations of the many levels of conclusions needed to identify health concerns accurately.

As is illustrated in Display 6-1, there may be one or many related factors for each problem or response. There is no magic number, but it is important to identify all possible related factors. Otherwise, when care is planned, something important may be left out. Think about this situation. If weight loss occurs because a person has problems preparing meals, a nurse might help that

---

DISPLAY 6-1. Examples of Diagnostic Statements

ACTUAL PROBLEM	**RELATED TO**	**RELATED FACTORS**
Altered Oral Mucous Membrane	related to (R/T)	irritation from dentures that no longer fit properly
POTENTIAL PROBLEM	**RELATED TO**	**RISK FACTORS**
High Risk for Ineffective Airway Clearance	related to (R/T)	17-year history of smoking two packs of cigarettes a day, impending surgery with 3 hours of general anesthesia
WELLNESS RESPONSE		
Family Coping: Potential for Enhanced Growth		

person adapt to alternative methods for meal preparation. But if another related factor exists, for example, the person's income does not allow for adequate food purchase, then dealing only with the meal preparation issue will not solve the problem.

Relationship Between Related Factors and Planning

One of the primary roles of related factors is to start the nurse thinking past assessing into the planning phase of the nursing process. A plan to alleviate or eliminate the problem must be developed. The factors related to the problem must be identified so something can be done about them. Doing something about the related factors allows for resolution of the problem.

To appreciate this close relationship among the problem, its related factors, and planning, read the following description of two different patients with the same problem but different related factors. Patient A has a sleep problem related to worries about school and inability to relax. Nursing care should focus on helping the patient relax and deal with the worry to alleviate the sleep problem. Patient B also has a sleep problem. This patient's problem, however, is related to frequent urination at night, secondary to excessive intake of fluids late in the day. Nursing care must focus on helping this patient change the fluid intake to alleviate the sleep problem.

The goal is identical for both patients—improved sleep patterns—yet what needs to be done for each patient is quite different. Examine Figure 6-3 to visualize this situation.

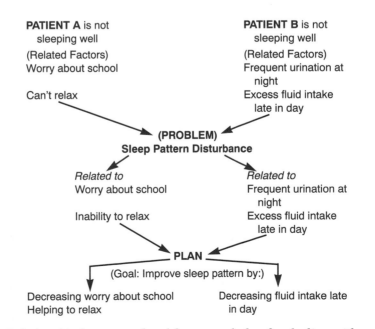

Figure 6-3. Relationship between related factors and plan for dealing with problem.

Nursing Diagnosis Taxonomy: How it Helps With Conclusion Making

Chapter 3 introduced readers to the NANDA Taxonomy of Nursing Diagnoses that is included in Appendix A. There have been several references to that taxonomy in the intervening chapters. As a review, remember these points: About 20 years ago nursing began developing a taxonomy of nursing diagnoses so that a common language could be established for those patient responses with which nurses deal. The taxonomic work of revising and adding diagnostic categories and labels continues today through the professional organization, NANDA. The taxonomy is a classification scheme of labels for actual problems, problems for which patients may be at risk (potential problems), and wellness responses.

The list of diagnoses in the taxonomy is most helpful when it is used with a book that cross-references the label with the usual data that "define" the problem, potential problem, or wellness response. (Examples of such books are given in the reference list of this chapter.) The data are the signs and symptoms (defining characteristics) that nurses usually find when that particular diagnostic label is valid. An example, "Impaired Skin Integrity," was discussed earlier in this chapter. Another example of an accepted label for an actual problem is "Impaired Verbal Communication." This label means the patient is experiencing one or all of the following conditions: "unable to speak dominant language; speaks or verbalizes with difficulty; does not or can not speak; stuttering; slurring; difficulty forming words or sentences; difficulty expressing thought verbally; inappropriate verbalization; dyspnea; disorientation." (NANDA, 1992, p. 36).

▶▶▶▶▶▶ Action Learning #29: Becoming Familiar With Labels, Definitions, and Defining Characteristics

Find a book that has nursing diagnoses accompanied by lists of defining characteristics and related factors.

Pick two diagnoses that you are interested in.

Study the defining characteristics. Do they "paint a picture" of the diagnostic label?

Study the related factors. Can you think of other factors, not on the list, that might contribute to the health concern identified by the diagnostic label?

Finally, get together with a classmate. Read the lists of defining characteristics for the diagnoses you studied to your classmate and see if she or he can identify from the list what diagnoses you are describing.

DISCUSSION Depending on your familiarity with nursing diagnosis books, you may have found this exercise easy or difficult. If you have not used such books much yet, you probably gained an appreciation for how helpful such resources can be. How easy was it to find the label for the defining characteristics listed by your classmate?

Ordering labels in the form of a taxonomy helps nurses find diagnoses easily and consider differential diagnoses (other possibilities) with increased accuracy. For example, the response category of elimination has labels for problems with bowel elimination and urinary elimination. When a nurse finds a cluster of data that may indicate "Functional Incontinence," the nurse can look for that label in the elimination group and find other labels (differential diagnoses) to consider as well. The alternative diagnostic labels to consider would be Reflex Incontinence, Stress Incontinence, Total Incontinence, or Urge Incontinence.

Because building the taxonomy is a relatively recent endeavor, it is not yet complete. Nurses may not always find the label for their independent nursing conclusions in the taxonomy. When no appropriate label is found, nurses develop the best label themselves. As nursing students, the best rule for using the taxonomy is to check it first and use the accepted label if possible, but, if no appropriate label is found, develop one that best summarizes in a word or two the patient response. Developing labels not currently on the taxonomy, which calls on the NEW IDEAS AND CREATIVITY mode of thinking, is particularly useful in the areas of mental health, community health, maternal–child, and wellness nursing. Most of the current NANDA labels are more geared to the area of medical–surgical nursing.

▶▶▶▶▶ **Action Learning #30: Finding an Appropriate Diagnostic Label for Priscilla**

Look again at the story about Priscilla Domphopper presented in Action Learning #26. Search the list of diagnostic labels in Appendix A and use a nursing diagnosis textbook to find the label that seems to fit best with the data on Priscilla. Write down that diagnosis label along with the data you used to arrive at that conclusion. Remember to identify both the data that "define" the problem, wellness response, or high-risk response, *and* the data that are related factors. Share your conclusions with a classmate.

Diagnostic label:

Supporting data (defining characteristics):

Related factors:

DISCUSSION   How similar were your conclusions to those of your classmate? If your conclusions were similar, how did your supporting data compare? How sure are you of your final conclusion?

This exercise shows how the taxonomy can help with conclusion making. The taxonomy can be used to stimulate thinking about differential diagnoses, it can remind the nurse of items to include in directed data collection, and it can validate the conclusion by showing how that conclusion usually accompanies that particular set of data.

▼ THINKING-LEARNING CHECK

The last several pages have addressed some very critical information about strengths and health concerns. Nursing diagnoses, a major category of health concern conclusions, has consumed most of the discussion. Pause here for a thinking-learning check. You should be able to elaborate on these ideas:

- ▼ The major conclusions of the assessment phase of the nursing process: identification of the patient's strengths and health concerns (nursing diagnoses and related factors, interdisciplinary problems, and problems for referral).
- ▼ Finding patient strengths: importance to planning care.
- ▼ Identifying strengths: need to get patient's perspective because of the very subjective nature of these responses.
- ▼ Nursing diagnoses: health concerns within the domain of independent nursing practice.
- ▼ Differentiating types of nursing diagnoses: wellness responses, actual problems, and high-risk responses (potential problems).
- ▼ Conclusions about related factors: part of the diagnostic statement and importance to planning.

▼ Format for writing nursing diagnostic statement.

▼ The Taxonomy of Nursing Diagnoses: how it is used in developing accurate diagnoses.

The rest of this chapter addresses the last two health concerns about which nurses need to make accurate conclusions—interdisciplinary problems and problems for referral. Both of these aspects of nursing require a strong knowledge of the other health professions.

▶ INTERDISCIPLINARY PROBLEMS

Interdisciplinary problems comprise those conclusions about patient problems that are in the interdependent domain of nursing. (For a review of independent and interdependent nursing domains, refer to Chapter 2.) Interdisciplinary problems, as the words imply, require collaboration with another health care professional (physician, physical therapist, nutritionist, social worker, clergy, and so forth). Depending on the setting and the patient population, there may be more or fewer interdisciplinary problems than there are nursing diagnoses.

The line between a nursing diagnosis and an interdisciplinary problem often is very fuzzy. There are few clean distinctions between what one health care provider does and what another does. Clear differences can be seen only at the extremes; for example, a patient recently diagnosed with renal failure may have the following interdisciplinary problem:

High risk for hyperproteinemia related to lack of knowledge of renal diet.

This patient needs assistance from a dietitian as well as from a nurse because renal diets are quite complex. In many cases, nurses deal with diet issues independently, but as the complexity increases, as in the example above, it is a good idea to collaborate with the diet expert.

In the fuzzier arena, consider a second example, which compares two patients with skin problems:

Impaired skin integrity related to immobility and incontinence.

At first glance this looks like a straightforward nursing diagnosis, not an interdisciplinary problem. However, it is not that simple. With one patient, the nurse may be able independently to diagnose and care for this problem by turning the patient and cleaning the skin frequently. For another patient, this problem may have become so severe that several layers of the skin are involved, and the area has become infected. In that case, the nurse needs to collaborate with the physician because medication and treatments may need to be ordered. In this example, the severity of the problem makes a difference; when the problem gets so severe that medical intervention is needed, the nursing diagnosis moves into the realm of interdisciplinary problems. The written diagnostic statement is the same, but one falls into the independent nursing domain and the other into the interdependent domain.

The above two patients with skin breakdown are a good illustration of how all the diagnostic labels have not yet evolved to their most descriptive level. As the taxonomic work continues, there may be labels that will better differentiate, for example, the severity of the patient's response. Whether or not interdisciplinary problems will be added to the NANDA Taxonomy remains to be seen.

A broad knowledge base and sharp thinking skills are necessary for nurses to make accurate conclusions about interdisciplinary problems. Not only do nurses need to know nursing's specific body of knowledge, they need to know quite a bit about the biomedical, social, psychological, and spiritual bodies of knowledge that are the primary foci of other disciplines such as physicians, social workers, psychologists, and clergy. Without that knowledge, conclusions about interdisciplinary problems may be missed or inaccurate.

▶ PROBLEMS FOR REFERRAL

Because nurses assess in a holistic manner ("holistic" means looking at all aspects of the person—biological, psychological, social, cultural, spiritual), they frequently find problems that fall completely into the domains of other health professionals. Here is an example: A nurse working in an emergency room, while assessing a patient brought in by a spouse, finds that the patient has not been eating for the past week, refuses to come out of her bedroom, won't talk to anyone, and has not been sleeping very well. The nurse recognizes that this patient is very likely depressed, but so severely that the problem requires more intensive therapy than the nurse is qualified to provide. The nurse would refer this patient to a psychiatric clinical nurse specialist, a psychiatric social worker, a psychologist, or a psychiatrist.

The specific person to whom the nurse refers the patient, and the referral process itself, vary from institution to institution. Sometimes there are chains of communication that must be followed, such as the nurse calling the primary physician, who calls the consultant. At other times, the nurse makes the referral directly, such as to a nurse practitioner or to a physician. It is very helpful to know the appropriate ways to refer within the organization; this saves a lot of time for the staff and the patient as well as improving the quality of care for patients.

Pause here for another thinking-learning check. You should be able to elaborate on these ideas:

▼ Interdisciplinary problems: health concerns within the domain of interdependent nursing practice.

▼ The importance of a basic knowledge about many health care professions in effectively identifying and planning care for interdisciplinary problems and problems for referral.

▼ Knowing an organization's specific referral system is very time saving and quality care focused.

▶ CONCLUSION ABOUT CONCLUSIONS

This chapter has examined the major nursing conclusions of the assessing phase of the nursing process. One reading of the chapter may not be enough to integrate all of the ideas and concepts into existing thinking about conclusion making. This chapter's Thinking Log has been designed to foster integration of the chapter's content. Creating a personalized visualization of the relationships among the concepts nurtures a higher level of thinking and understanding than that needed simply to read.

▶▶ *THINKING LOG #6*

Complete Figure 6-4 by creating an illustration of the process that occurs between data collection and the major conclusions of assessing. It may be helpful to review Chapters 5 and 6. Be sure to include the following concepts in your diagram:

Hunch	Ruled in
Data gaps	Ruled out
Data cluster	Directed data collection
Independent nursing practice	Interdependent nursing practice

(Note—There are lots of good ways to do this. The purpose is to engage your thinking in visualizing some of the more "hidden" aspects of thinking required for developing the multiple levels of conclusions that lead to the major conclusions of assessment.)

Have fun! Show your diagram to a classmate and explain it.

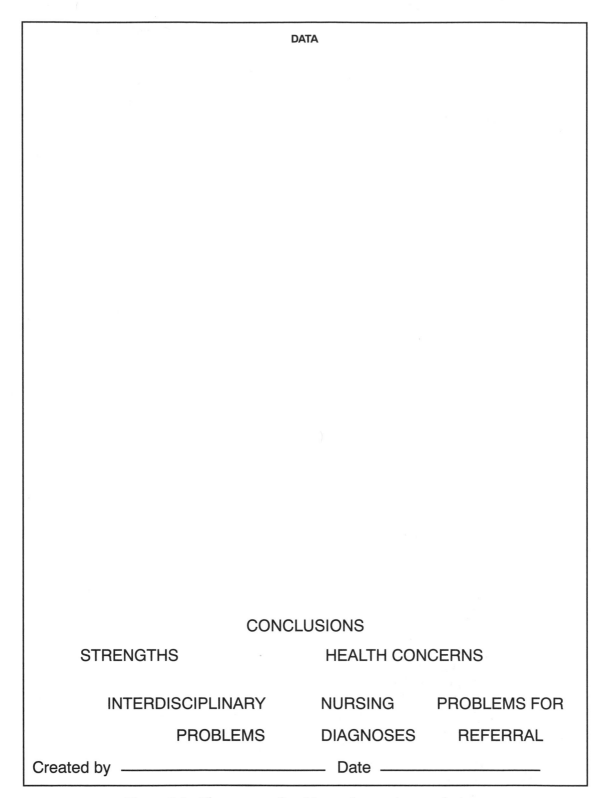

DATA

CONCLUSIONS

STRENGTHS   HEALTH CONCERNS

INTERDISCIPLINARY   NURSING   PROBLEMS FOR

PROBLEMS   DIAGNOSES   REFERRAL

Created by ———————————————— Date ————————————————

Figure 6-4. The process of making major nursing conclusions.

REFERENCES

Alfaro, R. (1994). *Applying nursing process: A step-by-step guide* (3rd ed.). Philadelphia: JB Lippincott.

Carpenito, L. J. (1993). *Nursing diagnosis: Application to clinical practice* (5th ed.). Philadelphia: JB Lippincott.

Carroll-Johnson, R. M. (Ed.). (1991). *Classification of nursing diagnoses: Proceedings of the ninth conference North American Nursing Diagnosis Association*. Philadelphia: JB Lippincott.

McFarland, G. K., & McFarlane, E. A. (1993). *Nursing diagnosis and intervention* (2nd ed.). St. Louis: Mosby-Year Book.

North American Nursing Diagnosis Association (1992). *NANDA nursing diagnoses: Definitions and classification 1992*. Philadelphia: Author.

Details of Thinking and the Nursing Process

7

Health Detectives: Data Collection and Data Analysis

LEARNING OUTCOMES

After reading and doing the activities in this chapter you will be able to:

Appreciate the role of the nurse as a health detective.

Demonstrate ability to find clues (data collection) and make sense out of them (data analysis).

Explain the thinking required to be a great nurse health detective.

▶ NURSES AS HEALTH DETECTIVES: OVERVIEW

Collecting and analyzing data and arriving at conclusions comprise the activities of the assessment phase of the nursing process. The thinking that occurs during assessment allows nurses to make accurate conclusions about a patient's strengths and health concerns. Determining what a patient needs from a nurse and what information the nurse needs from the patient is very much like detective work. The nurse looks for clues to health issues and problems. Once the clues are found, they are validated (check for accuracy) and put together into meaningful patterns. Like detectives, nurses keep their eyes, ears, noses and hands open to discover those clues. They also constantly question the validity of the clues; that is, they are careful not just to accept things at face value. Nurses think about what clues they are finding and confirm the accuracy of the clues with other data or other sources of data — just as good detectives validate their information to solve cases.

The purpose of this detective work is to arrive at accurate conclusions about the patient's strengths and health concerns. Those major nursing conclusions of assessment were described in Chapter 6. Keeping the purpose of detective work—making conclusions—in mind helps the nurse engage all five

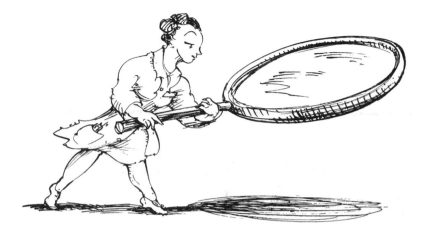

Figure 7-1.   Nurse health detective.

modes of thinking to find relevant clues and make sense of them. If this purpose of assessment is not in clear focus, it is easy to fall into an assessment rut; data collection becomes a mindless HABIT, in which the nurse simply asks questions and writes the patient's comments on a form without paying attention to the importance of the data or to the connections among them. If nurses slide into this rut, the information comes in through the ears or eyes and goes straight out the fingers to the paper, without passing through the brain in the process.

To avoid this assessment rut, it is extremely important to recognize that data collection and data analysis **must** occur simultaneously. Data collection is finding clues, and data analysis is making sense of the clues. Both activities must occur in unison, and all five modes of T.H.I.N.K. must be engaged to reach accurate conclusions of assessment.

This chapter focuses on the details of data collection (finding clues) and initial methods of data analysis (making sense out of the clues). The thinking used to analyze data as they are collected is described. The next level of analysis, clustering data (grouping clues that "fit" together) and making conclusions from those clusters, is described in Chapter 8.

▶ FINDING CLUES (DATA COLLECTION) AND MAKING SENSE OUT OF CLUES (DATA ANALYSIS)

The best detectives use a systematic approach to finding and interpreting clues. The classic approach asks six questions, *who, what, where, when, how,* and *why.* A similar approach is useful for nurse health detectives. *Who* are the

DISPLAY 7-1. The WHO, WHAT, WHERE, WHEN, HOW AND WHY of Finding Clues (Data Collection)

WHO are sources of data?
Patient
Significant others
Other health care providers

WHAT are the types of data?
Subjective raw data
Objective raw data

WHERE are the data or where is the patient?
Acute and long-term inpatient settings
Clinics and health care provider offices
Schools and workplaces
Homes and communities

WHEN are data collected?
All the time (during all phases of the nursing process, assessing, planning, implementing, evaluating)

HOW are data collected?
Observation
Measurement
Interaction

WHY collect data?
To make conclusions (back to the purpose of data collection)

sources of data? *What* are the types of data? *Where* are the data? *When* are data collected? *How* are data collected? *Why* collect data? Some answers to these questions are listed in Display 7-1, and are discussed in the following pages.

▷ Who

The patient is always the primary source of data and needs to be listened to and observed carefully, using all five senses. Although that seems like an obvious statement, the issues can be complex. The patient's level of consciousness, cognitive ability (memory and intellectual functioning), mental status, degree of comfort, desire to cooperate, and many other such factors can add to or detract from the amount and quality of data collected. Thinking nurses always keep these factors in mind as they collect data.

Significant others, an additional source of data, include family members, friends, companions, housemates, neighbors, and so forth. These sources can be valuable for validating information provided by the patient, filling in patient information gaps or guiding the nurse to explore additional health concerns not mentioned by the patient. When the patient is unable to communicate because of age, decreased level of consciousness, altered mental state, or other communication deficits, significant others serve as the primary source of verbal data.

Other health care providers also are sources of data and a means to validate data. Although they are generally very objective sources, they, like nurses, have human biases and value systems that can influence their perception and interpretation of information. Nurses need to be alert to the biases and validate these data as well. Other providers also may validate data collected by the nurse.

Except for first-encounter situations, when no one has seen the patient before, data collected by other providers frequently are documented in the patient's record. Most patient records contain past history, laboratory reports, medical orders, consultations by other providers, and progress notes. It is important to read records to avoid frustrating the patient by asking for the same information over and over. A word of caution, however: Do not always assume that something in the record is valid. Verify with the patient anything that seems inconsistent with what you observe directly or hear the patient say. For example, a nurse might say to a patient, "I noticed in your record that you are allergic to strawberries, but you are eating them with your lunch. Can you tell me about this discrepancy in information?"

Making Sense out of "Who" Clues

The thinking modes required for *who* are primarily H (HABITS) and I (INQUIRY). Going directly to the patient and significant others for information can and should become a HABIT. The best nurses combine that HABIT with INQUIRY as they gather data directly from patients and hear reports from other nurses about the patients. Again, nurses should not blindly accept everything they hear about patients, but validate data with the patients. Most nurses will directly assess patients as soon as possible. In hospital settings, nurses usually get a report from previous shift nurses and, before acting on anything, go on "rounds" to assess their patients directly. This example of INQUIRY thinking does not mean nurses do not trust the data collected by others. Rather, it is a double-check (validation) that is vital for safe, high-quality care. The same principle of checking and rechecking is used here as is used with the administration of medications. Validation also reflects the nurse's constant awareness of change.

▷ What

What types of data are available to the nurse health detective? There are different ways of classifying types of data. The first way makes a distinction between raw data and inferences. The second way divides raw data into subjective and objective categories.

Raw Data and Inferences

Raw data (as in "straight facts," not as in "uncooked") are those clues that are subjective (told to the nurse by the patient or significant other) and those clues that are objective (nonverbal data collected with the nurse's five senses). Inferences are judgments made about the data; they are miniconclusions.

Sometimes the distinction between data and inference becomes blurred because, in the real world, there are many degrees of interpretation. For example, two typical pieces of information about urine include its amount and its color. If 250 mL of urine is measured, there is little doubt that this is a piece of objective raw data (straight fact). But if a nurse says, "The color is amber," is that a fact (a piece of raw data) or is it a judgment (an inference)? A case could be made that "amber urine" is an inference, which depends on the nurse's ability to judge color. However, describing urine as "amber" is generally seen as a piece of raw data because currently there is no more precise way of measuring urine color other than visually examining it. "Amber" becomes a "necessary inference" that is acceptable in clinical practice. Necessary inferences are those inferences for which no practical way of better measurement exists. If, however, the nurse were doing research on urine color, a much more precise measurement would be demanded, requiring the use of expensive color analysis equipment.

Examples of some inferences that are commonly used but really *do need* supporting data include healthy appetite, good activity level, and noncompliance with medication regimen. All of these inferences (judgments) are mini-conclusions that nurses make about groups of data. Each inference needs raw data to support the conclusion. For instance, the data to support "healthy appetite" might include: "Patient consumes 100% of all meals within 15 to 20 minutes, occasionally asks for seconds and evening snacks."

Usually it is best to list the raw data, and not the inference, as a safeguard against making premature judgments. The important thing to remember is that whenever possible, the data should be measured and described as raw data. If too many inferences are showing up in the data base (the total of the information collected on one patient), the nurse may be making premature conclusions that can lead to inappropriate or unsafe care.

Objective and Subjective Data

Objective data, also called "signs," are all those clues (data) that the nurse sees, hears, smells, palpates (feels), or tastes directly. Few data are found through taste, but there are some examples, such as the salty taste when kissing a baby with cystic fibrosis.

Objective data also include descriptive observations and measurements collected by other health care providers and recorded in the patient's record. Objective data generally are acquired through observation and measurement, which are discussed later under "How" data are collected.

Subjective data, also called "symptoms," include direct quotes from patients or significant others. Subjective data are valuable information that provide the patient's personal perspective and interpretation of the concerns. Without subjective data, it is impossible to individualize nursing care. Subjective data are obtained through interaction with the patient and significant others. More details on interaction are given in the "How" section.

Two additional points about distinguishing between subjective and objective data are important. First, the hearing used to collect objective data (heart sounds, breath sounds, and so forth) is the same hearing used to listen to the patient or significant others talk about something. The data, however, are categorized differently. The heart or breath sounds heard by the nurse through a stethoscope are objective data; when the patient says, "My heart is beating too fast," the nurse hears subjective data.

Second, one might ask, "What difference does it make to distinguish signs from symptoms, objective from subjective data? They are all data." The importance is that, if no distinctions are made, the overall data base may be lopsided. If only objective data are collected, the patient's perceptions and ideas are being overlooked. If there are only subjective data, important signs (objective data) may be missed. Both objective and subjective data are needed for a complete picture of the patient's health status and concerns.

▶▶▶▶▶ **Action Learning #31: Distinguishing Types of Data and Inferences**

Part 1: Examine the pieces of data listed below. Label each according to the following criteria:

"R" for items of raw data

"I" for items that are inferences

"S" for items of subjective data

"O" for items of objective data

"*" for items that are inferences that have no better way of being measured, and are acceptable for clinical practice

Temp. = 98.6°F

Height = 68"

"I feel cold"

Patient's feet cool to touch

Overweight

Had orange juice, toast, and coffee for breakfast

Patient said he slept from 11 PM–6 AM

Patient anxious about surgery

Normal bowel movement

Eating well

Skin over left knee red, warm to touch, and shiny.

"My son has these awful ear infections every fall"

Part 2: Select two items you labeled as inferences with *no* "*." Write down what data could be used to validate and support that inference.

> *Data that could support this inference*
> Inference #1
>
>
>
>
> Inference #2

Part 3: Briefly describe your thinking to a classmate as you completed the above tasks.

DISCUSSION   How did you make your determinations? Were some very obvious and others less so? What standards did you use to make your decisions? Where did you find those standards? How did you describe your thinking?

Making Sense out of "What" Clues

The thinking modes used with *What* clues are primarily TOTAL RECALL, HABIT, and INQUIRY. One valuable HABIT should include making sure that a balance of subjective and objective data is collected. Obtaining accurate raw data and validating any inferences also should become HABITual.

To determine the relevance (importance) of the clues, TOTAL RECALL and INQUIRY are needed. Nurses need a good understanding of people and health, and what is normal. For example, when trying to determine if urine is "normal," the nurse needs to know what is normal for color, specific gravity, and output in a 24-hour period; it also is important to know the frequency with which the patient voids, and if there is any discomfort or pain during elimination. Determining "normal" requires the use of TOTAL RECALL of this factual information, or at least recalling where to look for the "normals" of urine. It also requires the use of the INQUIRY mode to make comparisons between what is found and what should be found.

Determining if a piece of data is normal signals the initial thinking required for data analysis. If it is normal, it could be a patient strength or just interesting information. However, if something is not normal, it is considered "relevant" and becomes significant in developing accurate conclusions.

Look at the following three pieces of information. Knowing nothing else about the patient, what do you *think* is relevant?

Eyes = two in front of head

Skin = green color with purple spots and neon stripes

Toes = 10, 5 on each foot

What made you say that the second item was relevant? Because it is not normal. How did you know it was not normal? Because nobody (on our planet, at least) has skin like that. So, in this situation, you compared the available data to a population norm (standard). You used TOTAL RECALL and probably thought about whether or not you had any memory of seeing, hearing, or reading about people with green, purple-spotted, neon-striped skin. More discussion on population norms (standards) is presented in Chapter 8.

This first level of data analysis, which used TOTAL RECALL and INQUIRY to distinguish relevant data from nonrelevant data, was accomplished by comparing data to population norms. There is another type of norm that must be used for further analysis—the individual's norms. When a nurse looks at separate pieces of information, the only comparison that can be made is with population norms. To find out if this condition or situation is normal for the individual, however, the nurse must get more data, even if this amounts only to asking the patient, "Is this normal for you?" Here is an example of the distinction of the two types of norms: A patient sleeps 3 to 4 hours each night. Does this meet population norms? No, most textbooks indicate 6 to 8 hours of sleep per 24 hours is "normal" for adults. To find out if this is normal for the patient, the nurse has to collect another clue to compare with his individual norm. The patient may say "Yes, this is my usual pattern." In this case, the data, "sleeps 3 to 4 hours each night" *and* "this is my usual pattern," become a set or a cluster of data that is less relevant than the single datum might have been.

In that example, the nurse had to go beyond analyzing one clue to clustering that clue with one additional clue. This clustering process is discussed more fully in Chapter 8, but for now it is important to see that judgments about the relevance of one piece of information constitute only a first step in data analysis.

▶▶▶▶▶▶ **A**ction Learning #32: Looking for Relevant Data

Examine each item in the following list of data. Using TOTAL RECALL and INQUIRY, determine which may be relevant, based on population norms, for each item.

(Hint: As you check books, you will not find the words, "population norms." What you will find are descriptions of "typical findings" or what something "should look like." For example, "The usual range for hemoglobin for women is 12 to 15 g/dL," or "When examining the eyes, assess the pupils for roundness and symmetry, size, reaction to light . . . ")

> Pupils dilated and fixed
>
> Pedal pulses 2+ bilaterally
>
> Hematocrit 39%
>
> Rales in both lower lung fields
>
> Three bowel movements a day

DISCUSSION   How easy was it to find the "norms?" How many did you know without having to look them up? Do you see how, after determining the fit with population norms, you would also need to check individual norms to determine if some information is relevant?

▷ Where

Where data are obtained depends on the physical location of the patient and the surroundings. Different kinds of data are available when patients are in acute or long-term settings, clinics or providers' offices, schools, workplaces, or homes. Patients in hospitals, for example, do not have their "things" around them. A patient whose home is filled with books may not be recognized as a avid reader while in the hospital. On the other hand, hospital rooms are not devoid of information that reveal things about the person. Consider a patient who has a rosary on the bedside table; seeing that object in the environment could give the nurse information about the patient's religion. Would an inference (judgment) about the patient's religious preference be wise without collecting more data?

Seeing patients in their homes can provide a wealth of information that frequently goes uncollected in an inpatient setting. Most people surround themselves with things that are extensions of themselves and that reflect their interests. Also, patients on their own "turf" often act differently than they do when they are on nurses' "turf."

It is easy to miss data from the environment, no matter where the location, when the patient is such a strong focus of attention. The nurse's natural tendency is to talk to patients and rely on verbal reports of data instead of looking at the more subtle clues surrounding the patient. These subtle clues, such as plants, clutter, room temperature, lighting, music, and the like, reflect needs, likes, and dislikes.

In addition to asking questions directly about the environment (eg, "Tell me about your sleeping environment, where and how you sleep, and how it helps or hinders your sleep patterns"), the nurse health detective must develop a keen sense of environmental observation. No matter what the setting, the nurse health detective must constantly observe for data about environmental hazards (eg, loose throw rugs in the home, bedrails not locking properly) and environmental impediments (eg, only bathroom is on the second floor of patient's home, patient's call light is not in reach).

Making Sense out of "Where" Clues

Again, the first three modes of T.H.I.N.K. are required to collect *where* clues. Finding clues in the patient's environment requires a HABIT of constant awareness of the "big picture," or seeing the patient as a unique individual within a larger system. The larger system includes, among other things, the physical space, the family, and the community. How the patient relates or does not relate to the larger system also is important. A broad understanding of people and how they interact with their environments is necessary to recognize clues and make sense out of them. This understanding comes from TOTAL RECALL of information learned in courses such as sociology, psychology, and nursing science. INQUIRY helps nurses question the environmental data and their relevance to the patient's health status.

To see how you measure up, test your current environmental awareness with Action Learning #33. Keep in mind that this skill, like any other, can be nurtured and improved with practice. Environmental awareness should become a useful HABIT.

▶▶▶▶▶▶ **Action Learning #33: Testing Environmental Awareness**

Select a TV show that you do not usually watch. Watch it for 10 minutes with the sound off. Pay attention to the environment and the nonverbal behaviors of the people. Write down what you observed that you might not have noticed had the sound been on. If you write down an inference, also write down the raw objective data you observed to support (validate) your inference.

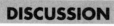 **DISCUSSION**   How acute was your awareness? Have you discovered a strength—that you are very aware of environmental clues—or is this an area that needs work? What can you do to enhance your environmental awareness?

Pause here for a thinking-learning check. You should be able to elaborate on these ideas:

▼ Nurses are health detectives who need to find clues and make sense out of the clues.

▼ Data collection and data analysis *must* occur simultaneously.

▼ Finding clues is focused on questioning *who, what, where, when, how,* and *why,* and using all five modes of thinking to make sense out of the data.

▼ Patients are the primary source of data.

▼ Raw data are subjective or objective, and a balance of both provides the best information.

▼ Some inferences are necessary, but most need to be supported (validated) with raw data.

▷ When

Data collection occurs at every patient encounter from start to finish. In fact, data collection (finding clues) occurs before the nurse encounters the patient, through verbal reports and records, during patient encounters, and after patient encounters through validating data with other data, or with other people. The bottom line on *When* is "always."

Making Sense out of "When" Clues

The T, H, I, and the N are all needed. Observing and listening need to become well-tuned HABITs. But habitually collecting data at all times is ineffective unless the nurse is putting pieces together and making sense out of them using INQUIRY. NEW IDEAS AND CREATIVITY are used when the nurse takes advantage of less obvious opportunities for when to collect data. For example, when accompanying a patient to the cafeteria or when facilitating a patient's leisure activity, the creative nurse may find clues that the less creative nurse would miss. These are not "usual" times for collecting data, but patients may be more relaxed and may reveal information that might not be shared in more formal situations.

▷ How

There are whole courses on *how* to collect data; traditionally, these courses are titled "Health Assessment." Although health assessment courses provide the foundation for *how* to collect data, all nursing courses add to the repertoire of data collection techniques. The basic categories of techniques are **interaction**, **observation**, and **measurement**.

Interaction

Interaction is the method for collecting subjective clues. Most beginning students know more about *interaction* than about other techniques because everyone interacts with people every day. Therapeutic interactions, however, require not only everyday experience, but nursing skill in knowing what promotes or blocks communication. Anybody can pick up a form and ask questions from it. Finding the best wording for questioning individual patients, however, takes thought and practice. Also, knowing when and how to ask for more specific information or expand on existing information is important. Most nursing textbooks cover the topic of therapeutic communication very well and should be read carefully. Reading about therapeutic communication before working with patients helps the beginning nurse plan how to ask questions efficiently. Role-playing a patient interaction, with a classmate playing the patient role, is very helpful. An even better learning technique is to videotape the interaction, play it back, and evaluate it for strengths and areas needing further development.

Because of time and space limitations, this text highlights only two specific interaction techniques that demonstrate good thinking skills. Both techniques are similar in that they provide for expansion and elaboration of information. The first is called "branching," and the second is called "DETAIL."

Branching is very descriptive of the technique itself. A patient's verbal response stimulates a thinking nurse to ask sequential questions that, when answered, clarify or validate the first piece of information. Branching is extremely helpful for collecting related pieces of data, organizing data, finding patterns, and making sense out of the data. Chapter 8 illustrates how important branching is to clustering data in the next level of analysis.

The second useful interaction skill designed for data collection is D.E.T.A.I.L. D.E.T.A.I.L. is a another mnemonic that generates even more branching-type questions when a patient has an identified area of concern. For example, D.E.T.A.I.L. helps to zero in on key pieces of data regarding a patient's complaint of pain. The categories of data collection in the D.E.T.A.I.L. mnemonic are as follows:

"D," date of onset and course, provides historical data and chronologic data that are useful in determining the chronic or acute nature of the concern. Typical patient responses to questions in this category include: "It started yesterday," "It started three years ago," "It was worse in the beginning," "It is gradually getting worse," or "It is OK in the morning but by noon I have the most trouble."

"E," exact location, provides anatomic data. Typical patient responses include: "The whole top of my head hurts," "Just one very sore spot right here," "It is just sort of all over my body," or "Right behind my knee."

"T," terms (patient's) for description of quality and quantity, provides the patient's perceptions of what the issue or problem is like and its severity.

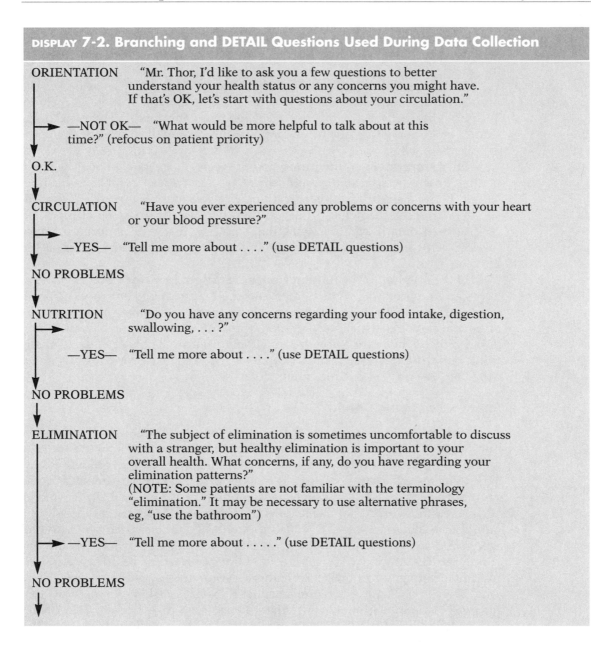

DISPLAY 7-2. Branching and DETAIL Questions Used During Data Collection

ORIENTATION   "Mr. Thor, I'd like to ask you a few questions to better
understand your health status or any concerns you might have.
If that's OK, let's start with questions about your circulation."

—NOT OK—   "What would be more helpful to talk about at this
time?" (refocus on patient priority)

O.K.

CIRCULATION   "Have you ever experienced any problems or concerns with your heart
or your blood pressure?"

—YES—   "Tell me more about . . . ." (use DETAIL questions)

NO PROBLEMS

NUTRITION   "Do you have any concerns regarding your food intake, digestion,
swallowing, . . . ?"

—YES—   "Tell me more about . . . ." (use DETAIL questions)

NO PROBLEMS

ELIMINATION   "The subject of elimination is sometimes uncomfortable to discuss
with a stranger, but healthy elimination is important to your
overall health. What concerns, if any, do you have regarding your
elimination patterns?"
(NOTE: Some patients are not familiar with the terminology
"elimination." It may be necessary to use alternative phrases,
eg, "use the bathroom")

—YES—   "Tell me more about . . . . ." (use DETAIL questions)

NO PROBLEMS

Typical patient responses include: "Its stabbing," "It's a dull ache," " It is like being jabbed with a burning hot poker," or "On a scale of 1 to 10, with 10 being the worst, it's a 12."

"A," aggravating and alleviating factors, help identify what makes the problem worse and what makes it better. Typical patient responses include: "Bright lights really make it worse," "The medicine the doctor prescribed helps some," or "A hot bath really helps," or "Small rooms with smoke are the hardest places to be."

"I," intersystem connections, provides information on what else is happening to the person at the same time. Typical patient responses include: "When I have a sinus infection everything else gets messed up too," "I get constipated from the medicine," "I get so tired because I can't sleep at night because I can't breath when I'm lying flat," or "I get a stiff neck because I have to sleep with three pillows to breath and my nose gets so sore from all the blowing."

"L," listening to the patient's interpretation, is always good advice. Patients are the primary source of data, but their perceptions of causes of problems and what might help alleviate problems can be overlooked easily. Patients often will not offer their interpretation, thinking the nurse knows best. When asked directly, however, patients can supply useful insight, such as, "I really think I'm just too stressed out to sleep well," "It feels like I have a sinus infection," or "My baby is coming **now**!"

Example of Using Detail

Nora Dakota, SN, is doing a home visit with the Peters family, who have requested help with new baby care and when to add solid foods to the formula feedings. Before getting started with the planned baby bath, Nora asked how Mrs. Peters was feeling, because this was her fifth day postpartum (after delivery). Mrs. Peters smiled and said she was fine except for a bad stomachache.

Nora thought, "A stomachache is not normal." (She was comparing the data to population norms.) She also thought, "A stomachache for a woman who is 5 days postpartum could be an indication of more serious problems." (She was RECALLing what she knew about postpartum health care issues, uterine bleeding, infections, constipation.) Nora's first question to Mrs. Peters was, "Do you normally have stomachaches?" (She was asking for an individual norm to compare with the data.) When the patient's response was "No," Nora proceeded to use the DETAIL format to collect more specific information. The following dialogue occurred:

> **Nora:** Tell me when you first noticed the stomachache and if there have been any changes. Is it getting worse or better?
> **Mrs. P.:** Well, it started 2 days ago. It does seem worse today.
> **Nora:** Show me where you are actually feeling the stomachache
> **Mrs. P.:** It's right here [she rubs the right side of her abdomen below her ribs].

Nora: Does it hurt anywhere else?

Mrs. P.: Mostly just right here, although sometimes it seems to move a bit over to the left.

Nora: Describe for me how it feels, and on a scale from 1 to 10, with 10 being the worst, how bad it is.

Mrs. P.: Well, it feels like a block of lead is sitting in me. I can't wear anything tight or it really hurts. I guess I would say it's about a 3 sometimes and a 6 at other times.

Nora: Is there anything that makes it worse or makes it better?

Mrs. P.: Sitting for a while makes it worse, or if I lie on my right side at night. Sometimes taking a walk helps it feel better. And, this is embarrassing, but passing gas helps too.

Nora: Have you noticed this stomachache affecting anything else?

Mrs. P.: I don't have much appetite. I'm also much more irritable than I usually am but I just assumed that was normal for a new mother.

Nora: Irritability can be a concern, and we can talk about it too, because it's not necessarily normal. But are you noticing anything else related to your stomachache—for example, have you had much vaginal bleeding? Have you had any diarrhea or constipation? Have you had a fever?

Mrs. P.: Let's not forget to discuss the irritability. But, no, no unusual bleeding beyond what the doctor said was normal. I haven't had any diarrhea; in fact I can't remember when I had my last bowel movement. I've been so busy I haven't paid much attention. And, no, no fever.

Nora: How often did you have bowel movements before the baby was born?

Mrs. P.: Usually about every day or at least every other day.

Nora: Have you ever experienced this kind of pain before, and what do you think might be going on here?

Mrs. P.: Now that you mention it, I did have something like this several years ago, but a lot worse; I hope this isn't the same thing. I had such bad constipation after a bout with the flu that I almost had an impaction. I'll bet that is what is happening!

Nora: The information you are describing does fit that picture. What did you do the last time?

Mrs. P.: I had to take this terrible medicine and several enemas. I sure don't want to do that again.

Nora: Lets consult with your obstetrician and try some less drastic measures first, like extra water, prune juice, raisins, exercise, and any other things that normally stimulate your bowels to move.

Nora and Mrs. Peters continued their visit. The baby bath was completed, they had time to talk about not starting solid foods yet, and about irritability. After consulting with her obstetrician, who ordered a mild laxative, they worked out a plan to increase her fluids and exercise. By the next day, Mrs. Peters began to pass small amounts of stool and was beginning to feel better. By Nora's second visit, Mrs. Peter's stomachache was completely gone and her bowel elimination was within her personal norms. She was no longer feeling irritable and was very comfortable with safely bathing her new baby.

▶▶▶▶▶▶ **Action Learning #34: Collecting the DETAIL Clues on a Headache**

Find a person who recently had or currently has a headache. Use the DETAIL format to collect expanded information on the headache. Share your data with a classmate who did this same activity and compare responses.

D = Date of onset and course of the problem

E = Exact location of the problem

T = Terms (patient's) for description of quality and quantity of the problem

A = Aggravating and alleviating factors

I = Intersystem connections of the problem

L = Listen to patient's interpretation of the problem

D.

E.

T.

A.

I.

L.

| **DISCUSSION** | Did you get a full picture of the headache? Do you see how these details give you more direction for planning |

Did you get a full picture of the headache? Do you see how these details give you more direction for planning interventions than you would have had without them? Did you also see how different headaches produce different data?

Observation

Observation is one *How* method used to collect objective data. Like interaction, it is something that all people use daily. Some people are very attentive; others are not. Nurse health detectives must have very attentive, fine-tuned observation skills at all times. When with a patient, a nurse must look at the patient *and* the environment. Sensitive eyes and ears can pick up changes in patients and their environments that the patient may not yet be able or willing to describe verbally.

The things that nurses learn to observe are too numerous to list. A few examples include the patient's nonverbal behaviors (movements, body language, facial expressions, voice tone, gait, and the like), skin color, eating behaviors, sleeping behaviors, condition of teeth, ability to use call lights, environmental hazards, and on and on.

▶▶▶▶▶ Action Learning #35: Using Observation Skills

Find a picture in a magazine or at an art museum that includes people doing something. Describe everything you see that may be related to the health of the people in the picture. Ask your classmate to look at the same picture and do the same activity. Share your findings.

| **DISCUSSION** | What did both of you find? Were there many differences? What subtle issues did you notice, such as skin tone, un- |

What did both of you find? Were there many differences? What subtle issues did you notice, such as skin tone, unhealthy behaviors, unhealthy environments, and so forth?

Measurement

Measurement, the third *how* technique, is also used to collect objective data. It is generally considered the most precise of the three data collection techniques because it quantifies data (amount, size, and the like) through specific instruments that enhance the nurse's five senses.

It is always best to use a measurement instrument when one is available rather than guessing at measurements. This may seem obvious for things like blood pressure readings, but it is easily forgotten when one measures something like a skin lesion. A specific measurement (4 cm as measured with a ruler) is more descriptive than statements like the "size of a grapefruit." There are too many variations in grapefruit size.

Remember the discussion on inferences and raw data. A good nurse will not substitute an inference for raw data if a specific measurement is possible. For example, instead of documenting the inference, "large lesion on back," measure it and record a clear description such as "2.5-cm, round, flat, red lesion with defined borders on coccyx." The word "large" is too general and open to interpretation, as are the words "lesion" and "back." In the more descriptive example, the word "lesion" was used but clearly modified with descriptive words that narrowed the limits of interpretation. The other parts of the description are so specific that anyone reading it could visualize it.

Although the precision of measurements and numbers is highly respected, the nurse's intuitive "measurements" are equally valuable in the overall picture. Experienced nurses often can make very accurate measurements without tools, but beginners do not have the necessary familiarity with patient situations to rely on their "eyeballing" as experts do.

▷▷▷▷▷▷ **Action Learning #36: Practicing Your Measurement Skills**

Part 1: Ask a friend to work with you for this Action Learning exercise. You will need a tape measure calibrated in centimeters. Practice measuring the following items:

A fingernail

A mole

The circumference of the calf of your leg

The great toe

The distance around an ankle

Abdominal girth

Part 2: Study the back of your hand and your friend's hand and describe it in writing so anyone would be able to determine which hand was whose by comparing the written descriptions to the actual hands.

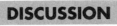 Can you think of patient circumstances where such measurements would be critical data? Check a nursing textbook for care of patients with ascites or deep vein thrombosis for examples. As you measured the calf and abdomen, did you think about the importance of specifying precisely where on the leg or abdomen the measurements were taken? What were the key differences in the backs of your hands?

Making Sense out of "How" Clues

All T.H.I.N.K. modes are needed to determine *how* best to collect and analyze data. TOTAL RECALL is important to organize the data collection and know what to ask, observe, and measure. Establishing therapeutic relationships before collecting data must become a HABIT. Just "jumping right in" and asking questions, observing, and measuring without establishing that relationship could alienate and possibly frighten patients. *How* to use data collection instruments, such as thermometers and blood pressure cuffs, appropriately and safely may become HABITS also. INQUIRY is important for branching and collecting DETAILs because the nurse must constantly mentally ask if the data need to be expanded. NEW IDEAS AND CREATIVITY are needed to determine *how* to get information in unusual patient situations. Use of the KNOWING HOW YOU THINK mode will help beginning nurse health detectives develop comfort with data collection and analysis. How each nurse thinks influences such things as *how* and *when* data are recorded, how structured the data collection process needs to be, and how easily relevant data are recognized.

▷ Why

The answer to the *why* question is found in the purpose of data collection. The reason for collecting data is to have raw data from which valid conclusions can be made. Data collection and analysis provide the building blocks for the thinking that leads to valid conclusions. Think about it! How productive and safe is it to pull conclusions out of thin air? Safe, great nursing demands thinking during data collection to develop accurate conclusions. Return to Chapter 5, if necessary, to review the thinking about conclusions.

▼THINKING-LEARNING CHECK

Pause here for a thinking-learning check. You should be able to elaborate on these ideas:

- ▼ Data are always collected during all encounters.
- ▼ Data are collected through interaction, observation, and measurement.
- ▼ Branching and D.E.T.A.I.L. are useful skills of interaction.
- ▼ Data are collected to develop the conclusions.
- ▼ All five modes of thinking are required during data collection and analysis.

▶ CLOSING COMMENTS

This chapter has covered a great deal of basic information that must be incorporated into the skills repertoire of the nurse health detective. These skills will not be developed overnight, but they are essential to great nursing. It takes practice and much repetition for many of these health detective skills to become useful HABITS. It also requires thinking in all five modes to avoid the assessment rut. The next chapter expands this thinking process of data analysis to cluster analysis, from which the major conclusions of assessment can be made.

▶▶▶ *THINKING LOG #7*

Think about how you learn best. Develop some strategies for remembering and being able to apply all the things you have just learned from this chapter. If you prefer the written word, you might outline this chapter on a 5 × 8 card. If you prefer a visual format, you might create a diagram or flow chart to illustrate all the concepts of the chapter. Use your creativity to enhance your learning and share your results with a classmate.

Making More Sense of Clues: Cluster Analysis

After reading and doing the activities in this chapter you will be able to:

Describe what clusters are and how to develop them.

Explain the need for clusters in developing conclusions.

Demonstrate all modes of T.H.I.N.K. in cluster analysis.

Chapter 7 focused on collecting data and the preliminary analysis that occurs as the nurse collects data. Analysis, however, must go much further before major conclusions of assessment can be made by the nurse health detective. This chapter shows how data are arranged and analyzed in groups so that the most accurate conclusions can be made.

To begin to appreciate this additional level of analysis, examine the following case study and the conclusions made by the nurse. Try to determine what the nurse did between point A (collecting the data) and point C (developing the conclusions); in other words, what constitutes point B (the additional level of analysis)?

CASE STUDY

CASE STUDY (POINT A)

Juanita Gomez, widow, age 76, has lived in nursing home for 4 months after she fractured her right hip and had open reduction and internal fixation surgery (ORIF). She is a former teacher. Mrs. Gomez was born in Puerto Rico but has lived in New York since age

5. She has adequate health insurance, with Medicare and supplemental insurance.

Her medical diagnoses are osteoarthritis, noninsulin-dependent diabetes mellitus (NIDDM), right hip ORIF. The scar on her right hip is pink and dry with no drainage. She is legally blind but can see shapes and light. Owing to neurologic changes, her hearing is slightly diminished.

She wears lipstick each day and gets her hair done every week in the beauty shop. Her hair is shiny and her clothes are neat and clean. She wakes each morning feeling rested. She wouldn't have chosen to live in a nursing home, but says "this one's not so bad." She usually sees her two children, who live out of state, about once a year. She has three grandchildren.

She spends lots of time alone in her room listening to the radio and "talking books" and crocheting potholders for the annual craft show. She says she feels alone and different from others because she is almost blind; she has not made friends.

Her vital signs are: B/P = 110/76, P = 86, Reg, R = 16, T = 97.8°F. She has 2+ ankle edema (swelling). She is 5′2″ and weighs 105 lbs. She follows a 1800-calorie diabetic diet. Her skin is dry, very thin, and translucent. She has bowel movements every other day. They are soft and brown, and she drinks prune juice daily to maintain regularity. She wears "Depends" because of some minor urinary dribbling. Her coccyx and elbows are reddened.

Mrs. Gomez sleeps through the night but has lots of trouble getting out of bed because of joint stiffness and limited range of motion of her right hip. She has a bruise on her left shin from hitting against the wheelchair during transfers from bed. She also has a skin tear on her left hand. She complains of discomfort and irritation of her buttocks from sitting in the wheelchair all day.

CONCLUSIONS ABOUT MRS. GOMEZ (POINT C)

Strengths:
  Vital signs stable
  Adequate nutrition
  Adequate bowel elimination
  Adequate sleep pattern
  Adequate health insurance
  Well groomed
Health Concerns:
  Nursing Diagnoses (actual problems and related factors)
    Impaired Skin Integrity related to mobility deficits, urinary incontinence, fragile skin, and compromised circulation

Social Isolation related to sensory deficits
Interdisciplinary Problems:
Impaired Physical Mobility (Physical Therapy)
Problems for Referral:
None at this time
Hunches to be Ruled In or Ruled Out:
Possible Knowledge Deficit regarding diabetic care
Possible problem for referral: vision deficits

▶▶▶▶▶ **Action Learning #37: Looking for "Point B"**

Write your responses to the following questions and share them with a class-mate. As you examined the data base, what was your first impression?

What could have been done with the data base to make it more understand-able?

Did the nurse's conclusions make sense to you? Why? Why not?

What other conclusions did you come up with?

Describe what you think the nurse might have done to arrive at the above conclusions.

DISCUSSION Did the data base provide adequate information from which to develop conclusions? How could the data have been presented differently to allow for some "natural" groupings of related in-formation? Would "natural groupings" have helped your thinking? If so, why? Did you sense the thinking piece between points A and C?

▶ **DEFINITIONS AND IMPORTANCE OF CLUSTERS**

The above data base and conclusions are realistic examples of what nurses process mentally every day. The mental processing required to get from point A (data collection) to point C (conclusions) is rarely discussed, let alone writ-ten down. This thinking is so important to great nursing, however, that all of this chapter is devoted to it. The major component of this thinking is the devel-opment and analysis of data clusters.

In general, a cluster is two or more similar pieces of anything. A peanut cluster is a tasty example. A data cluster is two or more pieces of information that fit together and have more meaning together than they do when examined separately. The nurse health detective finds clues, analyzes them for significance as described in Chapter 7 (comparing with norms), and then looks for patterns in those clues so that conclusions can be made. The patterns in the clues are clusters, and making sense out of those clusters is cluster analysis.

▷ Importance of Clusters

Making Accurate Conclusions

Clustering and cluster analysis occur simultaneously, as do data collection and data analysis, and are essential in making accurate conclusions. To make sound conclusions, nurses must look beyond individual pieces of data and how they compare to norms, to the relationships among the data and among the clusters. Nurses do not base care on a single datum because accurate conclusions rarely can be made with one piece of information. Think of this for a minute. A nurse finds a patient crying while talking to her husband on the phone. Would the nurse conclude that the patient and her husband are having marital problems? No, of course not. The nurse would certainly note that the crying is relevant, but would collect more data to develop a cluster before concluding anything. Later, the nurse learns that the patient was talking about her mother, who died 2 years ago in this same hospital, and listens as the patient describes her sadness. The nurse then develops an initial hunch that the patient is experiencing grief. (Of course, this conclusion would need to be validated with the patient.)

Taking Necessary Shortcuts

In addition to promoting accuracy of conclusions, appropriate clustering allows nurse health detectives to take necessary shortcuts by consolidating their thinking and communication with other health care providers. Think of the above example. It is much easier to say to another nurse (after validation), "This patient is grieving," as opposed to describing all the raw data that went into that conclusion: "The patient has been crying, talking about her mother who died 2 years ago in this hospital," and so forth. Hearing the diagnosis "grieving," other nurses can safely assume that the patient is experiencing certain signs and symptoms. They hear the word "grieving" and assume sadness and loss are being experienced. This does not mean the nurse couldn't describe all of the raw data; there simply aren't enough hours in the day to do that for all the patient responses that nurses find.

Avoiding Omissions

A third important aspect of clustering is that it prevents nurses from spending unnecessary time on data that "appear" abnormal on the surface, or from missing something important because the individual clues don't signal any concern. With clustering, something that seemed abnormal can be recognized as normal, and something that seems normal may be recognized as abnormal. Consider the following examples. Which of these situations is/are normal?

> A person:
> who wets the bed
> whose menstrual cycle hasn't started yet
> who sleeps only 2 or 3 hours at a time
> who has a bowel movement every 3 days
> who needs to have all his teeth pulled
> who is incontinent of urine

At first glance, a nonthinking nurse might say all these are abnormal and jump to premature conclusions. However, these single pieces of information, by themselves, should not be the focus of nursing care. Other data must be collected to round out the picture; there needs to be a cluster of data before any accurate conclusions can be made.

In the examples above, adding data about the age of the person might provide enough of a cluster to make some conclusions. If the person who wets the bed is 2 years old, it is not unusual; if the person is 11 years old, the same data cluster takes on new importance. In the second example, again, age and gender are important pieces of information to add before any conclusions can be made. In the third example, one more piece of information probably would not be enough. The nurse would want to find out how this person feels with this sleep pattern, what was waking the person, how long this was going on, if there had been attempts to change this pattern, and other data as well.

What these examples show is that data clusters may have two or any number of pieces of information in them. The amount of information depends on the area under study. Generally speaking, the more data in the cluster, the more accurate the conclusion can be, but that is not always the case. It depends on how critical each piece of information is. Look at the following clusters:

Grasping the throat	"I feel really strange."
Unable to talk	"I'm a bit dizzy at times."
	"My husband just left me."
	"I don't know what I'll do."
	"I can't seem to keep food down."
	Abdomen nontender
	B/P 130/88, P 92, R 24

The cluster on the left has two critical indicators of choking. The logical conclusion, which can be made quickly, is that the person is choking and needs a Heimlich maneuver. The cluster on the right, although it has more information, has fewer critical indicators. It is a larger cluster, but a conclusion based on those data would not be as easy to make and would have a lower probability of accuracy.

Taking Advantage of the Brain's Natural Memory System

Finally, clustering is important as a memory aid that is invaluable in health care. The human brain can store a great deal of information, but the way pieces are stored is the key to retrieval. Without effective retrieval systems the information is useless. Brains have a special short-term memory system for storing raw data as separate units of information. If people try to store too many separate units, however, their brains 'say', "Hold on, there is a better way to do this without using up so much short-term memory space." The brain starts looking for things that fit together into groups or clusters, and uses the

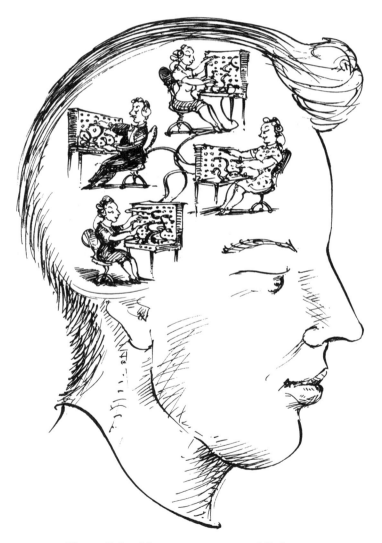

Figure 8-1. Memory patterns and linkages.

cluster labels as triggers to move deeper into its memory levels for storage or retrieval of the details. The brain's memory system seems to work in layers; each layer can hold only so much information. But remembering a label on one level can trigger the memory of the six or seven separate pieces of information (clues) on the level below it that were grouped together and summarized with that trigger label on the higher level (Hart, 1983; Carnevali & Thomas, 1993). This concept about memory and use of patterns was discussed originally in Chapter 1.

Neurophysiology notwithstanding, the important thing is that nurse health detectives can remember things more easily if they group clues (data) together than if they try to remember all the separate pieces. Because there is so much to remember and analyze in health care, it is impossible to practice great nursing without clustering.

▶ WHAT CLUSTERS LOOK LIKE

Clusters are the groups of data that support nursing conclusions. Some conclusions are simple phrases such as "vital signs stable," and other conclusions have more formalized titles, such as "Social Isolation related to sensory deficits," but all conclusions need to be supported (validated) with a cluster of data. Examine the clusters of data that support each of the conclusions for Mrs. Gomez.

▼ CONCLUSIONS AND SUPPORTING CLUSTERS OF DATA

Conclusion	Cluster of Data
STRENGTHS	
Vital signs stable	B/P 110/76, P 86, R 16, T 97.8°F
Adequate nutrition	Ht. 5'2", Wt. 105 lbs. Follows 1800-cal. diet, shiny hair.
Adequate bowel elimination	BM every other day, soft, brown. Drinks prune juice for regularity.
Adequate sleep pattern	Sleeps through the night and feels rested in the morning.
Adequate health insurance	Has Medicare and supplemental insurance.
Well groomed	Hair shiny, gets hair done every week, clothing clean and neat, wears lipstick daily.

HEALTH CONCERNS

NURSING DIAGNOSES

Problem

Impaired Skin Integrity	Coccyx and elbow reddened, bruise on left shin, skin tear left hand, complaints of discomfort and irritation of buttocks.

Related Factors

Mobility deficits	Wheelchair bound, stiff joints, trouble getting out of bed, limited ROM (range of motion) right hip, hitting wheelchair during transfers, osteoarthritis, right hip ORIF 4 months ago.
Urinary incontinence	Dribbles urine, wears "Depends."
Fragile skin	Skin dry, very thin, translucent.
Compromised circulation	Sitting in wheelchair all day, NIDDM, ankle edema.

Problem

Social Isolation	Spends a lot of time alone in her room listening to the radio, crocheting (noninteractive activities), says she feels alone and different from others because she is almost blind, has made no friends, sees family once a year.

Related Factors

Sensory deficits	Almost blind, hearing slightly diminished

INTERDISCIPLINARY PROBLEMS

Impaired physical mobility	Wheelchair bound, stiff joints, trouble getting out of bed, limited ROM right hip, hitting wheelchair during transfers, osteoarthritis, right hip ORIF 4 months ago.

HUNCHES TO BE RULED IN OR RULED OUT

Possible knowledge deficit regarding diabetic care.	Medical Dx: NIDDM Data gaps: Knowledge about NIDDM, knowledge about care needed to maintain health.

Possible problem for   Medical Dx: NIDDM
referral: vision   Legally blind
deficits.   Neurologic changes have already affected
                     hearing
            Data gaps: Actual visual acuity, use of
                     glasses, last vision exam, patient's
                     description of actual vision limits

Notice how the clusters "paint a picture" that can be summed up with the conclusion label. The type and quality of data in the clusters increase the probability of accuracy of the conclusions. Can you see how the pieces in the cluster logically fit together? Seeing the logic of the fit for some clusters may come from common sense, but, for other clusters it takes practice, experience, and study. Recognizing important data gaps (missing data) takes even more experience. Because this ability is so important, reexamine the clusters for Mrs. Gomez's data and then practice clustering.

▶▶▶▶▶▶ **Action Learning #38: Examining Clusters**

Examine the following clusters and explain why they do or do not fit together.

Cluster A: Runny nose
                Temperature of 101.2°F
                Watery eyes
                "I feel awful"

Cluster B: Sedentary job
                Occipital headaches
                Recently married
                Good health insurance

Cluster C: Bowel movements every 3 days
                Stools hard, dark brown
                Strains with bowel movements
                "I really feel bloated and I can't even button my pants
                    anymore"
                Drinks two cups of liquid a day
                Sedentary job
                Taking calcium and Tylenol #3 for back pain from
                    arthritis

Cluster D: Wringing hands
                Sweaty palms
                Wide-eyed stare
                Pacing floor
                "I can't think and I don't know what to do"
                "I think I'm going to throw up"

Cluster E: Sleeps 8 hours a day
Does not have vegetables in daily intake
Able to take care of all daily needs
Has high school education
"Every time I go to the bathroom it burns so bad, I get
tears in my eyes"

What preliminary conclusions (labels) should be considered for the clusters that appear to fit together? Try to make two or three hunches for each cluster.

Conclusion Hunches
Cluster A:

Cluster B:

Cluster C:

Cluster D:

Cluster E:

DISCUSSION Do you see how each item in the cluster, taken by itself, takes on a new meaning when it is combined with other items? How did you know which clusters had data that fit together? How easy was it to select preliminary conclusions for the clusters? Why was it easy or difficult to make conclusions for these clusters?

▶ HOW TO CLUSTER

Clustering skill varies greatly, from the beginning nurse health detective to the expert. Examining the thinking and teasing out the details provide some guidance for improving one's existing skills in this area. The primary tasks include determining what data fit together and what data are missing. After these basic tasks are completed, the nurse must choose the best clusters and the best labels for the clusters.

▷ Determining What Fits Together

Sometimes clustering data is fairly easy because one has current knowledge and experience in that area. If a person is 5′2″ and 200 lbs., it doesn't take a Ph.D. in nutrition to conclude this person is overweight. Most people have read or heard something about height and weight being related; if one is a certain height, one is healthiest in a certain weight range. In Western cultures, it is nearly impossible not to have come in contact with such information. To be really sure, one could check a book (probably a nutrition text) for height and weight proportion range norms. Comparing the norms to the actual height and weight would validate the conclusion that this person was overweight. Coming to that conclusion meant putting two pieces of data together and comparing them to norms to reach a judgment about what they mean together. Neither piece of information is important on its own, but together they take on new meaning.

For the beginning nurse health detective, however, what fits together often is not so obvious. Luckily, there are tools and aids to assist in this activity. These will be discussed shortly.

▷ Determining Data Gaps

These same tools and aids (to be discussed shortly) are also useful in determining what data are missing from the cluster. Figuring out what is missing is just as important as figuring out what fits together. The missing pieces are called "data gaps." In the case of Mrs. Gomez, the list of conclusions included some "data gaps" when the nurse was ruling in and ruling out the hunches about knowledge deficit and vision problems.

▶▶▶▶▶▶ **Action Learning #39: Looking for Data Gaps**

Look at the example below. For conclusion #1, the data cluster and data gaps are listed. For #2 and #3, the conclusion and the data clusters are given but the data gaps are missing. Write out two or three pieces of data that, if known, would help you develop a better cluster and, therefore, a more accurate conclusion. It might be helpful to use a nursing diagnosis text or nursing theory text to identify data gaps. (Hint: Look at the defining characteristics of the conclusion labels.)

Conclusion	Cluster	Data Gaps
Example: #1 Low self-esteem	Patient very timid Little eye contact Unable to identify any personal strengths	Verbalizes feeling unworthy Believes not worthy of being cared for
#2 Ineffective airway clearance	Abnormal breath sounds Productive cough	
#3 Adequate nutrition	Height = 6′ Weight = 191 lbs.	

DISCUSSION How did you decide what data were missing? What sources helped? Were there some missing data that were more important than other missing data?

▷ **Filling Data Gaps**

Filling in data gaps usually is accomplished by using "directed data collection" (discussed in Chapter 5). To set up directed data collection, the nurse's thinking might follow a pattern like this:

> The preliminary cluster of data is: straining with stool, complaints of stomachache, states needs laxative every day to have bowel movement.
>
> **Hunch #1 is: Constipation**
>
> **Hunch #2 is: Perceived constipation**
> (The above two hunches are **differential diagnoses**)
> The nurse then thinks," I don't have enough data to be comfortable with either hunch just yet; there are too many **data gaps**."
> "I need to direct my data collection to fill the gaps with useful data and not waste time collecting irrelevant data."

"**To rule in or rule out Hunch #1**, I know from experience that the additional data might be: hard, formed stools; feeling pressure in the rectum; and decreased frequency in bowel movements."

"**To rule in or rule out Hunch #2**, the textbook indicates that the following defining characteristics might be present: patient expects to have bowel movements at the same time every day, patient has been using laxative for extended period of time to maintain proper timing and amount of stool."

With this knowledge, the nurse would go to the patient to collect the necessary data.

Becoming skilled at identifying data gaps and using directed data collection to fill those gaps is a very positive sign that the beginning nurse health detective is moving in the direction of great nursing.

▼ THINKING-LEARNING CHECK

Pause here for a thinking-learning check. You should be able to elaborate on these ideas:

- ▼ Clusters of data: two or more pieces of information about patients that fit together and have more meaning together than separately.
- ▼ Cluster analysis: making sense out of the patterns of data.
- ▼ Clusters: increase accuracy of conclusions, allow for necessary shortcuts, help avoid omissions, take advantage of the brain's natural memory system.
- ▼ Clusters are formed by determining what fits together, determining data gaps, and filling gaps.

▶ AIDS TO FORMING CLUSTERS

The challenge of clustering for beginning nursing students lies in figuring out what fits with what. TOTAL RECALL and INQUIRY are the primary thinking modes used. With experience, some clustering of data becomes HABIT—the nurse knows that when one thing is present, another usually accompanies it. For example, if a nurse observes dark circles under a patient's eyes, it becomes automatic to watch for frequent yawning. Until those HABITS develop, INQUIRY must be used to ask "What is usually associated with this?" That ongoing use of INQUIRY is essential to seeing the complete picture of the patient situation. TOTAL RECALL (memory or looking it up) helps answer many INQUIRY questions. What beginners have to work with to develop clusters are knowledge from courses (nursing courses and all those other "-ology" courses), life experience, assessment instruments, and the taxonomy of nursing diagnoses.

▷ Content Knowledge From Courses

One of the reasons novice students find the thinking process in nursing a challenge is their limited knowledge base. Students are asked to put information together and act on it while they are still learning the importance of the information. Nursing and supporting courses continually provide a wealth of information about patterns of human responses. In physiology courses, nurses learn about the body's biologic processes; in psychology courses they learn about emotional responses; in nursing courses they learn about health and illness responses, and so forth. Each of these courses obviously adds to the nurse's knowledge of what usually fits with what, but it takes time to reach a "critical mass" of information. The challenge is to pull all of that knowledge together and quickly retrieve what is needed in each patient situation. INQUIRY thinking keeps nurses asking what other information is needed, and TOTAL RECALL thinking sends them back to the books or to whatever part of their minds the relevant information is stored. For beginners, INQUIRY is more of a challenge because they have less first-hand nursing experience to use as a thinking stimulus. This is where life experience can help.

▷ Life Experience

Remembering that patients are people just as nurses are people may seem like a simplistic notion; however, it merits some thought. As beginners, students may get so caught up in trying to sort through all they have to know that they forget what they do know—all that valuable information not taught in classrooms. Everyone has been sick at some time and can relate to things like lack of sleep and irritability, decreased appetite and anxiety, weight loss diets and frustration, stress and stomachaches, nausea and vomiting, and so forth. To stimulate your thinking about what you have learned from life experience, try this Action Learning:

▶▶▶▶▶▶ Action Learning #40: Tapping Your Life Experience

From the experiences listed below, circle those that you can relate to, either because you experienced them yourself or because you were around someone who did. For each one circled, list what signs and symptoms (objective and subjective data) went along with the item listed.

	Signs	**Symptoms**
Constipation		

	Signs	**Symptoms**
Stress reaction		
Anxiety or fear		
Nutrition problem		
Sleep disturbance		
Parenting issue		
Loss or grief		
Mobility deficit		
Situational crisis		
Other (add your own)		

DISCUSSION Do you see how you have identified clusters of data that go along with situations? Some of you probably had experience with many of these; others perhaps have experienced fewer. These and other such life experiences provide valuable information that will help you think. Obviously, you would not base nursing care just on your personal experience, but these experiences can help your INQUIRY by reminding you of questions to ask and leading you to the appropriate resources to help you build from the life experience to professional nursing interventions. Life experiences, by the way, also are very valuable in helping nurses relate to patients as human beings.

▷ Assessment Tools

Assessment tools, also called assessment instruments, usually are organized to enhance clustering. Such tools generally are developed from some theoretical model that indicates how human responses are seen as patterns with labels, and which patient behaviors are part of which responses. For example, Roy's model (Roy & Andrews, 1991) considers patient responses to be outputs (patient behaviors) in four modes, physiologic, self-concept, role function, and interdependence. Assessment tools based on her theoretical model are arranged according to those four modes. Other models, such as Orem's Self-Care Framework (Orem, 1991), and assessment tools based on her model, categorize patient responses as universal self-care demands. The North American Nursing Diagnosis Association (NANDA) considers response categories with the Unitary Person focus. A nursing assessment tool using the NANDA approach is presented in the following section.

Assessment tools often are used to collect data from patients in a systematic, organized way during first encounters. On repeated encounters with patients, depending on how tools are used in the particular setting, additional data may be added to the tool.

Once data are recorded on a tool, clusters emerge because data from observations, interactions, and measurements of each human response pattern are in one place. Look back to the data base on Mrs. Gomez. It would have been easier to see the clusters if the data had been arranged in more appropriate categories.

▶▶▶▶▶▶ **Action Learning #41: Using the Assessment Tool to Find Preliminary Clusters**

Use the blank assessment tool provided here. Refer to the data base for Mrs. Gomez on the first pages of this chapter. Put all the data into the tool format.
(text continues on p. 163)

Name _____Age _____Sex _____Admit Date _____
Medical Diagnosis _____
Allergies _____
Medications _____
_____
Persons/groups involved in care _____
_____

COMMUNICATING: Sending messages
[Nsg. Dx.: Impaired Verbal Communication]
English (circle)   read,   write,   understand
Other languages _____
Speech impairments _____
Alternate form of communication _____

VALUING: Assigning relative worth
[Nsg. Dx.: Spiritual Distress]
Spiritual orientation _____
Important religious practices _____
Cultural orientation _____
Cultural practices _____

RELATING: Establishing bonds
Role
[Nsg. Dx.: Altered Role Performance, Altered Parenting, High Risk for Altered Parenting*, Sexual Dysfunction, Altered Family
Processes, Caregiver Role Strain, High Risk For Caregiver Role Strain, Parental Role Conflict, Altered Sexuality Patterns]
Marital status or significant relationship _____
Age and health of significant other _____
Number of children _____Ages _____
Role in home _____
Financial support _____
Occupation _____
Job satisfaction/concerns _____
Recent losses _____
Sexual habits _____
Relationships (satisfactory/unsatisfactory)
  Effects of illness on relationship _____
  Sexual Concerns_____
Socialization
[Nsg. Dx.: Impaired Social Interaction*, Social isolation]
Relationships with others _____
  Patient's description _____
  Significant others' descriptions _____
  Staff observations _____

KNOWING: Meaning associated with information
[Nsg. Dx.: Knowledge Deficit (Specify)*, Altered Thought Processes]
Perception of current health issues _____
_____
Perception/knowledge of medications, treatments, procedures _____
_____
Previous illnesses/hospitalizations/surgeries _____
_____

Figure 8-2.   Blank nursing assessment tool.

KNOWING (cont.)
History of the following:

	Patient	Family		Patient	Family
Anemia/Blood disorder	_____	_____	Kidney Disease	_____	_____
Cancer	_____	_____	Stroke	_____	_____
Diabetes	_____	_____	Tuberculosis	_____	_____
Heart Disease	_____	_____	Alcohol/Substance Abuse	_____	_____
Hypertension	_____	_____	Smoking	_____	_____
Peripheral Vascular	_____	_____	Other	_____	_____

Readiness to learn _____
   Requests information about _____
   Education level _____
   Learning impediments _____

Orientation
[Nsg. Dx.: High Risk for Injury]
Level of alertness _____
Orientation: Person_____Place_____Time_____
Appropriate behavior/communication _____
_____

Memory
Memory intact: yes/no Recent _____Remote_____

Feeling: Subjective awareness of information
Physical Comfort
[Nsg. Dx.: Pain*, Chronic Pain]
Pain/discomfort: yes/no If yes:
Date of onset/course _____
Exact location _____
Terms for quality and quantity _____
Aggravating and alleviating factors _____
Inter-system connections _____
Labeled by patient as: _____
Emotional Comfort
[Nsg. Dx.: Dysfunctional Grieving, Anticipatory Grieving, High Risk for Violence: Self directed or directed at others, High Risk for Self-Mutilation, Post-Trauma Response, Rape Trauma Syndrome, (Compound Reaction, Silent Reaction), Anxiety*, Fear*]
Recent stressful life events _____
_____
Verbalization of feelings of: _____
_____
Physical manifestations of emotions _____
Fears or concerns _____
_____

MOVING: Activity
Activity
[Nsg. Dx.: Impaired Physical Mobility*, High Risk for Peripheral Neurovascular Dysfunction*, Activity* Intolerance, Fatigue*, High Risk for Activity Intolerance]
History of physical disability _____
Use of device _____
Limitations in daily activities _____
_____

Figure 8-2.   Continued

MOVING (cont.)

Exercise habits _____

Physical symptoms with activity _____

_____

Rest

["Nsg. Dx.: Sleep Pattern Disturbance]

Hours slept/night _____   Feels rested yes/no   Sleeps alone: yes/no

Position preference _____ Naps during the day _____

Sleep interruptions (number and type) _____

Sleep aids (pillows, meds, food) _____

Difficulty falling/remaining asleep _____

Recreation

["Nsg. Dx.: Diversional Activity Deficit]*

Usual leisure activities _____

Usual social activities _____

Illness-related changes _____

_____

Home Maintenance

["Nsg. Dx.: Impaired Home Maintenance Management*]

Size & arrangement of home (stairs, bathroom) _____

_____

Safety issues _____

Ability to maintain home _____

Health Maintenance

["Nsg. Dx.: Altered Health Maintenance]

Health insurance _____

Schedule of health exams _____

Access to health care _____

Self exams (breast, testicular) _____

Self Care

["Nsg. Dx.: Feeding Self Care Deficit*, Impaired Swallowing*, Ineffective Breastfeeding, Interrupted Breastfeeding, Effective Breastfeeding, Ineffective Infant Feeding Pattern, Bathing/Hygiene Self Care* Deficit, Dressing/Grooming Self Care Deficit*, Toileting Self Care Deficit]

Ability to perform ADLs (Indicate I for independent, D for dependent)

Feeding _____, Infant feeding (as applicable) _____, Bathing/Hygiene _____, Dressing/Grooming _____ Toileting _____

Specific deficits _____

_____

_____

Types of assistance needed _____

Growth and Development

["Nsg. Dx.: Altered Growth and Development*]

Developmental stage _____

Ability to meet developmental responsibilities _____

_____

Relocation

["Nsg. Dx.: Relocation Stress Syndrome]

Recent move: yes/no, description_____

Adjustment to move_____

Figure 8-2.   Continued

PERCEIVING: Reception of information

Self-Concept

[Nsg. Dx.: Body Image Disturbance, Self-Esteem Disturbance, Chronic Low Self-Esteem, Situational Low Self-Esteem, Personal Identity Disturbance]

Presenting appearance _____

Patient's description of self _____

_____

Effects of illness _____

Meaningfulness

[Nsg. Dx.: Hopelessness, Powerlessness]

Verbalization of hope/hopelessness _____

Verbalization of control/loss of control _____

Nonverbal cues about hope/control _____

Sensory/Perception

[Nsg. Dx.: Sensory/Perception Alterations (Specify) (Visual*, auditory, kinesthetic, gustatory, tactile, olfactory), Unilateral Neglect]

History of restrictive environment _____

Vision deficits _____ Glasses _____

Hearing deficits _____ Hearing Aid _____

Other Sensory/Perceptual changes _____

EXCHANGING: Mutual giving and receiving

Circulation

[Nsg. Dx.: Altered (Specify Type) Tissue Perfusion (Renal, cerebral, cardiopulmonary, gastrointestinal, peripheral), Fluid Volume Excess, Fluid Volume Deficit, High Risk for Fluid Volume Deficit, Decreased Cardiac Output]

Cerebral:

Neurological changes/symptoms _____

_____

Verbal response _____

Motor response _____

Cardiac:

Heart rate and rhythm _____ Blood pressure: R_____ L_____ Position _____

Peripheral

Pulses _____ Skin temp. _____

Color _____ Moisture _____ Capillary refill _____ Edema_____

Physical Integrity

[Nsg. Dx.: Altered Protection, Impaired Tissue Integrity, Altered Oral Mucous Membrane, Impaired Skin* Integrity, High Risk for Impaired Skin Integrity]

Tissue Integrity _____ Turgor _____ Rashes _____

Lesions: _____ Peteciae _____ Bruises _____

Other (specify) _____

Past history/treatment of skin breakdown _____

Pressure sores (site/grade) _____

Treatment _____

Oxygenation

[Nsg. Dx.: Impaired Gas Exchange, Ineffective Airway Clearance, Ineffective Breathing Pattern*, Inability to Sustain Spontaneous Ventilation, Dysfunctional Ventilatory Weaning Response (DVWR)]

Complaints of Dyspnea _____ Precipitated by _____

History of pulmonary problems _____

Smoking: Y/N Pk Yrs._____ Respiratory rate _____ Rhythm _____ Depth _____

Labored/unlabored; use of accessory muscles _____

Cough: (Productive/nonproductive) _____

Figure 8-2. Continued

EXCHANGING: Oxygenation (cont.)

Sputum: Color _____Amount _____Consistency_____

Need for suction (frequency) _____Breath sounds _____

Oxygen percent and device _____

Physical Regulation and Protection

[Nsg. Dx.: High Risk for Infection*, High Risk for Altered Body Temperature, Hypothermia, Hyperthermia, Ineffective Thermoregulation, Dysreflexia, High Risk for Injury*, High Risk for Suffocation, High risk for Poisoning, High Risk for Trauma, High Risk for Aspiration*, High Risk for Disuse Syndrome, Alt. Protection]

Temperature _____Route _____

Menstrual Period: Last _____Frequency _____Duration _____

Immune Status _____

White blood count _____Differential _____

Clotting: PT _____ PTT _____ Platelets _____

Intermittent unusual sensations _____

_____

Immunizations up-to-date _____

Alcohol/caffeine/narcotic use _____

Environmental/personal safety conditions _____

_____

Nutrition

[Nsg. Dx.: Altered Nutrition: More than body requirements, *Altered Nutrition: Less than body requirements, Altered Nutrition: Potential for more than body requirements, Impaired Swallowing*, High Risk for Aspiration]*

Eating patterns:

Number of meals/day: Usual _____Current _____

Special diet _____

Food preferences/intolerances _____

24-hour recall of food intake _____

Fluid intake/Type _____Amount _____Preferences _____

Appetite changes _____

Swallowing difficulty _____

History of ulcers _____Indigestion _____

Anorexia/nausea/vomiting _____

Condition of mouth/throat/teeth _____

Height _____ Weight _____ Ideal Weight _____

Current diet therapies _____

Lab values (place * by abnormal values):

Hemoglobin _____Hematocrit _____RBC _____Na_____ K_____ Cl_____

Glucose (fasting/not fasting) _____Cholesterol _____Triglycerides_____

Total protein _____Albumin _____Iron _____Other_____

Elimination

[Nsg. Dx.: Constipation*, Perceived Constipation, Colonic Constipation, Diarrhea, Bowel Incontinence, Altered Urinary Elimination, Stress Incontinence, Reflex Incontinence, Urge Incontinence, Functional Incontinence, Total Incontinence, Urinary Retention]

Gastrointestinal/bowel:

Usual bowel habits _____Changes from normal _____

Last BM _____Remedies used _____

Bowel sounds _____Abdominal examination _____

Stool Color _____Amount _____Consistency _____

Renal/Urinary:

Usual urinary patterns _____Changes from normal _____

Urine: Color _____Odor _____Amount _____per_____

Output for last 24 hours _____Avg. hourly _____Bladder distension: yes/no

Urinalysis _____Urine C&S_____

Figure 8-2.   Continued

CHOOSING: Selection of alternatives
Coping
[Nsg. Dx.: Ineffective Individual Coping, Impaired Adjustment, Defensive Coping, Ineffective Denial, Ineffective Family Coping, Disabling, Ineffective Family Coping: Compromised Family, Coping, Potential for* Growth]
Patient's usual problem-solving methods _____

Family's usual problem-solving methods _____

Patients method of dealing with stress _____

Family's method of dealing with stress _____

Patient's affect _____
Physical manifestations of emotional state _____
Support systems available _____

Participation
[Nsg. Dx.: Ineffective Management of Therapeutic Regimen (Individuals), Noncompliance (Specify), Health Seeking Behaviors (Specify)
Compliance with past/current health regimens _____

Willingness to comply with future health regimen _____
Perceived barriers to compliance _____

Judgment
[Nsg. Dx.: Decisional Conflict* (Specify)]
Decision-making ability
Patient's perspective _____
Others' Perspectives _____

PATIENT'S PRIORITIES FOR CARE

1.

2.

3.

4.

5.

6.

7.

8.

9.

10.

Tool adapted from: Guzzetta, C.E. Bunton, S.D., Prinkey, L.A., Sherer, A.P. & Seifert, P.C. (1989). Clinical assessment tools for use with nursing diagnosis. St. Louis, Mosby. (used with permission)

Figure 8-2.   Continued

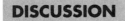

DISCUSSION   Did the data form any natural clusters? What conclusions could you see more easily with the tool format? Is this all the clustering that will be needed?

By using the assessment tool, it should have been easier to recognize how some data fit together. In a sense, some of the preliminary thinking, in the form of sorting, is done for the nurse as data are recorded on the assessment tool. However, not all the thinking is done. As mentioned before, human responses rarely fit into tidy boxes; any categorization of responses is somewhat artificial. Consider a patient who has a mobility deficit. Data about the mobility also are relevant to elimination responses (people who decrease their mobility often get constipated and may have urinary retention), skin responses (decubitus ulcers form when there is prolonged pressure on body parts), and many other responses. Therefore, assessment tools, although they provide a start to clustering, also can provide a false security; a nurse must rely on *thinking* to find the less obvious clusters.

▷ Taxonomy of Nursing Diagnoses

The NANDA taxonomy (Appendix A) can help nurses cluster data that lead to nursing diagnosis conclusions by reminding them of the various diagnostic labels grouped within response patterns. If one piece of information seems to indicate a particular diagnosis such as urinary incontinence, examining the taxonomy will remind the nurse that there are several types of incontinence. Referring to a book that has the defining characteristics of the diagnoses will trigger the nurse's search for data that can be added to the cluster. Directed data collection can be used, or the nurse can refer back to the data base to find the data and form the best cluster. The list of nursing diagnoses, along with the defining characteristics and related factors, can help fine-tune the clusters. Guidelines for ruling in and ruling out hunches (differential diagnosis) can be found in Chapter 5. Ruling hunches in or out is really a process of clustering data more and more specifically until the final cluster "paints" the best picture of the conclusion label.

▶ CHOOSING THE BEST CLUSTERS

Clusters have certain characteristics besides being groups of data. There are pure and mixed clusters. In addition, there are different types of clusters for nursing diagnoses that are actual problems and those that are potential ("high risk for") problems. It is important to recognize these subtle differences to select the best clusters for the major conclusions of assessment.

▷ Pure and Mixed Clusters

The clusters shown in the Mrs. Gomez example are "pure" clusters; they contain only the specific data for each conclusion. Some nurses used "mixed" clusters, especially when they are forming nursing diagnosis conclusions. They use mixed clusters because they feel it is more logical or easier to include all data supporting the problem statement and all data supporting the related factors in the cluster. For example, nurses who prefer mixed clusters would develop the following cluster for the nursing diagnosis of Impaired Skin Integrity related to mobility deficits, urinary incontinence, fragile skin, and compromised circulation:

▼ DATA CLUSTER

Coccyx and elbow reddened, bruise on left shin, skin tear on hand, complaints of discomfort and irritation of buttocks. Wheelchair bound, stiff joints, trouble getting out of bed, limited ROM right hip, hitting wheelchair during transfers, osteoarthritis, right hip ORIF 4 months ago. Dribbles urine, wears "Depends." Skin dry, very thin, translucent. Sitting in wheelchair all day, NIDDM, ankle edema.

There is nothing "wrong" with forming this type of mixed cluster; indeed, the mixed format may seem more logical at times. One must use this approach with care, however. Remember, there are two conclusions being made—one is the conclusion about the health concern, and the other is the conclusion about the related factors. When a cluster is mixed (supporting two conclusions), it is easy accidentally to have adequate data supporting one conclusion but only limited data supporting the other, and not readily recognize this situation.

The other problem is that this approach can lead to confusion in planning because the pieces haven't been clearly examined. A mixed cluster can decrease the probability of finding all the related factors. The related factors are less evident because there are so many data that the patterns get lost. For example, examine this mixed cluster and its accompanying conclusion:

▼ DATA CLUSTER

▼ Patient is 76 years old, has fourth-grade education, lives alone

▼ Recent diagnosis of diabetes mellitus

▼ Anticipated need for insulin injections

Conclusion: Knowledge Deficit regarding self-care with diabetes.

At first glance this seems logical. A person of that age with limited formal schooling, living alone, and recently diagnosed with diabetes would need to be taught how to give injections and so forth. However, the conclusion of "Knowledge Deficit" has no data to support it. It could be that this patient gave injections to his mother for years. So, what that cluster needs is information about the person's actual knowledge or deficit, if there is one. What the patient does or does not know is critical information to support a diagnosis of Knowledge Deficit.

▷ Clusters for Actual and Potential Problems

There also is a difference between clusters of data supporting actual problems and those clusters supporting potential problems (those problems for which a patient is at high risk). Again, consider the Mrs. Gomez case. She had a nursing diagnosis of an actual problem, "Impaired Skin Integrity." One can see why this was an actual problem. The data (defining characteristics for the problem of impaired skin integrity) were there to support the problem. Those data were reddened elbow and coccyx, bruise on shin, skin tear on hand, and complaints of discomfort and irritation of buttocks. These data *actually* existed for the *actual* problem. There also were data that showed the related factors for the skin problem—mobility deficits, urinary incontinence, fragile skin, and compromised circulation.

If the data that supported the problem did not exist (the reddened elbow and coccyx, bruise on shin, tear on hand, discomfort and irritation of buttocks), it seems one could assume there was no problem. The related factors, however, are still there. Mrs. Gomez still has incontinence; she is still immobile; she still has dry, fragile skin; and she still has poor circulation. Probability indicates that it will be only a matter of time before something happens to her skin. Sooner or later, her skin integrity will break down, and there will be an actual problem to deal with.

Should a nurse wait and see what happens? Of course not; nurses want to prevent health problems before they happen. The way to do this is to draw a conclusion about the risks and design care either to maintain the current status or promote a higher level of health that puts the patient at less risk. The conclusion in that case would be:

> High Risk for Impaired Skin Integrity related to incontinence, immobility, fragile skin with poor turgor, and compromised circulation.

This can be confusing, so think about it in this way. The "problem" portion of the diagnostic statement, **High Risk for Impaired Skin Integrity**, is not an actual problem yet. It is a "potential" problem, one that will become an actual problem if the risk factors are not dealt with soon.

Because it is not an actual problem yet, there obviously are no data and no cluster of data to support a conclusion that a problem exists. In other words, there are no defining characteristics such as "disruption of skin surface; destruction of skin layers; invasion of body structures" (NANDA, 1992).

The "related factors" portion of the diagnostic statement—**incontinence**, **immobility**, **fragile skin with poor turgor**, and **compromised circulation**— is the key to this type of diagnosis. These four related factors do exist and do put the patient at "high risk for" development of an actual problem if left unattended.

The related factors for a potential problem (or an actual problem) can be single pieces of data (fragile skin) or they can be labels for clusters of data (compromised circulation).

Diagnosing potential problems effectively generally requires a greater amount of content knowledge and experience. Knowing what relationships to anticipate among pieces of data and data clusters is the result of sophisticated, high-level thinking. More discussion of potential problems is presented in Chapter 14.

▶▶▶▶▶▶ Action Learning #42: Another Look at Clusters for Actual and Potential Problems

This Action Learning is similar to Action Learning #28 in Chapter 6. Consider this as more practice for differentiating data clusters. Using nursing diagnosis books or nursing theory texts, examine each cluster. This time, select a label and write it appropriately. For example, if it is a potential problem, write it as "high risk for . . . ."

Cluster #1:

Three-day-old infant with hyperirritability; mother addicted to cocaine; infant has great difficulty coordinating sucking, swallowing, and breathing.

Diagnostic Label
_____

Actual/Potential (circle one)

Cluster #2:

Thirty-three-year-old alcoholic in alcohol rehabilitation program; verbalizes feelings of guilt and anger toward husband; admits to diminished interest in sexual activity over the past 5 years; rape victim in early 20s.

Diagnostic Label
_____

Actual/Potential (circle one)

Cluster #3:

Fifty-nine-year-old wife of a 58-year-old man with Alzheimer's disease; caring for husband at home for 6 months; currently eating and sleeping well but notes that she is gradually getting less sleep because husband wakes and wanders through house several times a night; oldest daughter, who is major support system, was recently promoted to company president and had to move out of state; wife is hesitant to use local Alzheimer's' support organizations.

Diagnostic Label

Actual/Potential (circle one)

DISCUSSION   How did the nursing diagnosis manuals and nursing theory texts help in selecting appropriate labels? What additional data would be helpful in validating your selections? Could you identify the data that supported the problem and the data that supported the related factors?

▷ Using the Big Picture to Find the Best Clusters

Clustering data and eventually attaching labels that represent the conclusions made about the data are not governed by rigid rules. This is especially true with nursing diagnosis conclusions. There are few "right" or "wrong" ways to go about these tasks. The ideal for which nurses aim is to have as complete a picture of the patient's health issues as possible so that nursing care can be planned and implemented in an efficient, yet thorough, manner.

"Efficient" and "thorough" are key words here. As patient data are analyzed, one can see many, seemingly equally valid, conclusions that could be reached. In Mrs. Gomez's case, other nursing diagnoses could have been made. For example, "Sensory Impairment related to decreased hearing and sight," could have been a nursing diagnosis. There is a clear data cluster "painting a picture" of this actual problem. The reason why this conclusion was not listed as a nursing diagnosis is that the nurse cannot really do much about it. The nurse can, however, do something about the social isolation that is the result of the sensory deficit. Putting the sensory data together with other data led the nurse to a conclusion that, ultimately, will lead to more efficient and thorough care. If the focus were just the sensory problems, the social isolation could go unnoticed. By broadening the view a bit, the nurse can do everything possible for the sensory problem while trying to decrease the social isolation.

As well as showing that there are no right or wrong approaches to clustering and conclusion making, this example demonstrates that thinking ahead to the planning phase of the nursing process helps with finding the best clusters.

The value of looking toward planning as an aid to clustering is also illustrated in the nursing diagnosis, "Impaired Skin Integrity . . . ." The conclusions made from the related factor clusters also could be seen as conclusions about problems. In addition to that one diagnosis, these diagnoses and others could have been made from the same data:

Urinary Incontinence related to (possibly) neuromuscular changes 2°
   to diabetes and decreased circulation

Impaired Physical Mobility related to osteoarthritis and right hip ORIF
Altered Peripheral Tissue Perfusion related to immobility and diabetes

Actually, a long list of nursing conclusions could have been generated by clustering the data in various ways.

The decision to cluster in the way it was done for Mrs. Gomez was based on a projection toward planning care. When care is planned for the skin problem, the nurse will automatically deal with the mobility, urinary, fragile skin, and circulation problems because all of these contribute to the skin impairment. Making four or five conclusions by clustering another way would be redundant and inefficient.

Clearly, this is high-level thinking using the INQUIRY mode. the nurse tries out various clusters and thinks about relationships among them. This is a bit like the chicken and egg problem—which comes first? The nurse not only must look at the data and various clusters, but must think toward planning and implementation. The "final" clusters of data will point toward conclusions that are as all-inclusive as possible without overlapping too much. Remember, one "problem" conclusion can be a "related factor" conclusion for another problem. All human responses are interrelated (more on this in Chapter 9).

▷ Differences Between Novices and Experts in Developing Clusters

The thinking described in the preceding section is very sophisticated. Even expert nurses do not make such judgments easily. Beginning students have less knowledge and past experience to tap, so this thinking is particularly challenging. The guidelines given in Display 8-1 are useful in developing this thinking skill.

Novices should not fear redundancy as much as omissions. Trying to move too quickly through the thinking at this stage increases the likelihood of missing important issues.

Take the time to write things out. Do not assume your thinking can process such large volumes of new information without providing time to develop new patterns to add to old patterns of thinking.

▶ PITFALLS TO CLUSTERING

Clustering is seldom easy, and things can go awry when data are not clustered well. The fact that there are no right or wrong approaches to clustering, only acceptable, better, and best ways, should suggest why clustering can be challenging. Low-level thinking and intolerance for ambiguity (a factor hindering thinking that was discussed in Chapter 1) are the major contributors to the pitfalls of clustering.

The first pitfall, and the most serious one, is insufficient clustering so that premature conclusions are made. Data analysis and cluster analysis demand

DISPLAY 8-1. Guidelines for Choosing the Best Clusters

Write out all clusters and ask the following questions:
▼ How much overlap is there in my clusters?
▼ If there is overlap, can another way of clustering combine things and decrease the overlap?
▼ Of the conclusions reached about the cluster, which ones connect with each other?
▼ How are they connected?
▼ As I think about planning, will any of these problems be eliminated if I provide care for other problems?

serious INQUIRY work. Constant questioning of the relationships among the data and the clusters will help the nurse avoid premature conclusions.

The flip side of insufficient clustering is forming too many clusters without looking at relationships among the clusters. If this occurs, the nurse will make too many conclusions. As care is planned, there may be much redundancy, and trying to set priorities becomes a nightmare. If there are many repetitive parts of plans, other nurses will have insufficient time to read and implement them.

A balance between those two pitfalls is the best course. Form as many clusters as necessary to address all relevant data; but then analyze the clusters themselves, or cluster the clusters, to see what fits with what.

Not seeing the big picture or not projecting thinking toward planning is a third pitfall. Looking ahead to planning is one of the best ways to test out the usefulness of conclusions about clusters. If there is minimal overlap, and all of the patient's strengths, health concerns, and related factors are addressed, this is a good indication that the best clusters have been identified.

THINKING-LEARNING CHECK

Pause here for a thinking-learning check. You should be able to elaborate on these ideas:

▼ Aids to forming clusters: content knowledge, life experience, assessment tools, and the taxonomy of nursing diagnoses or nursing theory texts.

▼ Pure clusters: only the defining characteristics of the problem portion of the diagnostic statement and separate clusters for related factors.

▼ Mixed clusters: defining characteristics plus data to support related factors.

▼ Actual problems: supported by defining characteristics.

▼ Potential problems: supported by related factors; requires higher-level thinking to recognize relationships and patterns that could become actual problems.

▼ Seeing the big picture helps clustering.

▼ Pitfalls to clustering: low-level thinking, insufficient clustering, too many clusters.

▶ SELECTING THE BEST LABELS FOR THE BEST CLUSTERS

Selecting the best labels was originally introduced in Chapter 6 and is briefly expanded on in this chapter. The NANDA taxonomy, which was introduced in Chapter 3 and is in Appendix A, continues to be a primary source of diagnostic labels. The NANDA labels are used internationally to describe the types of patient responses that fall within the domain of independent nursing practice. The current labels on the taxonomy have been "accepted for testing," which means nurses are trying them out. Labels in the taxonomy are constantly being reviewed, researched, and adjusted. The *Proceedings* from each of NANDA's biennial conferences, as well as numerous nursing journal articles, report the ongoing work in refining and adding to the diagnostic labels.

Most (but not all) NANDA labels deal with nursing care in acute medical–surgical settings. For this reason, other professional nursing groups have developed labels more specific to their areas of practice.

For beginners, however, it is most important to be familiar with the NANDA labels. Each label is defined and has both a list of defining characteristics and a list of related factors. Several books, large and small, have been published to serve as references to all the current NANDA labels (see suggested references in Chapter 6). The following guidelines are useful in selecting the best NANDA label:

1. Study the list of NANDA labels to become familiar with all labels by name and the organization of the taxonomy.

2. Examine the cluster of data that needs labeling and develop a hunch as to which label may be appropriate. (This process may be simplified by using the assessment tool. For example, if relevant data are in the area of elimination, the nurse would focus attention on those labels that describe problems with elimination.)

3. Select one or more labels (differential diagnoses) that might work with the cluster.

4. Read the definitions of the labels to see which fits best with the problem or wellness issue the patient is experiencing.

5. Read the defining characteristics to see which ones currently exist (supporting data) and which ones would be appropriate to search for (data gaps). Note any defining characteristics that are identified as "critical indicators." These are particularly important to have in the data cluster.

6. Read the related factors (contributing factors). These usually are very general descriptions, such as "recent stress." Do any of the patient's data fit with the related factors? For example, a patient who was just fired from her job is experiencing recent stress.

7. If the definition, defining characteristics, and related factors have a good to very close match, there is a very good probability that the label is accurate.

8. Keep the label (write it down) for ongoing validation as the nursing process continues.

9. If no label fits well with the patient's situation, consider creating one using the Nursing Diagnoses Submission Guidelines from the NANDA *Proceedings* (Carroll-Johnson, 1991).

▶▶▶▶▶▶ **Action Learning #43: Selecting the Best Label**

Find a nursing diagnostic manual or nursing theory text to use as a reference. Read the following case study and complete the activities listed below.

CASE STUDY

Mr. Richard is 46 years old, has been hospitalized for ulcerative colitis, and recently had a colostomy. It is 3 days after his surgery, and he still refuses to help with the dressing changes or even look at his colostomy. When encouraged to participate in his care, he says, "I don't want anything to do with that 'thing.'"

The nurse considered the following as possible conclusions:

Ineffective Individual Coping

Dysfunctional Grieving

Situational Low Self-Esteem

Body Image Disturbance

Noncompliance with treatment plan for self-care of colostomy

Examine the definitions for each of these, and examine the defining characteristics and related factors. Which conclusion is supported best? What additional data would help to support further the conclusion you selected? Share your thinking with a classmate.

| **DISCUSSION** | Were you able immediately to rule out any of the original conclusions based on the case study alone? How confident are you that you have selected the best label at this point? How would you validate this label with Mr. Richard?

▶ **CLOSING COMMENTS**

If you have kept your Thinking Cap on for this whole chapter, it is probably time to take it off, rub your head, and get some nourishment. The content in this chapter required a lot of attention and thinking. Being able to cluster data and analyze the clusters, however, is vital to developing accurate conclusions. Without accurate conclusions, nursing care goes off on minor or major tangents that become a waste of time and energy for both the nurse and the patient. Take time to absorb this material; it probably will require some rereading or referring back to as care plans are developed. Take that time; your patients will appreciate it and you will be more confident in your nursing practice.

▶▶▶ THINKING LOG #8

Chapters 5 through 8 have focused on the thinking needed for the assessment phase of the nursing process. Review those three chapters together and look for the threads or essences of assessment thinking. In your own words, write down those essences. Thinking about how you think, consider what will help you engage all your THINK modes to make high-quality assessments: collect and analyze data, cluster data, analyze clusters, and develop the best conclusions.

REFERENCES

Carnevali, D. L., & Thomas, M. D. (1993). *Diagnostic reasoning and treatment decision making in nursing.* Philadelphia: JB Lippincott.

Carroll-Johnson, M. R. (Ed.). (1991). *Classification of nursing diagnoses: Proceedings of the ninth conference of the North American Nursing Diagnosis Association.* Philadelphia: JB Lippincott.

Hart, L. A. (1983). *Human brain and human learning.* New York: Longman.

North American Nursing Diagnosis Association. (1992). *NANDA nursing diagnoses: Definitions and classifications, 1992.* St. Louis: Author.

Orem, D. E. (1991). *Nursing concepts of practice* (4th ed.). St. Louis: CV Mosby.

Roy, C., & Andrews, H. A. (1991). *The Roy adaptation model: A definitive statement.* Norwalk, CT: Appleton & Lange.

Designing, Doing, and Determining Quality of Care: a.k.a. Planning, Implementing, and Evaluating

LEARNING OUTCOMES

After reading and doing the activities in this chapter you will be able to:

Describe the connections among planning, implementing, and evaluating.

Examine the conclusions of planning, implementing, and evaluating.

Describe how to plan, implement, and evaluate care.

Discuss the thinking used for planning, implementing, and evaluating.

The last of the details of the nursing process is the focus of this chapter. The nurse health detective must now expand *thinking* and *doing* from assessment to complete the cycle with planning, implementing, and evaluating care. It is now necessary to design care that is individualized to the patient, follow through on doing that care, and then determine the quality of that care.

Differing from many books on the nursing process that describe the phases of planning, implementing, and evaluating in relatively isolated segments, this text combines the phases into the same chapter to emphasize the interconnectedness of these phases of the process. This interconnectedness is demonstrated as the nurse, during planning, thinks ahead to how the plan will be carried out, if the plan can achieve its purpose, and how the outcomes will be evaluated. Likewise, as a plan is implemented, it must continually be adapted to the patient's changing circumstances through ongoing evaluation of its effectiveness. Doing all of this at once can be a monumental juggling act if careful thought is not a key ingredient. Continual assessment, which occurs simultaneously, compounds the task. Showing how to keep all these balls in

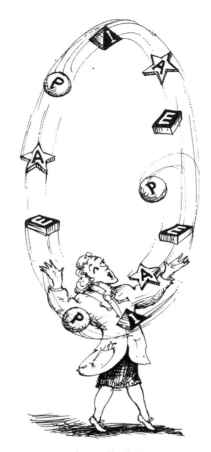

Figure 9-1. Juggling all of the nursing process.

the air at the same time to achieve great nursing is the overarching purpose of this chapter.

▶ COMPLETING THE CYCLE OF THE NURSING PROCESS

Great nursing is impossible without completing the cycle of the nursing process. Being skilled in one or some of the phases and not the whole is useless. It is like having the skill to survey a plot of ground **or** design a floor plan **or** construct walls **or** judge the soundness of a building, but not being able to do all four phases of home construction. The house will never be built.

To complete the cycle of the nursing process requires the use of all T.H.I.N.K. modes. Probably the best advice for planning, implementing, and evaluating care is to keep Thinking Caps on and well secured. For example, TOTAL RECALL of resources gives the nurse sound content knowledge to use for planning, but individualized plans that are unique to each patient cannot be copied out of books because they don't exist. To design individualized plans, the nurse must use INQUIRY and NEW IDEAS AND CREATIVITY. Implementing plans requires TOTAL RECALL of safe practice standards and HABITS for efficiency. Evaluating outcomes demands INQUIRY to determine quality and quantity of results and KNOWING HOW YOU THINK to analyze and make conclusions about planning, implementing, and evaluating.

▷ The Conclusions of Planning, Implementing, and Evaluating

As was discussed in the beginning chapters of this book, it usually is easier to understand how to do something if one knows what is suppose to be achieved at the end point. This section briefly examines the conclusions of planning, implementation, and evaluation before looking at the details of those components of the nursing process.

Chapter 5 described how the nursing process had many points where conclusions (judgments made after thinking) were made. The discussion of assessment focused on the conclusions the nurse made with patients about their strengths and health concerns. There are two more major areas of conclusion making in the nursing process—conclusions about the best nursing approaches to care for health concerns, and conclusions about how well those concerns have been cared for. Stated simply, the three major conclusions in nursing answer these questions: What is the concern (conclusions of assessment)? What should be done about the concern (conclusions of planning and implementation)? And, is the concern resolved (conclusions of evaluation)?

As was the case with assessment, there are many interim conclusions along the ways to these major conclusions. Before deciding on the best course of action, nurses work with patients to make conclusions about the best resources to use, the most creative solutions, the ideal time frame, the highest priority, and many, many other things. Likewise, as nurses implement care, they work with patients to make decisions about what to do first, what to record in the patient's record, which things require additional attention, and so forth. Each judgment and decision is a conclusion along the nursing process path.

Although all the components of the nursing process are intertwined, there is still a need to examine each component by itself to understand it best and how it relates to the other components. Studying the definitions, purposes, and the details of designing (planning), doing (implementing), and determining quality of care (evaluating) promotes this understanding.

▶ DESIGNING CARE (PLANNING)

Defined broadly, planning is time and resource management—a basic skill for any profession. In nursing, planning includes such things as organizing time to complete five patient home visits during the day, making sure *all* the equipment needed to do the catheter change properly is in the room, or having adequate, well organized information to support one's proposed suicide precautions policy change at the departmental meeting. Planning with the patient affects how one collects information, how one uses the information, how one delivers care, and whether or not one makes the time to evaluate the results of care. This broader view of planning as it relates to time and resource management is discussed in more detail in the section on implementation (doing) of care, because the two are so closely related.

The planning phase of the nursing process refers to working with patients to design care for all the conclusions of assessment, nursing diagnoses, interdisciplinary problems, and problems for referral. Although the resulting written plan of care is often equated with the "planning phase of the nursing process," it is essential to recognize that there is more to planning than a written care plan. The thinking behind the designing of care is much more indicative of the true definition of "planning."

▷ Definition of Designed (Planned) Care

Designed (planned) care is the most effective, efficient and safe approach to deal with all the patient's health concerns and promote the patient's strengths. The best plans reflect thinking by the nurse and the patient about setting priorities, establishing clear goals and objectives for the patient to achieve, and developing a specific course of action based on a sound rationale. Plans usually are documented (written) as part of a patient's record.

▷ Purposes of Designed Care

One of the primary purposes of designed care is to have an organized, systematic, safe, well thought-out plan before actually doing anything for or with the patient. This takes more time for beginning nurses than experienced nurses. But as beginners gain experience, their thinking and planning skills move more quickly.

The second major purpose of planning is to design criteria that will serve as guides for evaluation. It is not enough to design and provide care for patients; nurses and patients need and want results. Nurses and patients must have a way to determine if changes actually occur in patients' health conditions. The goals and objectives of the plan establish, in the beginning, parameters (criteria) for evaluation. For example, a goal followed by an objective might be, "By the end of 1 week the patient will have improved sleep patterns as evidenced by using relaxation techniques to fall asleep within 30 minutes." The planned nursing actions would center on helping the patient learn the relaxation techniques. When the week ends, the nurse and the patient determine whether or not the change (using relaxation techniques to fall asleep within 30 minutes) has occurred as planned. If it hasn't, then different approaches can be tried.

A third purpose of planning, that of having written plans of care, is to provide for continuity of patient care and for communication among health care providers. Think about that. In most health care settings, inpatient, outpatient, or home care, patients are cared for by several nurses. Without a written plan to serve as a guide to care, every nurse could be doing something different with each patient during every encounter. Patients would not get very good care, and the amount of wasted time and money would be unthinkable.

The fourth purpose of planning is to meet professional and legal expectations for accountability. The Professional Standards of Practice established by the American Nurses' Association (ANA) require that nurses plan care, not just haphazardly do things. Nurses who plan well are less likely to encounter litigation issues in their practice.

▶ DESIGNING CARE FOR NURSING DIAGNOSES

Care must be designed for all the conclusions of assessment. Later chapters focus more specifically on the care designed for interdisciplinary problems and problems for referral. This chapter addresses some of the general guidelines for designing care, but particularly addresses designing care for nursing diagnosis conclusions.

To design care effectively, nurses must constantly keep in mind the overview of designing care, as illustrated in the following outline:

▼ Set priorities about health concerns as they relate to the whole patient situation.
▼ Establish goals and objectives for each health concern.
▼ Develop nursing orders (actions) for all objectives.
▼ Identify sound rationales for all orders.

Like so many parts of the nursing process, there are no right or wrong ways to approach plans, but there are adequate, better, and best ways to plan. Learning what constitutes "best" gives one a head start. First, all diagnoses should be looked at collectively so that a sense of the whole patient and a general feeling about the interrelationships among the nursing diagnoses can be seen. Then, decisions must be made about what parts of the care should be implemented first. Those decisions must always involve the patient to the best of his or her ability.

▷ Setting Priorities

Setting priorities is the way that nurses and patients make the best use of their time, energy, and health care dollars. Nurses set priorities during many aspects of care, but it is particularly important in planning. Because nurses design plans *with* patients and their significant others, not *for* them, setting priorities can and should be done *with* patients. All conclusions from assessment must be discussed with the patient so that the conclusions can be validated and the patient can say which concerns are most important.

Setting priorities is no simple task because there are so many things that are unique to each patient and the situation. There are, however, general guidelines that help. Obviously, a life-threatening problem such as bleeding is a high priority and needs to be dealt with immediately. Next are safety issues. If the patient is at risk for injury, a plan must be made to decrease that risk. The other issues, however, do not fall into place so automatically. What the nurse thinks is a priority may not be what the patient thinks is a priority. If patients can communicate in any way, they should make the final decisions on priorities. The general guidelines for setting priorities, therefore, are: first, life-threatening issues; second, safety issues; third, the patient-identified priorities; and fourth, the nurse-identified priorities.

At first glance, these four guidelines seem straightforward, but they do not always work neatly. This is where INQUIRY thinking is needed. Within the guidelines nurses must make finer distinctions. They call on their TOTAL RE-CALL of ethical and moral reasoning, accepted models of human needs, and other knowledge of human behavior.

Sometimes the patient does not value something that, to the nurse, is such an important issue that it should be addressed. For example, suppose, in a community health nursing setting, the nurse finds parents who have not had their 2-year-old child immunized. The parents think the child's sleeping habits (waking twice a night) are more important. Should the nurse set the lack of immunizations aside and focus on sleep first? Suppose the reason the parents have not immunized their child is that they have religious beliefs against immunizations? Should the nurse try to change their beliefs?

In this example, most nurses would try to deal with both the sleep and the immunizations. Using principles of ethical and moral reasoning, the nurse would avoid criticizing the parents' beliefs, but make sure they were completely informed as to the pros and cons of immunizations. The nurse also might decide to focus initially on the sleeping issue for a week or two in hope of achieving the following: 1) resolving the sleep problem; 2) demonstrating willingness to focus on the parent's concern first; and 3) developing trust and rapport that will increase the parents' receptiveness to working with the immunization issue.

Further INQUIRY and TOTAL RECALL are needed when the nurse-identified priorities need to be rank-ordered, or when the patient is unable to participate in setting priorities. Suppose a patient is learning about wound care after a mastectomy and the nurse also identifies Body Image Disturbance and Diversional Activity Deficit as problems. Which should be dealt with first? Maslow's hierarchy of needs often is used in nursing as a method of determining priorities. Maslow (1970) promoted the idea that certain needs must be met before others, in this order: first, physiologic; second, safety and security;

third, love and belonging; fourth, self-esteem; and, finally, self-actualization. Using Maslow's scheme, the nurse would plan and implement care to teach the patient how to do safe wound care first, deal with the body image disturbance second, and the diversional activities deficit third. Suppose, however, that the body image problem was interfering with the patient learning the wound care? Wouldn't it make more sense to deal with the body image disturbance first?

To set the best priorities, the nurse must blend a standard system of establishing priorities with an overview of the individual patient's situation. The thing to remember is that knowledge about human needs and priority setting is useful, but setting priorities also must take into account the patient as a whole person, and not just as a list of problems. INQUIRY must be used.

Looking at the individual patient as a whole person means looking at the relationship among the conclusions. Sometimes, if care is planned and implemented for one health concern, other concerns, because of their interrelatedness, are taken care of. For example, if a patient has a Fluid Volume Deficit related to insufficient intake and excessive diuresis, and that same patient has Constipation related to insufficient fluid intake, caring for the first problem could automatically take care of the second (or vice versa). Looking at those types of interrelationships can save planning time, energy, and health care dollars as well as decrease repetition of care plans.

All priorities set during planning are significantly influenced by the length of time the nurse has contact with the patient. In an acute care setting, it is typical to plan care for two or three high-priority nursing diagnoses that will most quickly restore the patient to an acceptable health status for discharge. In long-term care settings, such as nursing homes or in the community, the list of planned priorities usually expands. The expanded time frame allows for planning in more areas.

In case anyone has started to think priority setting is linear, one final reminder is worthwhile. Setting priorities, as described on paper, may seem to imply that nurses work on one thing first, finish it, and then work on the second priority. This is neither true nor realistic. If there are no life-threatening concerns, the nurse may, for example, work on two patient-identified concerns and one nurse-identified concern during one shift or one encounter with the patient. Thinking and expertise allow the nurse effectively and efficiently to address several concerns simultaneously.

Taking into account the complexity of each patient situation, then, a revised summary of the guidelines for setting priorities is:

1. Life-threatening concerns
2. Safety concerns
3. Patient's priorities
4. Nurse's priorities based on:
   a. The overall picture of each health concern in relation to other concerns and the patient as a whole person
   b. Availability of time and resources

▶▶▶▶▶▶ **Action Learning #44: Setting Priorities**

Read the following situation and the initial nursing diagnoses. Using the NANDA taxonomy, see if you can find other diagnoses that would be appropriate. Record the data clusters to support the diagnoses you add. Add your new diagnoses to the list below and describe in writing how you would determine the order of priority for the diagnoses. Share your work with a classmate.

Mrs. Partridge is the mother of a 2-week-old baby girl. She had excessive bleeding because of a vaginal tear during the delivery, so she is anemic. She was told by her obstetrician to eat foods high in iron and take iron supplements, but she says the pills are making her constipated. She said, "I know I should drink more fluids because of the breastfeeding, but it is a real struggle to remember everything I should be doing." The baby is not sleeping well, waking several times each night. Mrs. Partridge is having difficulty breastfeeding, stating, "I don't have much milk yet and the baby seems to cry a lot. I'm so tired all the time, I barely have the energy to feed the baby, much less myself. I feel like my body is telling me not to breastfeed, but I know it's best for the baby. Everyone says I should just keep at it, feed the baby more often, and try to pump my breasts to increase the supply. All I do is lie around all day feeling tired, napping and feeding the baby. I haven't been out of the house or done anything physical for two weeks. I don't know how or when I'll ever return to my jogging and reading novels." Connie Ticket, RN, during a home visit to Mrs. Partridge, made the following nursing diagnoses:

Fatigue related to insufficient sleep, new mothering role demands, breastfeeding energy expenditure, and anemia

Decisional Conflict about breastfeeding related to conflicts between self-care and care of baby

Constipation related to iron intake, insufficient fluid intake and decreased mobility

Diversional Activity Deficit related to fatigue and time demands of new mother role

Added Diagnoses   *Data Cluster*

Order of Priorities of Nursing Diagnoses

1.

2.

3.

4.

5.

6.

DISCUSSION What additional nursing diagnoses did you find? How did yours compare to your classmate's? Was it possible to establish priorities in this situation? Did you find that some diagnoses overlapped others? How did the overlapping affect priority setting?

THINKING-LEARNING CHECK

Pause here for a thinking-learning check. You should be able to elaborate on these ideas:

▼ Completing the cycle of the nursing process requires that planning, implementing, and evaluating be added to the thinking begun during assessment.

▼ Planning includes designing the nursing care plan, day-to-day time management, and organization of resources.

▼ Planning (designing) addresses *all* conclusions of assessment (strengths and health concerns).

▼ Guidelines for setting priorities: looking at the whole patient in relation to life-threatening concerns, safety concerns, patient's priorities, and nurse's priorities.

▷ Establishing Goals

The next important part of planning is working with the patient to establish *goals*. Goals are broad statements of intent or what the patient should achieve to show that the health concern is resolved. Goals are always written as patient behaviors, not nurse behaviors: "the patient will . . . ," not "the nurse will . . . ." To develop goals, the nurse and the patient first determine a direction for care based on the nursing diagnosis itself. If the diagnosis is a problem, the goal would be to reverse the problem, or at least get it under control. For example, if the nursing diagnosis is "Ineffective Individual Coping," the goal would be for the patient to attain or regain effective coping or to increase coping skills. If the diagnosis is a wellness issue, the goal would be to maintain or promote that healthy behavior. For example, if the nursing diagnosis is "Effective Breastfeeding," the goal would be for the patient to maintain that effective breastfeeding. If the nursing diagnosis is a potential problem, the goal would be to reduce the risk of the problem occurring. For example, if the nursing diagnosis is "High Risk for Injury," the goal would be for the patient to decrease the risk for injury or to have no injury.

In the preceding examples, the words "attain," "regain," "increase," "maintain," "promote," "continue," and "decrease" are used. These verbs just about sum up the "directions" for care goals. If something about a patient's health response is altered, then the patient would want the usual response *restored* or would want to *regain* the usual response. Sometimes the patient needs to *attain* some new type of response or *improve* the present response. If a response is healthy, then the patient would want to *maintain*, *continue*, or *promote* that response. Sometimes, when there is an excess of something (usually risks), the patient needs to *decrease* the potential for the problem. When there is a lack of something, the patient would need to *increase* that something. These are useful verbs for the nurse to use habitually, because they cover the gamut of most ideal goals for most health issues or concerns for which nurses plan, implement, and evaluate care.

Most goals need a time frame. Exceptions to this are maintaining, continuing, or promoting responses, which imply something staying the same, so a time frame is unnecessary. But, when goals are to attain, restore, regain, improve, decrease, and increase a response, a time frame should accompany the goal. The time frames for goals may be long or short term, but these terms mean different things in different settings. Long-term goals in an acute care setting may be projected for a week or so, or until discharge, whereas in a long-term care setting, long-term goals could be achieved over months or years. Likewise, short-term goals may be defined in terms of hours to months. One

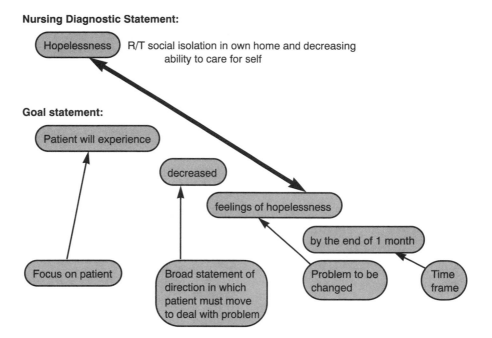

Figure 9-2.   Relationship between nursing diagnostic statement and goal statement.

value of short-term goals is that they divide up a long-term goal into more manageable increments for the patient.

The goal, whether long term or short term, provides general direction for the plan. It is the point toward which care is aimed. Most goals are not directly measurable, but are broad statements of intent; however, a word of caution about terminology is needed with regard to that last statement. Sometimes the terms "goals," "objectives," and "expected outcomes" are used interchangeably. When goals are written on a plan without accompanying objectives, they should be measurable outcomes. As such, they are more specific than broad statements of aim. In this text, the inclusion of both goals and objectives in care plans is advocated to see the direction for change (goal) as well as the specific behaviors that need to occur (expected outcomes) to determine if the goal was met and the problem resolved. Before preceding to Action Learning #45, study the example of the relationship between the nursing diagnostic statement and the goal statement given in Figure 9-2.

▶▶▶▶▶▶ **Action Learning #45: Establishing Goals**

What might the goals be for these nursing diagnoses? You will not be able to set time frames because you do not have the context of these diagnoses, but focus on the wording for each goal. Remember, goals are focused on the problem or wellness part of the diagnosis, not on the related factors. Also, remember that goals are patient goals, not nurse goals. Share your goals with a classmate.

Diversional Activity Deficit related to immobility secondary to fractured leg

GOAL:

Constipation related to low-fiber diet and immobility
GOAL:

Activity Intolerance related to extreme fatigue
GOAL:

High Risk for Aspiration related to neurologic deficits and impulsiveness during eating
GOAL:

Functional Incontinence related to difficulties transferring from chair to toilet
GOAL:

Family Coping: Potential for Growth related to effective communication
GOAL:

| **DISCUSSION** | Congratulations! You have mastered an important part of planning care. Hopefully, you have seen the link between |

the nursing diagnosis and the goal. How closely worded were your goals and those of your classmate?

▷ Establishing Expected Outcomes (Objectives)

Expected outcomes or objectives follow each goal statement. More than any other part of the plan, objectives are the key link to the evaluation phase of the nursing process. Objectives are established during the planning phase so that, later, the patient and nurse can judge if the planned outcomes were reached. Objectives (expected outcomes) are linked to goals by the words "as evidenced by" or the acronym, "A.E.B." These words imply that if the objectives are met, there will be evidence that the goal has been met.

The Structure of Objectives

Because of their use as evaluation criteria, objectives must be thought out and written as specifically as possible. They should be focused on patient behaviors, measurable, clear, and accompanied by a time frame. The focus on patient behavior means the patient, not the nurse, is the one who is expected to exhibit the behavior of the objective. For example, an objective written as, "Describe current understanding of diabetes," means the patient is the one who is expected to do the describing.

"Measurable" does not mean the behavior must literally be measured with a ruler or a scale. It means that precise terminology must be used that is descriptive enough that the behavior can be recognized, heard, or counted in some way.

▶▶▶▶▶ Action Learning #46: Finding Measurable Objectives

Listed below are some objectives, some of which are measurable, and some which are not. Circle those that are measurable and thus easiest to use as criteria for evaluating a patient's responses.

1. The patient will eat at least three quarters of all meals.
2. Mrs. Jones will feel better.
3. The decubitus ulcer will decrease to 1 cm in diameter.
4. The patient will have a better appetite.
5. The patient will be able to do self-care.
6. The decubitus ulcer will improve.
7. The patient will wash her hair unassisted.
8. Mr. Frank will describe his needs.
9. The patient will use an alphabet board to communicate his needs.
10. Mr. Smith will understand diabetic foot care.

DISCUSSION   If you were a nurse using a plan developed by another nurse, which objectives do you think would be easier to aim for? What makes some easier to measure? How could the others be changed to make them measurable?

In addition to objectives focusing on patient behaviors and being measurable and clear, objectives should be accompanied by a time frame. The time frame defines the point at which one could expect the patient to achieve that outcome. That is the time when that part of the plan should be evaluated. Time frames are highly individual. The nurse must know patients well to adapt standard time frames to them and their specific situations. This is where knowing the patient's strengths helps. Looking at the total picture of the patient's problems and available resources allows the nurse to determine a realistic time frame for the outcomes to be reached.

▶▶▶▶▶▶ **Action Learning #47: Adding Time Frames**

Go back to Action Learning #46 and identify two or three pieces of data you would need to make some reasonable conclusions about time frames for the objectives (outcomes) you selected as measurable.

DISCUSSION   What was the most helpful kind of information to determine time frames? How do the patient situation, setting, and resources influence time frames?

The "Content" of Objectives

Relationship of Objectives to Related Factors

Whereas goals address the problem part of the nursing diagnostic statement, objectives are designed to address, eliminate, or alter the related factors. Each related factor is considered an obstacle to the goal of getting rid of or controlling the problem. When objectives addressing all the related factors are met, then, logically, the problem should be resolved. Look at Figure 9.3, for a patient with the nursing diagnosis, "Sleep Pattern Disturbance related to worries about work and excessive intake of caffeine," the goal is to restore usual sleep patterns and the objectives are focused on reversing the worries and the caffeine intake. One objective could be "the patient will devise a plan to deal with the worries about the work situation," and another could be "the patient will decrease caffeine intake to one cup of coffee after 6 PM." In short, if the patient can do something to alter or eliminate the related factors, the goal can be met and the problem resolved.

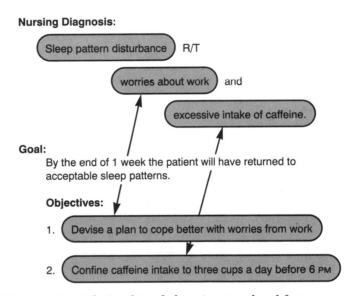

Nursing Diagnosis:

Sleep pattern disturbance   R/T

worries about work   and

excessive intake of caffeine.

Goal:
By the end of 1 week the patient will have returned to acceptable sleep patterns.

Objectives:

1. Devise a plan to cope better with worries from work

2. Confine caffeine intake to three cups a day before 6 PM

Figure 9-3.   Relationship of objectives to related factors.

When Related Factors Do Not Provide Guidance

Most of the time, the related factors provide guidance for establishing objectives, as illustrated above. But sometimes they do not. Consider the following situation and nursing diagnosis.

> Jennifer is 18 years old. She is confined to bed for 4 to 6 weeks in a body cast. She fractured both femurs and her pelvis in a skiing accident.

DISPLAY **9-1. Thinking Flow Sheet: Tracking Thinking From Assessment Through Establishing Objectives**

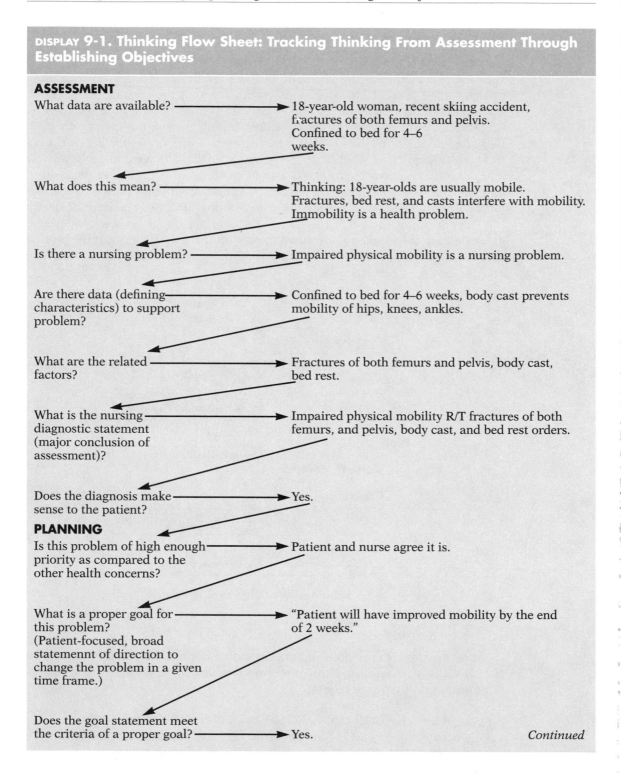

ASSESSMENT

What data are available? ⟶ 18-year-old woman, recent skiing accident, fractures of both femurs and pelvis. Confined to bed for 4–6 weeks.

What does this mean? ⟶ Thinking: 18-year-olds are usually mobile. Fractures, bed rest, and casts interfere with mobility. Immobility is a health problem.

Is there a nursing problem? ⟶ Impaired physical mobility is a nursing problem.

Are there data (defining characteristics) to support problem? ⟶ Confined to bed for 4–6 weeks, body cast prevents mobility of hips, knees, ankles.

What are the related factors? ⟶ Fractures of both femurs and pelvis, body cast, bed rest.

What is the nursing diagnostic statement (major conclusion of assessment)? ⟶ Impaired physical mobility R/T fractures of both femurs, and pelvis, body cast, and bed rest orders.

Does the diagnosis make sense to the patient? ⟶ Yes.

PLANNING

Is this problem of high enough priority as compared to the other health concerns? ⟶ Patient and nurse agree it is.

What is a proper goal for this problem? (Patient-focused, broad statemennt of direction to change the problem in a given time frame.) ⟶ "Patient will have improved mobility by the end of 2 weeks."

Does the goal statement meet the criteria of a proper goal? ⟶ Yes.

Continued

DISPLAY **9-1.** *continued*

Does the goal make sense? ——————→ Thinking: Decreased mobility has lots of problems
related to it (ie, skin breakdown, constipation,
muscle atrophy). So it isn't good to be immobile
and it's important to strive for improved mobility.
Yes, this part makes sense, but does the time frame
make sense? Maybe, maybe not; it may have to be
changed later if necessary.

What are appropriate objectives
(expected outcomes) for this goal?
(Objectives should be patient
focused, measurable, clear, have
a time frame, and **reflect how the
patient can fix or eliminate the
related factors**.)

SCREECHING HALT IN PLANNING!
The patient cannot eliminate or modify the
fractures, the cast, or the bed rest orders.

MORE INQUIRY THINKING

Does this mean that these are the wrong related factors?
Does this mean that the nurse should ignore this problem?
Does this mean that immobility really isn't a nursing problem?
What happens if the patient is left to be immobile?

Maybe it is time to go back to assessment and reexamine the data and the conclusions.

Data are unchanged, and nursing does need to address the issues of immobility.

Alternative conclusions (differential diagnoses) are considered:
1.   High risk for complications of immobility
        secondary to fractures, cast, and bed rest.
2.   High risk for disuse syndrome secondary to fractures,
        cast, and bed rest.

Nursing Diagnosis: Impaired Physical Mobility related to fractured pelvis, fractures in both femurs, body cast, and bed
confinement.

Now examine the thinking that the nurse used in moving from assessment to establishing objectives. Highlights of the nurse's thinking are illustrated in Display 9-1, the Thinking Flow Sheet. If this kind of thinking does not

occur, the care plan that eventually gets written on paper ends up being use-less.

▶▶▶▶▶▶ **Action Learning #48: Thinking Through to Establishing Objectives to Select the Best Nursing Diagnosis**

After reading the Thinking Flow Sheet, answer the following questions and share your answers with a classmate.

1. At what point do you think the nurse began to suspect something might not be on track?

2. Did the nurse's thinking follow a logical sequence? What, if anything, would you have done differently?

3. How does this illustrate the interconnectedness between the assessment, planning, implementation, and evaluation phases of the nursing process?

4. What are the next questions the nurse would ask to rule in or rule out the two differential diagnoses?

DISCUSSION   How easy or difficult was it to answer these questions? What happens to patient care if you don't ask these kinds of questions? A word of encouragement: The answers come more easily and more quickly with experience. Your thinking becomes HABITUAL and you probably suspect problems as soon as you develop the first hunch about the original diagnostic label.

Multiple Related Factors, Not All Providing Guidance

Another situation that affects the "content" of objectives occurs when there are multiple related factors, only some of which lend themselves to objectives. In those cases, unlike the impaired mobility example earlier, the nursing diagnosis (problem label) still may be the best one, but only some of the related factors lend themselves to objectives and interventions. In those cases, the objectives focus on those factors for which the patient can achieve change; other related factors are not addressed. A logical question might then be, should those "unfixable" related factors even be listed in the nursing diagnostic statement? Yes, they should, because they help to clarify the dimensions of the problem and indirectly help with the design of objectives. If a related factor to a patient's self-care deficit is his inability to grip because of a stroke, even though nothing can undo the stroke, objectives will be different than they would be if the inability to grip was because of arthritis. The patient with a stroke might be able to increase his grip with exercises, but the patient with arthritis might have to augment the grip with an assistive device.

Multiple Objectives for One Related Factor

There also could be more than one objective for each related factor, especially in long-term settings. A nurse and a patient dealing with a work-related stress problem might have as an objective for the first week that the patient would list the work problems, one for the second week to consider options for dealing with the work problems, and, for the third week, to devise a plan to change the work situation. The time frames in this example are appropriate when the patient is coming into a clinic weekly. If the patient were in an inpatient setting, the time frames would most likely be much shorter.

In addition to time frames necessitating multiple objectives for each related factor, objectives also can focus on different types of patient behaviors for one related factor. There are three general categories of patient behavior: affective (eg, sharing feelings), cognitive (eg, describing, explaining, listing, stating), and psychomotor (eg, doing an activity, demonstrating, participating). In reality, there is a lot of overlap among these three, but it is helpful to consider patient behaviors in all three categories. The following is an example of what this looks like:

> **Nursing Diagnosis:** High Risk for Injury related to knowledge deficit regarding daily insulin administration.
>
> **Goal:** Patient will decrease risk for injury with insulin injections by the end of the visit as evident by:
>
> 1. Sharing feelings about self-administered injections (affective)

   2. Explaining safe procedure after being taught (cognitive)

   3. Demonstrating safe insulin injection (psychomotor)

Objectives That Address Changes in Patient Conditions

To make life even more complicated, there is one additional area of content for objectives that reflect patient behavior but are not generally within the patient's conscious control. This deals with "pure" physiologic changes in patient conditions that are monitored by such things as vital signs, laboratory values, urine output, and the like. Some nursing diagnoses are very specific to the patient's physiologic status, for example, "Fluid Volume Excess related to fluid retention secondary to congestive heart failure." The goal is to decrease the fluid volume, and the ways to measure that change are with objectives that break down the goal into smaller increments. Objectives for the above nursing diagnosis could be stated as follows:

   1. The patient's body weight will return to its usual range within 3 to 5 days.

   2. The electrolytes will return to a normal range in 3 to 5 days.

   3. Dependent edema will decrease to no more than 1+ by 3 days.

   In the above case, the objectives are clear, measurable, and include a time frame. They differ from the earlier examples of behavioral objectives, however, because they are primarily matters of the patient's physiologic responses rather than behavioral control.

   In summary, objectives are patient-focused, measurable, clear outcomes with expected time frames for completion that usually focus on controlling the related factors of the nursing diagnosis. Collectively, they should help the patient meet the goal to resolve the problem. Objectives are also the basis for evaluating patient outcomes. They are preset in the plan as standards or criteria toward which the patient and nurse work. At the set time, the nurse and patient determine if the objectives have been met.

▶▶▶▶▶ **Action Learning #49: Establishing Objectives**

Review Mrs. Partridge's situation in Action Learning #44. For the nursing diagnosis, "Constipation related to iron intake, insufficient fluid intake, and decreased mobility," develop objectives with time frames for Mrs. Partridge to go along with this goal: By 1 week, Mrs. Partridge will restore her usual pattern of bowel movements, as evidenced by:

   Objectives:

DISCUSSION   Are your objectives patient oriented, clear, measurable, and accompanied by a time frame? Did you address all related factors? How did you address the iron intake?

THINKING-LEARNING CHECK

Pause here for a thinking-learning check. You should be able to elaborate on these ideas:

▼ Goals set the direction for care and objectives establish criteria for evaluating the outcomes of care.

▼ Goal statements are patient focused, flow from the problem part of the diagnostic statement, and include a time frame.

▼ Objectives (expected outcomes) are patient focused, measurable, include a time frame, and should address the issues of the related factors identified in the diagnostic statement.

▼ Clear, organized thinking about the structure and content of goals and objectives is necessary for great nursing care.

▷ Developing Nursing Actions

The nursing actions, also called nursing orders, on a care plan are written descriptions of those things the nurse will do to help the patient achieve the objectives to meet the goals and resolve the problem. The nurse who develops the actions must keep in mind that the actions as well as the overall plan in most health care settings will be used by other nurses. Therefore, nursing actions should be written with enough specificity that all nurses in that setting can understand and implement the plan. Keeping the purposes of continuity of care and clarity of communication in mind will help the nurse develop actions that are clear, specific, concise, and focused on what the nurse will do. Obviously, these actions must be based on sound principles of nursing care that maintain patient safety.

Each objective on the plan must be accompanied by one or more nursing orders. For example:

Objectives	Nursing Orders
1. Explaining how to self-administer insulin safely by the end of 1 week.	**1a.** Ask pt. to share what he already knows about insulin injections.
	1b. Add to current knowledge by teaching pt. about proper technique for holding equipment, maintaining sterility, selecting and rotating sites and injecting and storing insulin.
	1c. Demonstrate for pt. and ask pt. to repeat back what he learned, providing positive reinforcement, and correcting misunderstandings before he does own injection.

For more examples, refer back to the Sample Care Plan in Chapter 4.

The "Content" of Nursing Actions

Thinking Used

Deciding what are the best nursing actions (orders) for each patient requires all modes of T.H.I.N.K. TOTAL RECALL draws on memory of information or where to find information in books, journals, policy and procedure manuals, and so forth. HABITS allows for use of shortcuts and techniques that save time. INQUIRY asks key questions about how standard ideas can be adapted to fit with individual needs. NEW IDEAS AND CREATIVITY encourages developing orders oriented toward each patient's unique needs and strengths. And KNOWING HOW YOU THINK provides insight into how to do all this safely, efficiently, and effectively.

Resources Needed

Experienced nurses who know their area of clinical practice well can design appropriate nursing actions based on their experience and their ever-expanding knowledge base. Beginning nurses and nursing students, however, who have less experience and have a less developed knowledge base, generally rely more on external resources. These external resources include, but are not limited to, textbooks, journal articles, nursing diagnosis manuals, standardized care plans, mentors, preceptors, instructors, and other nurses.

Standardized Plans Used to Trigger Thinking

Using standardized plans does not mean copying the standard care plan from a book onto a sheet of paper and writing the patient's name at the top. Nor does it mean pulling a preprinted standardized form out of a drawer and writing the patient's name on it before inserting it in the chart. It means using only the parts of the standard plan that fit that particular patient's needs, and using the rest as a guide to trigger INQUIRY and NEW IDEAS AND CREATIVITY to develop the rest of the nursing orders. For example, most standard approaches for care of a patient with a nursing diagnosis of "Constipation" recommend that the nurse encourage the patient to increase intake of raw vegetables. This is good, safe care in most cases, but suppose the patient has renal problems and is on a low-potassium diet? The nurse must individualize nursing actions to specify which vegetables or foods would help with the constipation *and* maintain a low potassium intake to avoid making the renal problems worse.

The above example illustrates how standardized plans and standardized nursing orders, which are designed *only* to address the problem portion of the nursing diagnostic label, cannot be used exclusively if individualized care is desired. Standardized plans do not, nor can they be expected to, address the infinite number of related factors that make this problem unique for this patient. Standardized plans should be used only as guides to start the thinking required for designing individualized nursing orders to help the patient achieve the objectives (based on the individualized related factors) to meet the goal and resolve the problem. Standardized plans are a valuable tool if used appropriately, but not if they are used as cookbook solutions for all patients with similar problems.

▶▶▶▶▶▶ **Action Learning #50: Individualizing a Standardized Care Plan**

Find a book with some standardized care plans for nursing diagnoses. Review Mrs. Partridge's case in Action Learning #44 and, for the nursing diagnosis "Diversional Activity Deficit related to fatigue and time demands of new mother role," find a standardized plan and individualize it to Mrs. Partridge. Explain to a classmate how you changed the standardized plan and why.

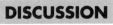 **DISCUSSION** What was the biggest challenge to doing this? Did you find the standard plan helped or hindered your thinking about what Mrs. Partridge needed? Do you see how easy it is just to copy plans from a book to a patient situation without giving it much thought? What are the benefits of individualizing a plan? If you were the patient, what would you want?

▷ Identifying Rationales

An additional part of a care plan consists of the rationales for the nursing actions. All nursing actions must be based on sound nursing principles. Answering the question, What is sound? is not always easy for novices. The only way to learn what is sound is to find written rationales for nursing actions. Initially, most nursing instructors will require that students literally write the rationales on the care plan. Later, however, it is assumed that the rationales are in the nurse's head. Examine the following example for one way to document an identified rationale. Refer to the Sample Care Plan in Chapter 4 for more rationales in the written plan.

> **Nursing Diagnosis:** High Risk for Impaired Home Maintenance Management related to fractured hip, living alone in older home.
>
> **Goal:** Patient will be able to maintain self safely in own home after discharge.
>
> **Objective #1:** Patient will identify potential barriers to care at home by end of week.

Nursing order:	*Rationale:*
Assess home environment for barriers to ambulation.	Physical barriers (especially stairs, bathrooms) may limit patient's ability to ambulate and care for self at home (Smeltzer & Bare, 1992, p. 1815)

As a summary of the many components of care planning for nursing diagnoses, the following guidelines are provided. Meeting the criteria for each care plan part will ensure that sound plans are designed. Study the guidelines below that highlight the criteria for each part of the written plan.

Criteria for Developing Written Plans

Care Plan Part	*Criteria*
Nursing Diagnostic Statement	1. Actual or potential problem or wellness condition that is clearly supported by data and is treatable by nurses.
	2. *All* related factors are connected to the first part of the statement with the phrase "related to" or "R/T."
Goal Statement	1. Patient centered
	2. Designates direction for change: restore, maintain, improve, and the like.

	3. Focuses on the problem part of the diagnostic statement.
	4. Includes a time frame for completion.
Objectives	1. Patient centered
	2. Measurable
	3. Focus on reversing or eliminating the related factors when possible.
	4. Focus on patient behaviors such as affective, cognitive, psychomotor, or patient physiologic conditions.
	5. Include a time frame for completion
Nursing Orders	1. Nurse focused, providing specific directions for nursing care.
	2. Specifically address each objective with one or more orders.
	3. Based on sound rationale.
Rationales	1. Sound, tested
	2. Referenced

Designing care for nursing diagnoses is no small undertaking if it is to be done well. Although there are minor variations in schools of nursing and health care agencies, the major issues as addressed above can be found in most well designed care plans. Before moving on to examining planning in other areas of care, complete Action Learning #51 to test your understanding of this important part of nursing care.

▶▶▶▶▶ **Action Learning #51: What's Missing in This Written Plan?**

Study the following abbreviated care plan and circle the things that do not follow the guidelines discussed above. Explain to a classmate why it is a problem. If you really want a challenge, try to fix the plan's problems and identify rationales for the appropriate nursing orders.

Nursing Diagnosis: Fatigue R/T anemia, depression, and sleep pattern disturbance.

Goal: The patient will feel better.

Objectives	*Nursing Orders*
Pt. will experience less anemia in 1 wk.	Pt. will follow doctor's orders and take iron pills.
Pt. will be less depressed	Develop trust with patient to encourage him to talk about his depression.
	Encourage pt. to identify things that help him feel good and feel depressed.
	Help pt. structure day to avoid long periods of isolation.

DISCUSSION   How many less-than-ideal things did you find? How easy was it to fix those areas? Would it have been easier to start from scratch? What is the best way to remember all these criteria for developing planning for nursing diagnoses?

▶ DESIGNING CARE FOR INTERDISCIPLINARY PROBLEMS AND PROBLEMS FOR REFERRAL

So far the discussion of plans has centered on plans the nurse develops for nursing diagnosis-type conclusions. It also is necessary to plan for other conclusions. With interdisciplinary problems, it may be the nurse, it may be the collaborator, or it may be both people together who design the plan. How this collaboration is done often depends on the setting and the usual types of problems addressed. Generally speaking, however, most disciplines take the same approach to planning that nurses take in designing plans for nursing diagnoses. There is usually a goal or objectives and some actions to be taken by health care providers. In some settings, such as mental health, these are called Interdisciplinary Treatment Plans or Master Treatment Plans.

Planning for problems for referral obviously is simpler. The nurse usually refers the patient to another health care provider for the identified problem. The other provider either plans the care or comes back to the nurse to design an interdisciplinary plan. Documentation that the nurse made the referral and for what reason is important. Where this information is documented depends on the agency or institution; generally, it is recorded in a progress note. The key is to remember to do it somewhere.

It is also important that, as priorities are established, nurses look at all conclusions collectively. It may be that an interdisciplinary problem or a problem for referral has a higher priority than a nursing diagnosis. Thinking and keeping the "big picture" in focus is of utmost importance in planning care.

▶ DOING (IMPLEMENTING) CARE

Now is a good time to return to Chapter 2 for a review of the *doing* part of nursing. Reconsider *all* the types of *doing* and the factors that affect those actions. Also, review the section on independent and interdependent nursing actions. With an expanded understanding of the nursing process gained through the several intervening chapters, do you see things in Chapter 2 that you did not see previously? How has your appreciation of the complexity of nursing changed?

The focus of this chapter is to examine only two key aspects of *doing*: first, doing as it relates to the implementation phase of the nursing process, and, second, doing as it is inseparably interwoven with the time management part of planning all areas of nursing, from patient care to delegation of care, to supervision and leadership.

▷ Doing (Implementing) as a Phase of the Nursing Process

Definition and Purpose of Doing

Doing (implementing) as it relates to the nursing process means carrying out the nursing actions in nursing care plans, and the nursing parts of the physician's plan and the interdisciplinary plans, while also assessing for new problems, evaluating previous care, and keeping an open mind for subtle or major changes that need to be made in the current plan. Doing is also documenting all parts of care so others on the health care team know what is happening.

The basic purpose of implementing is to provide the interventions that patients need to attain, maintain, and regain health or, in cases where the patient is terminally ill, maintain comfort and dignity in dying.

Guiding Principles for Implementation

The three guiding principles for implementing care are 1) maintain patient safety, 2) provide effective care, and 3) provide care as efficiently as possible. Safe, effective, and efficient care are professional standards.

Safety

No matter what actions are implemented, they must focus first and foremost on patient safety. Actions that jeopardize patient safety are not only ethically in violation of professional nursing standards, but are also subject to litigation, depending on patient outcomes.

Although maintaining patient safety sounds fairly straightforward, it is not always that simple. The simple version requires a good understanding of patient behaviors (confused patients tend to wander off), implementation of nonharmful interventions (soft restraints must not cause skin damage or decrease circulation), awareness of environmental hazards (hot liquids cause burns), and thinking about all those factors as they work together. A more complex version arises, however, in the attempt to decide individual safety priorities and quality-of-life issues. This is where T.H.I.N.K. comes into play.

In some situations, a balance is needed to maintain as safe an environment as possible without violating a patient's other needs such as growth and development, rights to freedom of movement, or quality of life. For example, Steven, age 11 months, is starting to walk and climb on everything in sight. He is being kept in a playpen all his waking hours to avoid falls and injuries. Or Adam, age 92 years, is confined to a chair several hours a day with a vest restraint because staff are worried about his falling because of his poor balance and his forgetting to use his walker.

Both of these interventions (confined to playpen and confined to chair) will maintain patient safety, but to the exclusion of other, equally important patient needs—growth and development and quality of life. This is where thinking becomes the critical ingredient in planning and implementing care. Thinking is required to achieve safe care within the context of the total needs of the patient. Discussing the overall care needs with patients and family members can provide guidance for implementing safe care.

Effectiveness

Effective care means the kind of care that does what it is supposed to do. For example, the nurse who is trying to help the patient sleep better must take actions focused on improving sleep, not on teaching how to inject insulin.

The better the content knowledge, the more likely the nursing actions are to be effective. One of the best ways to develop effective care is keep up to date with the nursing literature. For example, if the nurse is caring for a patient with a decubitus ulcer, he would not use a textbook that was 10 years old to find ideas for nursing actions. The thinking nurse would either find a more current text, consult with more experienced nurses, do a computer search of the literature, or better yet, do all of the above.

When nursing actions are effective they save time, money, and energy for the nurse, the patient, and the health care delivery system. Effective care is cost effective as well.

Efficiency

The third principle, providing efficient care, calls for making the best use of the nurse's time, which results in the best use of the patient's time. Efficiency sounds like common sense. The faster care is provided, the sooner the patient's problems are resolved and the more time the nurse has for other problems and other patients. Again, thinking is required to find the proper balance to attain efficiency as well as provide great nursing care. Efficient, poor nursing care or efficient, adequate nursing care usually are not acceptable goals for most nurses. The key to efficient, great nursing care is time management.

Time management is a complex efficiency issue. Dealing with that complexity is one of the great challenges of implementing care, and it requires planning—not just the type of planning done for the written care plan, but a day-to-day planning imbedded in the implementation process.

Each day nurses start work, they make some sort of time-line or plan for the day. If one asked 10 nurses how they did this, it is likely that 10 different responses would be given. Such differences are due largely to those nurses' differences in organizing styles, thinking styles, and working styles, as well as in what they believe is important and in their work environments. Some nurses do schedules in their heads; others write them down. Beginning nurses generally need to write them down because they are less familiar with the routines.

The following is a typical schedule jotted down by a nurse who works part time on weekend evening shifts at an inpatient rehabilitation unit. Note that the nurse's usual work schedule, the shift, and the type of setting are mentioned. That is because those three factors are strong influences on the type of schedule a nurse needs or uses. The schedule presented here has everything written out fully; most nurses would use some shorthand version of such a schedule. Also keep in mind that this is a schedule of things that the nurse knows ahead of time; all the incidental patient needs and nursing issues fill in the unplanned time. Those things are myriad; some examples are answering telephones and call lights, giving unscheduled medications, suctioning patients who cannot cough up secretions, assessing patients with new complaints, planning care for new problems, comforting patients and significant others, and on and on.

▼ A TYPICAL EVENING SHIFT NURSE'S SCHEDULE

1500–1600: Shift report; check med sheets; check current lab work; do rounds on patient; check med drawer; check physician order sheets; read care plans; develop schedule for specific interventions such as tube feeding, IVs, splint schedules, patient exercises, check supplies in each patient's room.

1600–1700: 5 PM meds; do q2h interventions such as turning and repositioning patients, changing splints, casts, ICDs; help patients out of bed for dinner; check incontinent patients; vital signs on some patients.

1700–1800: Cover for first staff dinner; Help or supervise patients eating dinner.

1800–1900: Dinner; do q2h interventions; implement nursing care plan actions.

1900–2000: Continue implementing nursing care plan actions [these might be reviewing patient's communication book, helping a patient exercise, walk, teaching self-care practices, teaching or doing intermittent catheterizations]. Give evening bowel program meds, such as suppositories, that take time to work.

2000–2100: 9 PM meds; do q2h interventions; charting; revise plans.

2100–2200: Do q shift interventions such as tracheostomy care, PEG tube care, dressing changes, etc.; help patients get ready for bed; assess patients returning from day passes.

2200–2300: Give HS medication; check IVs, tube feedings, etc. to make sure enough up for next shift; total and record end of shift intake and output; check on patients in bed; do q2h interventions; charting; tape report.

2300–2330: Clean up rooms; charting; count narcotics; double-check work.

Looking at this schedule, one can see that many of the specifically pre-scheduled things are interdependent nursing actions (eg, giving medications, changing splints, tube feedings). The independent nursing actions are often more spontaneous and difficult to schedule ahead of time (eg, comforting patients, teaching families, assessing new complaints). That is because those things depend more on the individuality of each patient and are therefore more typical of great nursing actions. The interdependent actions that are known ahead of time are usually more task oriented.

The question beginning students may ask is, "How do I develop my skills for implementing safe, effective and efficient care?" Experience is a big help, but there are also many books and workshops dealing with these issues. Reading, listening, watching, asking questions, and keeping those thinking caps on are equally useful. To learn about some real-life examples, complete Action Learning #52.

▶▶▶▶▶▶ **Action Learning #52: Finding Safe, Effective and Efficient Ways to Implement Nursing Care**

Ask a practicing nurse the following questions and write a short summary of your findings to share with a classmate.

1. What things do you routinely do to provide for safe patient care?

2. What things do you routinely do to provide effective patient care?

3. What things do you routinely do to provide for efficient patient care?

4. What do you think are the three most important things to remember when implementing care?

5. What tips do you have for me on good time management?

DISCUSSION   How did the responses of "your nurse" compare to the responses of your "classmate's nurse?" What words of wisdom will you take with you as you develop your practice of implementing safe, effective and efficient nursing care?

▶ DETERMINING QUALITY OF CARE (EVALUATING)

Evaluation is the "checking" part of any activity that provides feedback as to how well the activity worked and if the desired results were achieved. In daily life, evaluation occurs rather informally. If you are doing a load of wash with extra stains, you might try a new stain-removing product that just came in the mail. After the wash cycle, you check the stains to see if they are gone. That's evaluation.

In nursing, evaluation is done in more formal ways. The classic method includes evaluation of outcome, process, and structure. Most nurses are not regularly involved in structure evaluation because it includes evaluation of the physical building (eg, room sizes, classroom space), the physical environment (eg, ventilation, room temperature), and resources that support direct care (eg, equipment, supplies, computer terminals). When these structural elements directly affect care, however, they become necessary areas for all nurses to evaluate.

Process evaluation focuses on what and how things are done. In nursing, that generally means nursing actions. Policy and procedure manuals describe ideal nursing actions and may be used as a standard for process evaluation. Employment evaluations for pay raises and promotions also fit in this category. Some process evaluation occurs with the nursing process, but it is secondary to outcome evaluation.

▷ Definition and Purpose of Outcome Evaluation

Outcome evaluation is just as it sounds, a determination of whether or not a desired result has occurred.

Evaluating is often seen as an end point, but in actuality it is a way of constantly updating nursing care. Outcome evaluation, commonly called simply "evaluation" within the nursing process, is the way of measuring whether or not the patient is meeting the goals and objectives of the care plan.

To see the purposes of evaluation clearly, think what nursing is all about. Nurses try to help improve patient responses to their health conditions. There must be a way to determine if that is happening. Evaluation is the nurse's ever-present, internal quality control device. Because of professional accountability, evidence of evaluation must be written in the patient's record. Written documentation is discussed in more detail in Chapter 10.

▷ Guidelines for Outcome Evaluation

Outcome evaluation consists of a series of steps and questions. It starts with the establishment, in the planning stage, of the expected outcomes (objectives) as evaluation criteria. Another word for expected outcomes and evaluation criteria is "indicators." Indicators or expected outcomes become the measurement tools to determine whether or not patients have achieved their goals. This is particularly important for quality assurance, which is discussed in Chapter 11.

Evaluation continues as nurses assess patients to determine if the objectives are met within the designated time frames. Evaluation is a process of moving back and forth among the parts of the whole nursing process. If needed, modifications are made and evaluations continue until the patient problem is resolved or discontinued. Figure 9-4 illustrates the outcome evaluation process (a process within the nursing process).

The outcomes planned for each health concern are continually evaluated. The first question to ask is, did the patient meet the expected outcomes? If objectives were met, the patient has achieved what was expected. The nurse can assume that data collection for that issue was complete, the analysis was accurate, the goals and objectives were realistic, and the nursing actions were sound and well implemented. If those patient outcomes have not been met, then the nurse must go back through the steps of the process until the point of breakdown is found. That backtracking process requires lots of INQUIRY

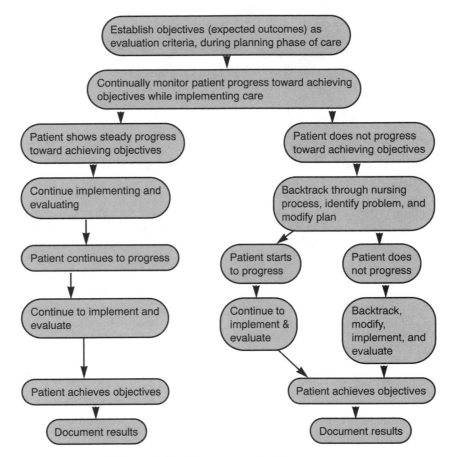

Figure 9-4. Outcome evaluation process.

thinking in which all phases of the nursing process are examined. That is where outcome evaluation becomes a process evaluation.

Study the tracking patterns shown in Display 9-2. The first one is the ideal situation in which everything works as planned. The second one provides the questions to ask along the way to find the point of breakdown. That point is where the nurse would then start to revise the process. This revision process is called modifying.

▷ **Modifying Plans**

Modifying plans is a significant part of evaluating. If outcomes are not achieved by the designated time frames, it is often an indication that some part of the nursing process was not completed—something broke down in thinking and doing. The hunt begins to locate the process "breakdown." The hunt in-

DISPLAY 9-2. Evaluation Tracking Patterns

TRACK # 1: PATIENT RESPONSES FIT WITH EXPECTED OUTCOMES

Evaluation Question Sequence	Answers
1. Patient objectives met?	Yes
2. Patient goal(s) met?	Yes
3. Problem or issue resolved?	Yes

TRACK # 2: PATIENT RESPONSES DO NOT FIT WITH EXPECTED OUTCOMES

Evaluation Question Sequence	Additional Questions
1. Objectives not met? or partially met?	Were they realistic? Was time frame OK? Complete (all related factors addressed)?
2. Goal(s) not met? or partially met?	Were they realistic? Time frame OK? Linked to problem (conclusion or Dx)?
3. Problem or issue not resolved?	Did it change? Was it validated or not validated by the patient? Priority or not?
4. Implemented actions done fully? or partially?	Reasons why not done as planned?
5. Planned actions	Sound? Realistic? Fit with objectives and goals? Complete?
6. Analysis of data and clusters	Accurate (conclusions fit with data)? Complete (all possible conclusions considered)? Clusters of data logical?
7. Data	Complete? Accurate?

volves methodically backtracking through the process to find the problem or problems. Once it is discovered, the breakdown can be corrected. Sometimes the "fix" is simple, such as when a time frame needs to be adjusted. Sometimes the fix is more complicated, such as when the nurse discovers that he or she did not validate a problem with the patient but proceeded to plan care anyway.

Consider the following situation. A nurse concludes that the patient is overweight and needs a reducing diet. The nurse develops a goal and an expected outcome that the patient will lose 2 pounds by the end of 1 month. The nurse teaches a new diet and helps the patient develop meal plans for 2 weeks. The nurse evaluates to see if the patient is halfway toward achieving the objective by the end of the 2 weeks of meal plans (it is a good idea to do interim checks). The patient is not progressing toward achieving this objective; in fact, he has gained 3 pounds. What happened? The expected outcomes (goals and objectives) were not achieved, even though they were realistic, had appropriate time frames, and addressed all of the related factors identified as contributing to the problem (numbers 1 and 2 of the evaluation checking sequence). What about number 3 on the evaluation checking sequence? Bingo, there's the breakdown—validation of the problem with the patient. The patient did not see his weight as a problem. What the nurse needs to do in this case is explore why the patient does not think it is a problem. By revisiting assessment and collecting more data, the nurse may discover the patient has a culturally related desire to be overweight and sees no reason to change; he was just being "polite" when he agreed to the plan initially.

Evaluation may be humbling at times, especially when nurses find that they were off target in their conclusions. The purpose of evaluation, however, is not to place blame, but rather to ensure that the patient is getting the best care possible and is moving toward healthy responses. No one is perfect, neither nurses nor patients. Both can learn much from each other in the process of achieving great nursing.

▶▶▶▶▶▶ **Action Learning #53: Tracking One's Method of Evaluating**

If you are working in a practice area now, evaluate your last episode of care using the evaluation tracking patterns in Display 9.2. If you are not in a practice area now, describe how you used evaluation in some recent life event.

DISCUSSION How does your current system for evaluating fit with the Evaluation Tracking Patterns method? How can you modify either or both versions to achieve effective evaluation of your care and your patient's outcomes?

▼ THINKING-LEARNING CHECK

Pause here for a thinking-learning check. You should be able to elaborate on these ideas:

- ▼ Nursing actions (orders) assist the patient in achieving the objectives to meet the goal and resolve the problem.
- ▼ Standardized plans trigger thinking for developing individualized nursing actions.
- ▼ All nursing actions must be supported by a rationale.

▼ Interdisciplinary problems and problems for referral also require planning by the nurse.

▼ *Doing* (Implementing): actions taken with the principles of safety, effectiveness, and efficiency in mind.

▼ Effective time management produces efficient nursing care.

▼ Determining quality of care (Evaluating) works best when its value is appreciated and it is completed with systematic INQUIRY.

▶ THINKING WITH PLANNING, IMPLEMENTING, AND EVALUATING

Throughout this chapter, there have been many references to the importance of thinking. Actually, it is just about impossible to plan, implement, and evaluate care without high-level thinking. It is, however, possible to "go along" and do a minimum level of nursing without great thought—carry out medical orders, do the routine nursing tasks without accepting the responsibility to help patients get better, prevent their problems, or reach their highest potential. Such behavior is potentially dangerous to patients and certainly not professional. Accepting the professional responsibility for consistently thinking must become firmly implanted in the nurse's brain as a good HABIT; otherwise, nursing becomes a cookbook routine. (Authors' note: In case the readers think the authors don't like cookbooks, they are only partially correct. It is cookbook nursing that is the focus of all the negative comments in this text. Cookbooks for food preparation are really great. Yet, even good recipes need a bit of "tweaking" occasionally to best suit the user's individual palate.)

One way to develop that good habit of high-level thinking is again to put oneself in the patient's situation. If you were the patient, what would you want? Would you want a nurse who pulls a standardized plan out of a file drawer, puts it on your chart, routinely implements only predetermined care, and occasionally checks to see if you are progressing? Put that way, just about everyone would say, "Of course not." Most people want a nurse who uses high-level thinking, and that means using all thinking modes.

Throughout the earlier discussions, TOTAL RECALL was shown to be necessary—to use knowledge and resources for planning, to know how to implement a variety of nursing interventions, and to recognize reasonable expectations for evaluation. Several thinking HABITS were important—putting patient safety first, including the patient in all planning, respecting the individuality of each patient, and habitually using INQUIRY. INQUIRY was the key to continual questioning of what was best in each situation—how each health issue affected others, how priorities were set, how realistic goals and objectives were established, how the best ways to promote patient strengths were developed, how constant evaluation of the patient's progress was achieved, and what the best ways to manage time were. In short, INQUIRY forces the nurse to ask, "Is there a better way to accomplish the task at hand?" NEW IDEAS

AND CREATIVITY was described as the driving force of individualized care; creative nurses expand the standardized approaches and make each patient feel unique. The final mode, KNOWING HOW YOU THINK, merits a bit more consideration as this chapter draws to a close because it brings thinking back to its core for each individual nurse.

Accomplishing the simultaneous tasks of designing and doing care and determining its quality can be seen as an insurmountable obstacle or an exciting challenge. Choosing the obstacle or challenge options depends on the quality of the nurse's thinking in all five modes, but especially in the KNOWING HOW YOU THINK mode. Three areas in particular are critical in successfully accepting the challenge. The first area involves the environment for thinking, the second area covers skill in convergent thinking, and the third returns to the concepts of dualistic and relativistic thinking that were addressed in Chapter 1.

The working environment of nurses frequently includes noise, confusion, constant interruptions, time pressures, and downright chaos. Yet thinking and decision making still must occur. Identifying what environmental factors help and hinder thinking is an important step in KNOWING HOW YOU THINK and applying the nursing process. If the environment itself cannot be altered to enhance thinking, certain parts of the environment, or the nurse's ability to cope with the environment, must change.

Convergent thinking is the ability to bring pieces of information together to create a whole. It is like putting the puzzle together from all the separate pieces. In nursing, effective convergent thinking allows the nurse to bring all the phases of the nursing process together to make sense out of the patient's health response puzzle. It is the dynamic blending of assessing, planning, implementing, and evaluating all rolled into one. KNOWING HOW YOU THINK with regard to convergent thinking will give you some clues about how to see the big picture, and will show if this aspect of thinking needs enhancing.

Relativistic thinking is the ability to accept the fact that most things in this world are not simply "right" or "wrong," nor do they fit in neat little boxes. In nursing, relativistic thinking is accepting the fact that patients, their health responses, and the solutions to those responses do not usually fit into those well-defined boxes. KNOWING HOW YOU THINK relativistically provides understanding and guidance for growth in this area of thinking.

To get a better idea about your "KNOWING HOW YOU THINK" regarding the environment, convergent thinking and relativistic thinking, answer the following questions about your thinking in general:

Are you a person who needs absolute quiet to think through a problem?
Does your thinking become energized in the midst of chaos, excitement, noise, and confusion?
Do you like to talk things through with others before making decisions?
Do you prefer thinking things through privately before involving others?

Can you think on your feet quickly or do you like to mull things over?
Does chocolate help you think?
How threatening is it to share ideas with others before you are "sure" of your ideas?
How do you feel if you can't find the "right" answer?
Does lack of time pressure you into decisions you might not make otherwise?

This very brief self-evaluation of your thinking is designed only to trigger your further exploration. It is very important for beginning nurses to return continually to this thinking mode. Regular attention to KNOWING HOW YOU THINK allows beginning nurses to recognize the "hindrances" and to identify the "helps" of putting together the planning, implementing, and evaluating phases of the "big picture."

Here are some suggestions for dealing with one of the major hindrances (chaos and confusion) to effective thinking about planning, implementation, and evaluating as a whole.

Find a quiet room to work.
Jot down ideas before working with patients.
Identify a trusted colleague with whom to talk things over.
Develop and write care plans at less chaotic times, such as at the beginning of a shift.
Eat chocolate (or popcorn, for those who are more diet conscious) if it helps.
Practice saying, "I need time to think about this," and then say it.
Think out loud and tell patients and other staff what you are doing (you'll be a great role model for other nurses).
Keep paper and pencil handy for jotting down ideas and organizing thoughts.
Monitor your behavior, your thinking, and your communication style when you feel pressured.
Try to select a work environment that is suited to your thinking style (ie, busy, fast-paced, quick-changing; or slower, in-depth, long-range approach to care).

Unfortunately, nursing has been portrayed as an action-oriented rather than as a thinking- *and* action-oriented profession. This misconception makes it very difficult for beginning nurses who do not always "think on their feet" as quickly as they would like. This situation also promotes less useful thinking HABITS that hinder great nursing. If beginning nurses learn to value higher-level thinking, especially KNOWING HOW YOU THINK, *and* build in "think time" to their practice, the results are inevitable: great nursing through simultaneously designing and doing care, and determining its quality.

▶ **CLOSING COMMENTS**

First of all, congratulations. This was a long chapter and it took high-level thinking and concentration to persevere. Designing care, doing it, and determining its quality are all important components that must be appreciated for their own unique contributions to the nursing process. However, it is only when designing, doing, and determining quality are applied as a dynamic whole, in collaboration with assessing, that great nursing is possible.

TOTAL RECALL and HABITS will instill the knowledge gained from this chapter into memory, but then all five thinking modes must be used to apply it in practice. The remaining chapters provide more guidance and practice activities to continue to nurture your thinking skills as you incorporate planning, implementing, and evaluating skills into your repertoire of great nursing.

▶▶▶ *THINKING LOG #9*

The first nine chapters of this text have been full of many ideas about nursing and thinking. It is very likely that your thinking has been modified to accommodate all this learning. To illustrate the changes that have occurred, redraw your Thinking Cap. Describe to a classmate the changes that have occurred since the first drawing, and write out a brief description of how your thinking has changed.

REFERENCES

Maslow, A. (1970). *Motivation in personality.* New York: Harper & Row.
Smeltzer, S. C., & Bare, B. G. (1992). *Brunner and Suddarth's textbook of medical–surgical nursing* (7th ed.). Philadelphia: JB Lippincott.

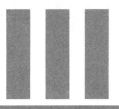

Communicating Thinking
and the Nursing Process

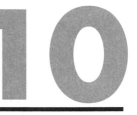

Written and Verbal Communication of Thinking and Doing

LEARNING OUTCOMES

After reading and doing the activities in this chapter you will be able to:

Appreciate the importance of clear verbal and written communication.

Document the results of thinking and care during assessing, planning, implementing, and evaluating.

Describe several methods of documentation.

Explore the finer points of clear communication.

Thinking and doing great nursing are not enough—the thinking and doing must be communicated to others. Because the doing can be seen, but the thinking cannot, it is especially important that the thinking be communicated. Nurses often are, and need to be, more skilled communicators than other people. The information communicated by nurses can be significant to the well-being, even the life of patients. To add to the challenge of communication, nurses often have to organize their thoughts and communicate them clearly in the midst of busy schedules, overwhelming demands, and, sometimes, even chaos.

In this chapter you will examine your present written and verbal communication style and judge how well it works in nursing situations. Methods to enhance communication are explored. Selected methods of written communication in nursing and how they are used in various phases of the nursing process are examined. Finally, this chapter will whet your appetite for some of the finer points of written communication.

▶ DESCRIPTION OF CLEAR COMMUNICATION

Clarity of communication is not automatic. It requires thinking. In all communication, there is a sender and a receiver of information, each of whom exchange roles throughout an interaction. The receiver must listen, see, read, or sense the message. Hopefully, the receiver gets the message from the sender in the way the sender meant it to be. There is a better chance of that occurring if the sender is clear.

This chapter focuses on the sender role and the importance of clarity. "Clarity" means that the message is descriptive of what is in the sender's mind. It is organized, specific, and to the point. In nursing, it also means that the communication is professional, which is different from social communication. Professional communication portrays respect for the the receiver and for the person who is the subject of the communication (usually the patient) and for that person's privacy.

▶ PURPOSES OF CLEAR COMMUNICATION

There are several purposes of clear communication, some of which are quite obvious. The first is to promote continuity and consistent quality of care. Nurses must coordinate their care with that of others. If care issues are not well communicated, patients get disjointed, sporadic care. Accurate and specific verbal and written reports from one nurse to another or between nurses and other health care providers will decrease duplication of efforts, ensure that important issues are not missed, and save time, energy, and resources.

A second purpose of clear communication is that it provides evidence of the thinking that accompanies the nursing process. All parts of the nursing process must be communicated verbally or in written form. Notes and oral reports reflect the thinking that guided data collection and analysis, which resulted in well designed and implemented care, and the thinking that judged changes in patients' conditions.

A third purpose of clear communication is to establish credibility and legal accountability for care. Nurses are legally accountable for the care they do *and* do not provide. Written communication, in particular, is a tangible way to validate that legal responsibility. Records are legal documents, and as such, may be called into court. What a nurse writes in a patient record could make the difference between winning or losing a lawsuit. The legal issues are discussed more fully in Chapter 11.

There also are some less obvious but equally important purposes of clear communication. Effective verbal communication with patients and their significant others enables the nurse to obtain information that might otherwise remain unknown. Clear verbal communication also plays a major role in developing the nurse–patient relationship, which is based on trust. Studies have shown that health care providers who are classified as "good communicators" are less likely to be sued by patients and more likely to have their treatment plans followed (Northouse & Northouse, 1985).

Clear written communications in the forms of well worded nursing diagnoses and well worded goals and objectives go a long way toward streamlining nursing care and achieving successful outcomes. Developing these finer points of written communication requires great thinking, and is explored at the end of this chapter.

▶ VERBAL COMMUNICATION

▷ Personal Styles of Verbal Communication

It is often said that it doesn't matter how smart you are; if you cannot communicate well, the world will not see you as smart. Regardless of the truth of that statement, it is worth some consideration. Great thinkers without great communication skills may make great eccentric hermits, but they do not make great nurses. Great nurses must be able to communicate their thinking.

Clear communication requires practice and thought. People vary widely in their abilities to communicate verbally. Verbal communication is affected by self-image, self-confidence, thinking styles, language background, and so many other personal factors that it is often difficult to pin down where each person's strengths and weaknesses are. Because of the personal nature of communication skills, it is worthwhile for nursing students to do some self-assessment, or thinking about their communication abilities.

▶▶▶▶▶▶ **Action Learning #54: Evaluating Your Verbal Communication**

Tape-record yourself giving a 5-minute report on a topic about which you are well versed. (If you have access to a video recorder, videotape yourself.) Do not rehearse what you will say ahead of time or write it out; rather, mentally map your thoughts and main points. Then, listen (or watch, if you used video) to the tape and analyze your verbal skills. Answer these questions:

▼ Was I clear?

▼ Did I make my main point?

▼ Did I develop my ideas in a logical manner?

▼ Did I sound as if I knew as much about this subject as I really do?

▼ How often do I use speech hesitation mechanisms such as "er," "ah," "you know," "like," or "well?"

▼ Was my voice too loud, too soft?

▼ Did I vary the pace and tone?

DISCUSSION So, are you a clear communicator? Did you like what you heard? If you found things you did not like, what can you do about them? Based on listening to that tape, what do you think others would think of you, of your communication skills, of your thinking skills? Keep in mind that the point of this exercise is not to decrease your self-esteem, but to increase awareness so that you can identify what works, what does not work, and what you want to change. Some people have more skill in this area than others, but effective communication is learned; no one is born with it.

▷ Verbal Communication in Nursing

Nurses, of course, communicate with patients and their significant others as they assess, plan, implement, and evaluate care. "Therapeutic communication" is a term used in a variety of ways in nursing. Some refer to all nurse–patient communication as therapeutic, because it is focused on nurses helping patients deal with health needs. At other times, such as in the specialty area of psychiatric nursing, therapeutic communication is used to mean specific treatment approaches. It is beyond the scope of this book to describe in detail the elements of the varying definitions of therapeutic communication. To avoid confusion in terms, the focus here will be on clarity of communication.

Clear verbal communication by a nurse will put patients at ease and help them open up and share information with nurses during assessment. Nurses who communicate well with patients during planning will design the most individualized care. During implementation of care, nurses who communicate clearly will find patients more cooperative. During evaluation, patients will provide the most useful feedback on how their care is going when nurses are open and clear in their interactions. In all of these situations, clarity of expression is vital.

In addition to communication with patients and their significant others, nurses also communicate daily with other health care providers. Some of these interactions are preplanned; many others occur spontaneously. Change-of-shift reports and conference reports are two common preplanned events. Reports on changes in patients' conditions are examples of spontaneous interactions.

It often is easier to recognize unclear communication techniques than to practice clear ones. One example of an end-of-shift report is presented below to illustrate the problems with unclear, ineffective communication. An end-of-shift report was chosen as an example because those reports are a good test of clarity and concision. Also, those reports are a type of communication that beginning students must practice early in their nursing programs. In these short reports, nurses highlight important information, but do not have time to fill in large amounts of detail. They must be organized, specific, clear in their directions to others, and must address the components of the nursing process they have used, and do all of this in a professional manner.

> ▶▶▶▶▶▶ **Action Learning #55: Evaluating Nurse Elie Norman's Communication**

Read this script of a taped end-of-shift report by a nurse, Elie Norman R.N. After reading it, make a list of things that you think are problematic with this communication.

Hiya guys. This is Elie reporting on the new patient in 51. He was admitted before lunch but I'm just now getting his stuff together. I'm so tired today, I'm just dragging around. Must be the late hours last night. Ah, well, let's see, this patient was in the ER for a few hours before coming up here. His family is floating around the hospital somewhere. They are quite the tribe; watch out for them. Let's see, his diagnosis is diabetes insipidus and he goes to the bathroom every time you turn around. I think we're supposed to watch his intake and output really carefully. I started assessing him and got some things written on the intake form, but I only have a few hunches yet. No one knows why he has this disease; the docs from urology are working him up. They wrote some orders that I think were processed; the lab should be getting his blood by now. One thing I do know is that he is scared. I filled in one column of a care plan dealing with his fears, but I don't have it finished yet. I'll try to get that done before I leave.

Problems With Elie's Communication:

DISCUSSION   What is interfering with clarity here? If you are appalled and unable to imagine a nurse communicating like this, think about having a hectic day at work after a busy night of socialization and ask yourself, honestly, would you do and say some of the same things that Elie did? Do you think Elie gave this patient good care? How can you tell? Does Elie give any evidence of her thinking about this patient and his needs? Giving Elie another chance, here is how she could have given the same verbal report:

> Mr. Packer was admitted to Room 51 from the ER at 11 AM, accompanied by his family, who went to the cafeteria at 2:30. His admitting medical diagnosis is diabetes insipidus of unknown origin. He is being worked up and should have his lab work done by now. Drs. Jones and Brown from urology have written orders, including a request for strict intake and output records. Mr. Packer has been urinating every hour since his arrival. From my assessment, which is still incomplete, I have found him to be fearful of this mysterious illness. My care plan includes some strategies to decrease his fears. My other conclusions are possible problems with fluid volume deficits, nutritional problems, and family conflicts. Please see my notes for details on these and for suggestions for further assessment today.

▷ Strategies for Clear Verbal Communication

The differences between Elie's first report and the revised one were the organization, specificity, clarity of direction to others, evidence of the nurse's thinking and use of the nursing process, and professionalism or the omission of social chit-chat and value judgments. Even though the second report included much of the same information as the first, it was professional and it exemplified the work of a thinking nurse, someone in whom one could put trust. Given the choice, which report would the next shift's nurses prefer? Now there's an easy answer. To develop the kind of style seen in the revised report, study and practice the following parameters of effective communication.

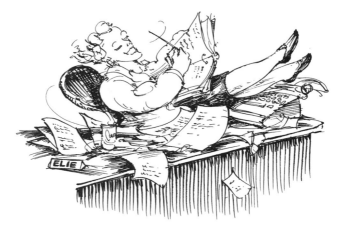

Figure 10-1A. Elie at her worst.

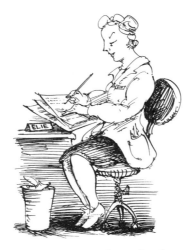

Figure 10-1B. Elie at her best.

Organization

Speaking in an organized manner requires organizing one's thoughts first. There are many ways to do that; most people have some personal approach that works for them. Some write notes to themselves, others use a scheme such as thinking about the who, what, where, when, why, and how of subjects. Whatever the method, INQUIRY thinking is needed to decide what is important and what is relevant to what. The actual method used to organize one's thoughts needs to become a HABIT. The method is less important than finding something that works and sticking with it. KNOWING HOW YOU THINK will help you find a system that works.

Specificity

Vague communication is both frustrating and potentially unsafe, not to mention a waste of time. In Elie's first report, although she had assessed the patient and made some preliminary conclusions, she was so vague about them that the nurse on the next shift would have had to redo what had already been done. Decisions about what areas need to be communicated specifically and which ones can be mentioned casually or omitted are not easy to make. A good report is not necessarily a long one with detail on everything. Listeners start to ignore the report when it gets overdone. As with organization, the nurse needs INQUIRY thinking to make decisions about relative importance of details.

Clarity of Direction to Others

Many verbal reports that nurses give are meant to let the next nurse caring for the patient know what needs to be done next. Without clear directions, the next nurse has to second-guess the first one. In the revised report, the nurse hearing the report would know that some directed data collection was needed to verify Elie's hunches that Mr. Packer had fluid, nutrition, and family problems. The second nurse could pick up where Elie left off with the nursing process. The revised report specified the need for accurate intake and output records, an interdependent nursing activity critical to the medical care. Elie's flippant comment in the first report ("I think we're supposed to . . . ") lacked clear direction and could have caused harm to the patient, or, at the very least, would have delayed his care.

Evidence of Thinking and Use of the Nursing Process

It was unclear in the first report what Elie's thinking was and how it fit with her assessing, planning, implementing, and evaluating. Because the patient had been recently admitted, other nurses could guess that some assessment had been done, but how much of it was completed was not clear at all. In the revised report, Elie showed that she had collected data, had some hunches, and knew that other data were needed to verify those hunches. Others could tell that she had been thinking. In the first scenario, she was not focused on the data as much as she was on filling out the intake form, or getting things written in the right place. Likewise, with the plan, it appeared that she was more focused on what was written in the columns of the plan than she was on the significance of the whole approach. The revised report showed her thinking within the framework of the nursing process much more clearly. She was focused on thinking about the significance of data rather than on filling out forms.

Professionalism: Omitting Social Chit-Chat and Value Judgments

Nurses are educated to appreciate diversity and the uniqueness of each person; however, nurses are people just as prone to value judgments as others. The difference is that nurses do not act on those judgments or communicate them to others. Nurses are also social people, but they need to keep their social lives separate from their professional lives. That doesn't mean that Elie should not have told other nurses about her socialization the night before. It's just that she should not include it in a report about a patient. When referring to other health care providers, she should identify them by their names, not as "the docs from urology."

Patients have the right to be respected and identified accurately in reports. Their names, rather than some other designation such as a room number or a medical diagnosis, should be used. In the revised report, Elie called the patient by name, not by a room number designation.

Clear communication takes practice and should not be taken lightly. A good rule of thumb to help in deciding what constitutes a professional report is this: If you would be comfortable with the patient and significant others hearing the report, then it is probably appropriate. Another guideline for deciding if a report is organized, specific, and clear is to ask yourself this: If I were hearing this report, would I know the important aspects of care for this patient, and would I know what needs to be addressed next?

THINKING-LEARNING CHECK

Pause here for a thinking-learning check. You should be able to elaborate on these ideas:

- ▼ The importance of clear communication: promotes continuity and consistent quality of care, provides evidence of thinking, establishes credibility and legal accountability, and enhances rapport and trust with patients.
- ▼ Personal verbal communication styles: analyzing them for clarity.
- ▼ Verbal communication in nursing occurs with patients and significant others, other nurses, and other health care providers
- ▼ Strategies for effective verbal communication include organization, specificity, clarity of directions to others, evidence of thinking and use of the nursing process, and professionalism.

▶ WRITTEN COMMUNICATION: DOCUMENTATION

There are many forms of written communication in nursing. Nurses write policies, procedures, letters, reports, self-evaluations, articles, chapters, and books, to name only a few. This chapter, however, focuses on one type of written communication—documentation of nursing care in a patient's record. Next to verbal communication, written documentation may seem a more daunting task; however, the same principles of organization, specificity, clarity, thinking, and professionalism apply to written communication as to verbal communication.

Written documentation is a necessary part of nursing because storing information in one's head is neither safe nor practical. In many professions, as in nursing, writing notes in a patient's record is referred to as "documentation." As the term implies, documenting is a formal recording of events. A patient's record, or chart, is a formal, legal record of health care.

Today, documentation must be interpreted to include computerized "writing." With computer programs, the nurse gets some assistance with organization because certain things can be entered only in certain ways. Computer programs also help with wording because multiple-choice options are available to describe what is being reported. Computers are organized, logic-oriented machines. Their programs provide basic patterns for recording data in pre-established, organized ways. This can be very helpful and time saving. But computers do not think. (Some might argue that "artificial intelligence" is approaching some degree of thinking, but systems used for daily documentation in most health care settings are not that sophisticated.) Because computers don't think, nurses must continue to decide what information is important, what it means, and what to do about it. Whether entered into a computer or written on paper, it is the nurse's thinking that must get communicated to promote good patient care. Because handwritten communication will continue in many settings even with computerization, the traditional issues of documentation continue to be relevant.

▷ Parts of a Patient Record

The specific things in a record vary from setting to setting, but, generally, records contain progress notes, assessment forms, care plans, physician order sheets, laboratory results, consultation records, and graphic sheets. Nurses need to be familiar with everything in a patient's record.

Sometimes records are divided by discipline, with nurses writing on one section of the chart, physicians on another, social workers elsewhere, and so forth. That format is less common today than it once was, especially in acute care settings. Today, for example, rather than having a section for the nurses's notes, there is a section for multidisciplinary progress notes. All health care providers write their progress notes in the same section of the patient's chart. They identify their disciplines at the beginning of their note or with the credentials after their names, so that those reading the notes can see who the provider was.

The way a record is organized and how a progress note is to be written usually are stated in the institution's policies. After a preliminary discussion of other elements of documentation, some examples of progress note styles are presented.

▷ Documentation Rules

There are certain universal "dos and don'ts" or rules of documentation. These rules, when used properly, provide consistency and clarity in documentation as well as legal protection. There also are some generally accepted "rules" that are important, but not quite so critical. The "dos" are that all entries should be legibly written in pen and accompanied by a date, time, signature, and professional title; when mistakes are made, one line should be drawn through the entry, and it should be signed and dated. The "don'ts" include recording unsupported value judgments or inferences, obliterating or trying to erase errors, and using pencils. Other generally accepted rules for documentation include using phrases instead of full sentences and making entries compact with no blank lines inside the entry or between the entry and the nurse's signature.

Computers have added a few dos and don'ts and eliminated a few. They replace the pen with an electronic entry system (keyboard, light pen, touchpad) and printer. The date and time may be recorded automatically, or the nurse may need to type them in. The nurse's signature is often coded into the computer. The rule of computer signatures is never to share one's code or chart under someone else's code. Computer programs have a method to correct errors that eliminates the need to cross things out.

▶▶▶▶▶ **Action Learning #56: Finding the Documentation Errors in a Progress Note**

Examine the following documentation entry in Mrs. Blake's record. Identify where documentation rules were not followed and discuss with a classmate how to fix them. Rewrite the entry and correct the problems.

Pt. looks terrible today. I sat with her for 30 minutes trying to get her to talk to no avail. B/P 220/80 124/70, P 80, R 16. Refused lunch. Slept Stayed in room all afternoon with the lights out and covers pulled over her head.

I. Smith, RN

DISCUSSION How many errors did you find? How easy was it to fix the problems? Did the note reflect any thinking or use of the nursing process?

▷ Documenting the Nursing Process

Parts of a record can be linked to the phases of the nursing process. This is more evident in the record systems some agencies use than it is in others. For example, first-encounter assessment data are recorded on assessment tools, nursing histories, and data bases. Planning is recorded on care plans and kardexes. Implementation is recorded on progress notes, graphic sheets, flow sheets, and critical paths. Evaluation is recorded on care plans, progress notes, and on discharge summaries. These places are not mutually exclusive, however. For example, after initial encounters, assessment data may be recorded as evaluation data. Documentation of implementation, once it includes conclusions about how a patient is progressing, becomes documentation of evaluation rather than implementation.

The complexity of documentation is the reason why nurses must continually use their T.H.I.N.K. modes. Documentation is more than merely writing things down; thought must go into deciding the best place to record things, the best things to record, and how to word what is to be recorded.

Documenting Assessment

In some settings, assessment data are written in narrative form on blank sheets of paper. More often, initial assessment data are recorded on assessment forms (usually a form with blank spaces for specific data collection identified, sometimes as checklists). The assessment tool in Chapter 8 is an example of this type of form. These forms are used to record a first assessment or the baseline data on a patient. These data provide the basis for initial conclusions of assessment and for care plans. As such, these forms should include only raw data, not inferences or conclusions, unless there are designated sections labeled "conclusions or impressions." These sections are usually at the end of the forms.

In acute care settings, data and conclusions from the second, third, and fourth encounters with a patient are usually recorded in the progress notes, rather than on the assessment tool. The progress notes are just what they sound like—a record of the patient's progress. As a patient's condition changes, new assessment data become significant for showing the progress. Sometimes, new problems are discovered; sometimes, the previous problems change. Data discovered through ongoing assessment may actually become evaluation data and are recorded as such. These methods of documenting assessment data are noted in the following sections, which describe documentation in the other phases of the nursing process.

In long-term care and community health settings, initial data collection tools may be used differently. In nursing homes, for example, a complete data base is redone annually in an effort to track over longer periods of time changing patient health status and needs. In community health, where the data base typically includes a whole family unit, data are added to the form over time.

Because the amount of data required for family care is extensive, it cannot all be collected at one time. This continual adding to the initial assessment allows for historical data, growth and development data, and the like to be analyzed in the ongoing plan of care for the family.

Overall, what is important during documentation of assessment is that data are raw data and conclusions are judgments based on the data. There should *never* be any conclusions recorded on a patient's chart that cannot be tracked to their supporting data.

Documenting Planning

The plan that is written on the patient's record (chart) is the result of much complex thinking on the nurse's part; the better the thinking, the better the plan. In reality, it is often the written plan and not the thinking behind the plan that is equated with the process of planning. As with many things in nursing and elsewhere, what gets written down takes on special significance because it is what everyone can *see*. Unfortunately, this gives beginning nurses a false impression about where to focus their energy. Great plans do not write themselves or get copied out of books; they require great thinking. A well-written, great plan, therefore, should be seen for what it truly is—clear evidence of the great thinking behind the written words.

Written formats for care plans vary somewhat from institution to institution. Most settings use some type of column format similar to that used for care plans in this book. There usually is a place for the nursing diagnosis or interdisciplinary problem, goals or objectives, and nursing actions. Some plans have a column for evaluation comments; some do not. All entries on a plan are dated and signed, either with the nurse's full signature or with initials that can be linked with a name elsewhere on the record.

With the increasing use of computers in health care, many institutions have computer programs for care plans. Sometimes standard plans for commonly found problems can be "pulled up" by indicating that the patient has one of these problems. These standard plans then can be adapted to the patient, just as preprinted standard plans are adapted.

Other parts of the patient record devoted to planning are flow sheets, critical paths, graphic sheets, and kardexes. These are shorthand plans that give direction for parts of the plan that are usually done repetitively. Part of a plan for a patient with diabetes might be to track the blood glucose levels. A kardex might say "BS QID," (blood sugar four times a day) or a flow sheet might be put on the record as a reminder to do this. Likewise, these quick references might be used for parts of the plan that cross over many problem areas. For example, if a patient does not communicate verbally, but uses an alphabet board to spell words, "Use alphabet board for communication" might be written on a kardex. That piece of information, then, does not need to be rewritten on all parts of the plan; it is automatically assumed in all other parts of the plan where communication is necessary.

Documenting Implementation

Documentation of interventions is the recording of activities done for or with the patient. When a conclusion about how a patient is progressing is included in a written note, then the nurse is documenting evaluation as well. Because nurses are expected to record actions and their effect on the patient's progress, intervention documentation is more often than not incorporated into evaluation notes. There are, however, some interventions that are documented solely as interventions, and need no comments about evaluation. The administration of medications, one of nursing's interdependent functions, is a common example.

Generally speaking, independent nursing actions are more often documented in evaluation notes, and interdependent actions are more often written as intervention notes. For example, many interdependent nursing actions are part of the medical plan of care. It makes sense that physicians would be doing most of the evaluation of the medical plan; nurses would be communicating that their part of the plan had been implemented. Likewise, nurses would be the primary evaluators of their independent plans. Their implementation notes also would include an evaluation of the patient's progress in the areas of nursing care. These are certainly only general rules, with many exceptions.

Documenting Evaluation

Documenting evaluation probably comprises most of the recording a nurse does, because nurses must constantly monitor and record changes in patient conditions. Some conclusions or judgments need to be made about those changes, and, when judgments are made, evaluation has occurred.

Evaluation notes usually are written in the progress notes section on a patient's record, although some care plan formats are set up with evaluation columns. Most documentation formats for progress notes have some element of evaluation built into them. The many formats for documenting evaluation are too numerous to explain in detail here; other nursing textbooks may be used to explore other methods. Three methods will be discussed here— narrative notes, SOAP (**S**ubjective and **O**bjective data, **A**ssessment and **P**lan) notes, and DAR (**D**ata, **A**ction, **R**esponse) notes. Of these three, SOAP and DAR have evaluation built in, so a well written note will contain some judgments about the patient's progress. Narrative notes do not have this built-in mechanism, but they often include judgments about patient progress.

▷ Documentation Formats

Most institutions or units adopt a documentation format that is expected to be followed by all care providers in that setting. This format is shared with new employees during orientation. One of the purposes of newer documentation formats is to reflect thinking in all phases of the nursing process. When used appropriately, the newer formats are triggers for thinking.

With the advent of computer charting, the formats may be adapted to computer capabilities, or the usual format can be kept, with the staff simply typing in their notes rather than writing them by hand.

Narrative Notes

A narrative note is just what it sounds like—a narrative of what has occurred. This is the oldest format for charting and its effectiveness is highly dependent on the nurse's skill in writing clear, organized information. The order of recording is generally the order in which events occurred. For example:

> 11/20/92 1300 Ambulated with walker 20 feet once in AM and once in PM. Vital signs stable during ambulation. Complained of back pain after walking, relieved with massage and sitting with pillow at back for 30 minutes. Dry dressing changed over hip staples. Incision site clear, no signs of infection. Pt. states she is anxious to start physical therapy so she can get home before the holidays.
>
> J. Gold, RN

In this example, there is evidence of the nurse's data collection and conclusions about the data, implementation, and evaluation. There is not much on planning. This type of note allows a nurse to record all of the nursing process in any order desired. A problem with this format is that the parts of the nursing process are not automatically evident. Nurses who write narrative notes must give extra thought to the flow of ideas. What will make sense to the person reading it? There are many individual styles with narrative notes, some of which work better than others.

▶▶▶▶▶▶ **Action Learning #57: Writing a Narrative Note**

Read the following case study. Write a narrative note to report the information on today's visit. Compare your note to that of a classmate and discuss your different styles.

CASE STUDY

Ms. Jacob is a 48-year-old lawyer. She had polio at the age of 10 years. Two years ago, she suffered from post polio syndrome (a recurrence of some of the symptoms of the earlier disease). She was hospitalized for 6 months with progressive paralysis. After a respiratory arrest, a permanent tracheostomy was performed (a tracheostomy is a special tube inserted into the trachea through which a person breathes). Ms. Jacob is now home. She has had to quit her job, but is financially comfortable. She lives alone in a one-floor apartment and has a community health nurse visit twice a week to help her manage her tracheostomy care. She is a fast learner and is doing the care with no problems. Today the nurse watched her doing the tracheostomy care and only had to remind her of one thing—to wipe with strokes rather than in a back and forth motion. During today's visit (1 month after hospitalization) she has puffy, red eyes, avoids eye contact with the nurse, and finally admits she feels very alone. She says, "I hate going out in public; I can talk if I cover up the trach but people seem so uncomfortable around me and I don't like to make people uncomfortable. Even my friends don't visit very much; they're so busy, but really I think they don't know what to say or do. I can deal with the trach myself and I don't mind using the cane to walk, but I feel so isolated, I'm going crazy."

Narrative Note:

DISCUSSION Was this an easy type of note to write? Did you remember to use the "rules" of documentation? Do you think another person would have a good picture of the day's events by reading the note? On which part or parts of the nursing process was your note primarily focused?

SOAP Notes

SOAP notes are used with problem-oriented medical records, which have a central list of problems identified by the health care team. That problem list includes the conclusions reached by the whole health care team—medical diagnoses (eg, L. CVA, tuberculosis), interdisciplinary problems (eg, decubitus ulcers), nursing diagnoses (eg, Self-Care Deficit . . . , Social Isolation . . .), and diagnoses made by other providers (eg, recreational deficit). Each problem has a number and a plan of care. All progress notes refer to a problem by number.

SOAP notes are used to document all parts of the nursing process, but they are primarily focused on assessment *or* evaluation. Understanding this distinction makes learning the SOAP format much easier. In the following description, "A" designates how each component of SOAP is used to write an assessment note, and "E" designates how they are used for evaluation notes.

SOAP stands for Subjective, Objective, Assessment, and Plan. If this sounds strangely like the nursing process, that's because it is. Here is a closer look at the parts of a SOAP note:

Subjective: What the patient (or significant others) said (A and E).

Objective: What was observed or measured (A and E) **and** what the nurse did (E). "What the nurse did" does not obviously fit with the word "objective," so it is important to think of some way to remember this piece of SOAP.

Assessment: This is the tricky part. When nurses hear the word "assessment," they automatically think, "First phase of the nursing process, which includes data collection, data analysis, and conclusions." The only part of that traditional meaning that works with a SOAP note is the "conclusions" part. Other nurses think of the "A" in SOAP as meaning "analysis." This also is confusing and results in inaccurate SOAP notes. What is important here is that the "A" of "assessment" in SOAP stands **only** for one of two types of conclusions in the nursing process—assessment conclusions or evaluation conclusions. Assessment conclusions are judgments about patient strengths and health concerns. Evaluation conclusions focus on whether the goals and objectives were met, not met, or partially met. Therefore, **when writing the "A" part of a SOAP note, the nurse either makes an assessment conclusion about the strengths and health concerns (A) or makes an evaluation conclusion about how the patient is progressing toward meeting the plan's goals and objectives (E).**

Plan: This is just what it sounds like. It is what the nurse is going to do about the conclusions (A and E). Given the subjective and objective data and the conclusion reached based on those data, what is the plan for the **future**? The difference between plans made after assessment and those made after evaluation is that the plan is developed first after assessment, and it already exists and needs to be continued or modified after evaluation. If, as is the usual case, the plan is written on the care plan part of the record, then the nurse may refer to the plan in the SOAP note. "See plan" or "see plan for changes" may be written at the "P" part of the notes. The actual plan changes may be written in the note, but this should be done only if it does not duplicate what is written elsewhere.

Here are some examples of SOAP notes:

EXAMPLE 1. EVALUATION NOTE

11/20/92, 0900: #3, Pain:

S: "My back really hurts today. The pain is about a 6 (on a scale of 10). I barely slept last night. I feel better now" (1/2 hour after massage and medication).

O: Pt.'s face in a grimace. Lying on side with pillows behind back. Heating pad applied to lower back. Medicated with Darvocet. Area massaged. 1/2 hour after interventions, pt.'s face and body in relaxed position.

A: Pt. progressing toward goal of pain relief, but continues to need narcotic medication.

P: See additions to plan to offer heating pad and massage more frequently. G. Blakely, RN

EXAMPLE 2. FIRST ENCOUNTER WITH PATIENT (ASSESSMENT NOTE)

11/20/92, 1500: #1, Skin impairment:

S: "I know I shouldn't lie in one position so long; it makes my skin break down. I've had dry skin all my life."

O: Skin warm, dry, 4-cm circular, reddened, unbroken area on coccyx; right heel cracked, peeling in a 3-cm area. Pt. turned and sheepskin pads applied to heels.

A: Impaired Skin Integrity related to immobility and bed pressure.

P: See care plan #1. G. Blakely, RN

Notice how the "A" parts of the notes differ. The evaluation note "A" addresses how the patient is progressing toward the goal. The "P" comment mentions *additions* to the plan. In the assessment note, the "A" is a nursing diagnosis and the "P" refers only to the plan, without any changes (because the plan was just written).

In both notes, the date and time are recorded and the note starts with a reference to a numbered problem. Identifying the problem allows everyone reading the note to know exactly what aspect of patient care is being discussed.

Reading a series of notes on one problem allows a person to track the progress of a health concern.

►►►►►► **Action Learning #58: Sorting the Parts of a SOAP Note**

Examine the following pieces of data and sort them into the proper SOAP note categories. Indicate for each situation if it is an evaluation note or an assessment note.

SITUATION A:

See new objective and action on care plan.
"I'm walking much better."
Goal met.
Patient walked 30 feet independently with walker.
"I think I can walk further by myself."
Steady gait.
11/15/93, 3 PM, #3, Impaired Mobility

S.

O.

A.

P.

SITUATION B:

High Risk for Injury: falls R/T unsteady gait, use of area rugs in home and dim lighting.
Patient 93, CVA 3 months ago, lives alone, small apartment, hardwood floors with area rugs at entrance and in kitchen.
Recently ambulating with quad cane.

No overhead lights, table lamps in each room with 25-watt light bulbs (patient states to save energy and money).

"But I love my Oriental rugs, they're family heirlooms."

Patient stated she has had her rugs a long time and never had problems before.

Patient encouraged to purchase rug adhesive to stabilize rugs and keep the edges flat.

Taught patient importance of good lighting. Brochure from the Center for Independent Living on methods of improving indoor lighting given to patient.

#2 High Risk for Injury

11/18/93 1400

Follow-up visit arranged for next week to check on status.

S.

O.

A.

P.

DAR Notes

Notes that are organized by Data, Action, and Response are used with a system of "focus" charting. Similar to problem-oriented records using SOAP, where a problem is identified for each note, the "focus" is the problem or health issue that is being addressed each time a DAR note is written. The note is organized into columns—one for the patient data, one for the action taken by the nurse or other health care provider, and one for the patient response. Some agencies write out the DAR running down the page just as the SOAP note is written. This form of documentation, like SOAP, has evaluation built in. Making a judgment about the patient response focuses on the outcome of the care or changes in the patient condition.

Example of column format DAR note:

Focus: Reflex Incontinence: Self-Catheterization

Data	Action	Response
11/10/93 2100 Pt. reports she is still having difficulty finding meatus using mirror. After 3 position changes, pt. did cath. Urine clear, yellow, odorless.	Assisted pt. to try positioning knees; set up cath. equip.; reviewed importance of cleaning meatus thoroughly. Plan to review this next time.	Objective of self-cath not met yet, but pt. making progress.

G. Blakely, RN

Note the similarities of this method to SOAP notes and to the nursing process phases. Assessing, planning, implementing, and evaluating are all evident.

▶▶▶▶▶▶ **Action Learning #59: Writing a DAR Note**

Sort the following information into a DAR note:

11/16/93 1300

"I enjoyed the Bingo game especially because I could sit next to Mr. Jones."

Objective of attending one recreation program/day being met most days.

After some prompting, patient went to recreation room after Bingo game had started.

Prompt patient half hour before recreation program in future.

Patient returned to room, smiling.

Diversional Activity Deficit: Increase recreation activities

Helped patient choose recreation program from the day's schedule.

Focus:

Data   *Action*   *Response*

Pause here for a thinking-learning check. You should be able to elaborate on these ideas:

▼ Documentation: must be organized, specific, clear, and professionally done to represent great thinking.

▼ Documentation follows several rules and can be done on computer or through handwritten records.

▼ Documentation needs to reflect all phases of the nursing process: assessing, planning, implementing, and evaluating.

▼ Documentation formats: three examples and how they trigger thinking to address all phases of the nursing process.

▼ The "A" in a SOAP note means a "conclusion" in either the assessment phase or the evaluation phase of the nursing process.

▶ THE FINER POINTS OF COMMUNICATION

So far, this chapter has focused on the basic issues of communication that every nurse must master. As beginning students gain proficiency in these basic verbal and written communication skills, they will be able to move their focus to some of the finer points of communication. These finer points require even more thinking about the subtleties of word selection. The more clearly and concisely the patient's health condition is described with words, the better the chance of designing and implementing the best individualized care. Well-written plans of nursing care can increase the efficiency and accuracy of nurses' work and the quality of patient care.

As most readers will have deduced by now, there are few right and wrong answers to most nursing issues, but there are qualitative differences—adequate, good, better, and best. The following are two examples of how the wording of the nursing diagnosis and the wording of objectives result in qualitative differences in the plan and thus the nursing care.

▷ Well-Worded Nursing Diagnoses

In earlier chapters, descriptions of differential diagnoses showed how important it was to consider alternative options as labels for nursing conclusions. Some of the work of differential diagnosis has to do with making decisions about wording. A well-worded nursing diagnosis can make care planning much easier. What, then, is a well-worded nursing diagnosis? Look back to Action Learning #57 and Ms. Jacob's situation. There are several nursing diagnoses that could be equally valid as conclusions, based on the data. There is a definite data cluster in her emotional response pattern.

▼ DATA CLUSTER

Has tracheostomy
Lives alone
Quit her job
Puffy, red eyes
Avoids eye contact with nurse
Admits to feeling alone

"I hate going out in public; I can talk if I cover up the trach but people seem so uncomfortable around me and I don't like to make people uncomfortable."

"Even my friends don't visit very much; they're so busy, but really I think they don't know what to say or do."

"I can deal with the trach myself and I don't mind using the cane to walk, but I feel so isolated, I'm going crazy."

From these data, there are several possible nursing diagnosis conclusions that could be reached, each seemingly equally valid.

Possible Nursing Diagnosis Conclusions

A. Social Isolation related to living alone, recently quitting job, and perception that friends are uncomfortable with her.

B. Body Image Disturbance related to tracheostomy and mobility changes.

C. Diversional Activity Deficit related to excess time alone, recently quitting job, dislike of going out in public, and perceived discomfort of friends.

D. Impaired Social Interaction related to decreased contact with friends, perceived discomfort of friends, changed verbal skills with tracheostomy, living alone, and recently quitting job.

E. Ineffective Individual Coping related to situational crisis of illness (tracheostomy, impaired mobility) and change in roles.

These are five possible nursing diagnoses that are supported by the data in the cluster; there could be others as well. A nurse whose thinking led to these conclusions would need to decide which of these diagnoses was the most accurate label for the patient's situation. By focusing on the finer points of written communication, the nurse would be able to make the conclusion that is the most accurate, precise picture of the situation and the one that points toward realistic interventions that would improve the patient's situation. By using IN-QUIRY thinking, a nurse might ask and find answers to several questions. Answers to each question, some of which are found through TOTAL RECALL of nursing knowledge, will assist the nurse in making the final conclusion.

Question #1:

Which conclusions best reflect the data fully?

Answer:

Dx. A, C, and D

Rationale: B may be a less accurate label for the cluster because the patient stated she could deal with the tracheostomy and didn't mind using the cane. The body image issue may need to be addressed, but the patient is not primarily focused on that. E focuses on her inability to cope, but it is a very broad label. She is coping well with caring for the tracheostomy and using a cane, but she may not be coping with being alone. Therefore, ineffective coping is too broad to reflect best the specifics of the data.

Question #2: Of diagnoses A, C, and D, which ones reflect critical subjective data? In other words, what is the patient most focused on?

Answer: Dx. A and D

Rationale: The patient doesn't actually say she doesn't have enough to occupy her free time, and C is focused on activities. She specifically said, "I hate going out in public"; "My friends don't visit much"; "I feel isolated." She admits to feeling alone. Each of those comments is focused on aloneness and social interaction more than on not having enough diversional activities in general.

Question #3: Of diagnoses A and D, considering the difference between "Social Isolation" and "Impaired Social Interaction," which one is a better label?

Answer: Dx. A is better

Rationale: The North American Nursing Diagnosis Association (NANDA) definition of "Social Isolation" is "Aloneness experienced by the individual and perceived as imposed by others and as a negative or threatened state" (NANDA, 1992, p. 37). "Impaired Social Interaction" is defined as "The state in which an individual participates in an insufficient or excessive quantity or ineffective quality of social exchange" (NANDA, 1992, p. 36). The patient is focused on aloneness and she perceives it as imposed by others. Therefore, Social Isolation most closely matches this patient situation.

This fine-tuned level of thinking for selecting the best words to describe a health concern is not reached overnight. Beginning students have many things to think about; they may not develop this finer level of thinking and communicating for quite some time; however, it is an ideal toward which nursing students should aim. Before these skills get well tuned, an acceptance of their importance will trigger the nurse's thinking each time a conclusion is written in a patient's chart. The nurse will remember to ask, "Are these the most descriptive words for what I want to convey?"

This fine-tuned thinking about the wording of nursing diagnoses will deter nurses from overusing HABIT thinking about written communication. Excessive HABIT thinking occurs when the first label that comes to mind is the one that is recorded on the patient's record. Questioning those first words and thinking about how they can be refined will trigger the INQUIRY mode, promote more accurate documentation, and, ultimately, more efficient nursing care. The best-worded nursing diagnosis will almost literally lead to a great plan for care. In Ms. Jacob's case, the chosen diagnostic statement points to a goal of increased socialization as evidenced by such things as the patient considering alternatives to living alone, considering finding something to do with her time that has a social component, and openly discussing with her friends her perception of their discomfort. If those outcomes were achieved, the problem would very likely be resolved. If one of the other diagnoses had been chosen, the path to those outcomes might be more circuitous. It would not be wrong; it might even turn out to be just as helpful as the other path. The precision of the recorded label for Ms. Jacob's health concern, however, diminishes the chances for confusion among other providers, and ensures a more direct line from the problem to the resolution.

▷ How Well-Worded Objectives Affect Implementation and Evaluation

Chapter 9 provided extensive descriptions of how to formulate objectives for care plans. Many of the directions focused on wording issues—specificity, measurability and clarity. Review that part of Chapter 9 if you need a refresher. Now, bearing in mind this chapter's focus on clear communication, think about the actual written words of the objectives. A well-worded objective will simplify evaluation and clearly guide the way to developing great nursing actions; conversely, poorly worded objectives create confusion and result in sloppy evaluation. As an example, go back again to Ms. Jacob's situation and the final nursing diagnosis that was chosen, "Social Isolation Related to living alone, recently quitting job, and perception that friends are uncomfortable with her." Because Social Isolation was used as an example in an earlier chapter, it should be a familiar nursing conclusion by now, one to which the finer points of communication can be applied.

The goal for care would be for Ms. Jacob to increase her socialization within a month. (A month probably is realistic considering that she is at home and needs to do several things to meet that goal.) Using the general guidelines for formulating objectives, the nurse would look at the factors related to the isolation—living alone, recently quitting her job, and her perception of her friends' discomfort.

Assuming the patient has been a partner in the planning process, here are some options for objectives for the first week of the plan:

1. Objective options related to her living alone: Ms. Jacob will:
   A. Describe how she can compensate socially for living alone.
   B. Consider living with someone else.
   C. Accept how her living arrangements contribute to her isolation.
   D. Increase her socialization at home.

2. Objective options related to her recently quitting her job: Ms. Jacob will:
   E. Describe her feelings about quitting her job.
   F. Think of options for jobs to increase her socialization.
   G. Know her job options.

3. Objective options related to her perception of her friends' discomfort with her: Ms. Jacob will:
   H. Understand her friends' discomfort.
   I. Increase her friends' comfort with her.
   J. Role-play how she will confront her friends with her perceptions of their discomfort.
   K. Describe how she will deal with her friends' discomfort.
   L. Tell her friends how she feels.
   M. Invite at least two friends over to her house.

How would a nurse decide which were the best-worded objectives? Because nurses ideally try to address all related factors to a problem, one can assume that at least three objectives are needed for a start. There certainly could be more than that, however. Stop for a moment and review these options or develop some of your own. Which one objective option in each category would you use?

Here is how a nurse might choose the best-worded objectives:

A is measurable (the nurse can hear patient describe something); it seems automatically to show that nursing actions should be directed toward helping the patient explore options, and it involves the patient very directly. Keep this one.

B is narrow and may be too disruptive; because the patient has been managing on her own, there is no reason to ask patient to consider this. Not easily measured. Discard this one.

C is okay but it doesn't help her progress from where she is now. Consider discarding unless patient seems unrealistic about her living arrangements. Not easily measured either.

D is too vague and hard to measure. What would constitute an increase? Discard this one.

E is probably a necessary first step considering she quit her job recently and very little is known about her feelings about that. It is measurable and "points" to nursing care focused on feelings. Keep this one.

F is not measurable because one cannot see or measure another person thinking. Discard this one.

G is not measurable; how would anyone evaluate someone "knowing?" Unless the verb is changed to "describe," "explain," "list," or something equally measurable, discard this one.

H also is not measurable. "Understand" is like "know"; one needs a measurable sign to evaluate it. Also, Ms. Jacob seems already to understand her friends' discomfort; she was able to describe their behavior. Discard this one.

I is too vague. What would the nurse do to help? The nurse would need to work with the friends to know if this outcome occurred, and Ms. Jacob is the person of focus here. Discard this one.

J is very specific and leads directly to the nurse participating in role-playing. This objective specifies a tangible action for the patient and allows her to explore a potentially uncomfortable situation in a safe environment. Keep this one.

K is okay but not as good as J because it requires less involvement by the patient. This would also be a necessary part of J for J to work well. Would keep if J weren't better.

L does not help the patient in any specific direction. There is very little nursing care that automatically comes to mind with this objective. Discard because J is better and will accomplish the same thing and more.

M is very specific and measurable; it is a reasonable start, but it is not focused on the discomfort per se. Could keep it, but it is not very dynamic.

The nurse is left with is A, E, and J as the best-worded objectives. These are measurable, specific, relevant to the patient situation, and logically lead the nurse to specific nursing actions that would be individualized to Ms. Jacob. The final selection of wording would look as follows:

Nursing Diagnosis: Social Isolation R/T living alone, recently quitting job, and perception that friends are uncomfortable with her

Goal: By the end of 1 month, Ms. Jacob will increase her socialization A.E.B.:

1. Describing how she can compensate socially for living alone.
2. Describing her feelings about quitting her job.
3. Role-playing how she will confront her friends with her perceptions of their discomfort.

Obviously, to complete this plan, clear nursing actions are needed. Students generally have fewer problems wording nursing actions because there are many suggestions provided by textbooks. However, without clear nursing diagnoses and patient outcomes, the wording of actions can be more difficult. For beginners, the best use of their time in learning written communication is to hone their diagnoses and patient outcome wording skills. Then the nursing actions fall into place.

▶ CLOSING COMMENTS

It is hoped that this chapter has provided an appreciation of the thinking that must occur for clear verbal and written communication. It is easy, when learning communication, to focus on the structure, or the "how" of talking and writing. Nursing students may, for example, try to learn documentation formats by memorizing what goes where. Although that know-how can be learned and converted to HABITS, it will not help with deciding what should be recorded when, where, in what way, and in what order of importance. Nor will it help with verbal communication. Communicating the complexities and interrelationships of all parts of the nursing process requires the use of TOTAL RECALL, INQUIRY, NEW IDEAS AND CREATIVITY, and, most of all, KNOWING HOW YOU THINK.

▶▶▶ *THINKING LOG # 10*

If you are in a clinical area, examine several medical records. List several questions you have about the documentation. Then look at three nursing progress notes and evaluate them with regard to what you have learned in this chapter. Note: It is not appropriate to inform the staff verbally of any parts of the notes you perceive as errors; that can be shared confidentially with your instructor, who will also be able to explain the documentation in more detail for that particular agency.

REFERENCES

North American Nursing Diagnosis Association. (1992). *NANDA nursing diagnoses: Definitions and classification 1992*. Philadelphia: Author.

Northouse, P. G., & Northouse, L. L. (1985). *Health communication: A handbook for health professionals*. Englewood Cliffs, NJ: Prentice-Hall.

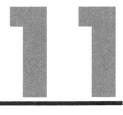

Consequences of Thinking and Not Thinking When Documenting

LEARNING OUTCOMES

After reading and doing the activities in this chapter you will be able to:

Discuss the relationships between the nursing process, thinking, documentation, quality assurance, and legal issues.

Identify errors and problems within several documentation examples.

Appreciate the value of documentation as a reflection of thinking and doing in nursing practice.

In Chapter 10, the purposes of clear communication, including documentation, were discussed. These purposes included promoting continuity and consistent quality of care, providing evidence of thinking, and establishing legal accountability for nursing care. When communication is unclear, the quality of patient care is severely compromised, nurses do not show their thinking, and they become vulnerable to legal action against them.

In this chapter, the nursing process and the documentation process are explored as sequential processes. Several case studies are used to illustrate how the nurse's thinking is reflected in documentation. The relationship of documentation to quality assurance is discussed, as well as the use of incident reports and the legal ramifications of documentation.

▶ RELATIONSHIP OF THE NURSING PROCESS TO THE PROCESS OF DOCUMENTATION

Remember, the nursing process and the documentation process are true processes. A process is a *continuous series* of actions that arrives at an *end result*. The nursing process is a series of actions—assessing, planning, implementing, and evaluating. The nursing process also is continuous; the nurse must con-

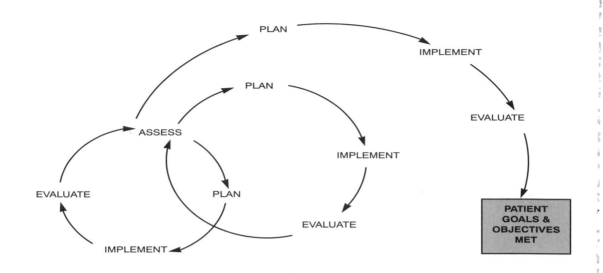

Figure 11-1.   Nursing process.

stantly reassess, replan, reimplement, and reevaluate as the patient's condition changes. The end result is reached when the patient's goals and objectives are met. Figure 11-1 is a schematic drawing of the nursing process.

Now, superimpose the word "documentation" over each word in the nursing process diagram, and the documentation process emerges. Every aspect of the nursing process must be documented; otherwise, the sequence of the process breaks down and thinking is not reflected.

▷ Process Characteristics of Nursing and Documentation

Because both nursing and documentation are processes, they work best when completed. If the process stops, nursing care stops, or looks like it stops. Compare this to a car being made; this is called an "assembly process." If the assembly line stops, does the car get built? No, the car remains in whatever state it is until the assembly line starts up again. The same problem occurs when the nursing process stops. If a nurse collects a data base, but fails to make conclusions about the strengths and health concerns of a patient, how can a plan of care be developed or action taken? The nursing process stopped short. Until the nurse identifies the patient's needs (makes conclusions as part of assessment), a safe, effective, and efficient plan cannot be formulated. In another situation, the nurse may assess, develop, and document a wonderful plan, but, if the plan is never implemented, the nursing process stops at planning. If nothing is done for the patient, there are no outcomes to evaluate and the nursing process is incomplete.

Now, again, add the word "documentation" to the preceding paragraph. If documentation does not accompany each part of the nursing process, there can be no high-quality nursing care except for very short-term interventions by one nurse. If one nurse does not communicate to other health care providers what has been done or what needs follow-up, the next person must start the process all over again. This results in sporadic care and inefficient use of the nurse's and the patient's time and energy.

▷ Sequential Characteristics of the Nursing and Documentation Processes

Both the nursing process and the documentation processes are sequential. "Sequential" does not mean strictly linear. The nurse constantly goes back and forth among the phases of the process many times before all the phases are completed. Sequence is important, however, in that some things must be done before others. For example, to change a flat tire on a car, one would first get the jack and tire iron out of the trunk, then remove the hubcap, loosen the lug nuts, raise the car on the jack, and so forth. The lug nuts cannot be loosened without first removing the hubcap, but they must be loosened before the car is jacked up. The tire-changing process illustrates the importance of certain things being done first. Examine the tire-changing process in relation to the components of the nursing process:

Assess: Recognizing the car doesn't steer quite right: "Oh, no, I've got a flat tire! I'll be late for class."

Plan: Thinking through what needs to be done efficiently and safely: "I guess I'd better change tires! What do I do first? Do I have everything I need? Do I remember how to do it safely? Will I need outside help? Should I have kept up my road service insurance? Where is the nearest phone? I need to get out the right equipment and do this in the right sequence."

Implement: Changing the tire: Get the jack and tire iron out of the trunk, remove the hubcap, loosen the lug nuts, raise the car on the jack, and so forth . . . until the tire is changed.

Evaluate: Determining if desired outcome was met and making changes in plan: "I did it; I changed the tire; good thing I had a spare with air. I'm going to have to buy some lubricant for those lug nuts so, if I get a flat again, I'll have something to help me loosen them. I'll also put a rag in here to wipe my hands when I'm done."

The point here is that one has to follow a reasonable, logical sequence of steps and document them (in the case of nursing care) along the way to achieve the desired purpose, whether it is changing a tire or caring for patients' needs. Otherwise, safe, efficient outcomes have a very low probability of occurring.

▷ Problems That Arise When Process and Sequence are Ignored

When the nursing process is not used in a sequential manner, the patient does not receive high-quality nursing care. This can result in prolonged hospitalization. Even worse, a problem may go unrecognized and untreated, which could result in serious complications or death for the patient. Consider the following examples of "partially processed nursing."

▶▶▶▶▶▶ **Action Learning #60: Mr. Schultz's Missing Care**

Read this case and answer the questions that follow:

CASE STUDY

Mr. Schultz had his gallbladder removed today and is now complaining of incisional pain. The nurse writes " Patient states pain is a 9 on a scale of 10. Patient is grimacing and holding abdomen." The nurse takes no action, however. She walks out of the room because she got paged for a phone call. Later, she comes back into Mr. Schultz's room and asks, " So, how are you doing?"

How do you think Mr. Schultz might respond?

If you were Mr. Schultz, how would you feel?

Which nursing process component(s) did the nurse complete? (Circle one or more.)

Assessing   Planning   Implementing   Evaluating

What should have happened to complete the nursing process for Mr. Schultz?

What else should the nurse have *assessed* in this case?

What should the nurse have *planned* to do?

What should the nurse have *done* (implemented) for Mr. Schultz?

How should the nurse have *evaluated* the care?

DISCUSSION   Clearly, this nurse began to assess Mr. Schultz's complaints of pain; however, there was no plan to do anything about his pain. Thus, poor Mr. Schultz continued having postoperative pain of uncertain origin.

▶▶▶▶▶ Action Learning #61: Mr. Fodler's Missing Care

Read about Mr. Fodler and answer the following questions:

CASE STUDY

Mr. Fodler had a CVA (cerebral vascular accident, or stroke) and has right-sided paralysis. The nurse enters Mr. Fodler's room, and starts feeding him breakfast. Mr. Fodler tries to interrupt the nurse, but, because he has difficulty speaking, he has trouble making his wishes known. The nurse speaks in a very loud voice to Mr. Fodler, telling him, "You must rest; you've had a stroke. Now let me do this for you." The nurse then proceeds to bathe, shave, brush his teeth, and dress him. Mr. Fodler simply gives up in disgust. The nurse finishes and can't understand why Mr. Fodler is so disgruntled.

Which component(s) of the nursing process did the nurse complete while caring for Mr. Fodler?

Assessing   Planning   Implementing   Evaluating

How do you think Mr. Fodler felt having this nurse care for him?

Which component(s) of the nursing process should have occurred *first* in Mr. Fodler's care?

DISCUSSION   You probably said the nurse needed to do some further assessment of Mr. Fodler's abilities to do his own care. Had the nurse done this, it would have become apparent that Mr. Fodler was able to feed, dress, and bathe himself. With a little more investigation, the nurse may have discovered that Mr. Fodler owns a business and has been self-sufficient since his early 20s, when he lost both parents. He is a very proud man and likes to do things for himself. He had made great strides in rehabilitation in adapting to his paralysis, but his strengths were being ignored.

With this additional information about Mr. Fodler, what more appropriate interventions could the nurse have tried? How would this additional information have saved the nurse a lot of unnecessary work and Mr. Fodler a lot of unnecessary frustration? What do you think of the efficiency and quality of nursing care this nurse delivered to Mr. Fodler?

In the last two examples, great nursing care was not given to these patients. The nurses did not demonstrate evidence of *thinking*. In the case of Mr. Schultz, the nurse assessed his pain, but did not seem to think about the patient's answers; hence, nothing was done to relieve his pain. In the case of Mr. Fodler, the nurse did not even assess his needs. Implementing nursing care that did not fit the patient's needs reflected a lack of thinking on the nurse's part. Thus, Mr. Fodler's strengths—being capable of performing some of his own activities of daily living—were not identified, and he was treated as an invalid unnecessarily.

► **CASE STUDIES ILLUSTRATING APPROPRIATE AND INAPPROPRIATE DOCUMENTATION**

Not only is it important to think to provide high-quality care to patients, it is equally important to document the care to reflect the thinking that occurred. The following case studies are from actual nursing malpractice suits (the names and cases have been altered to protect the privacy of those involved). Study the nursing care that was documented and analyze the documentation for evidence of thinking during use of the nursing process.

CASE STUDY

CASE STUDY #1: MRS. HENDRICKS

Mrs. Hendricks was admitted through the emergency room with a history of vaginal bleeding for several weeks. Her hemoglobin at that time was 4.0 (normal is 12 to 16). Her vital signs were stable and her only complaints were of being a little tired and cold (due to the low hemoglobin). She was admitted to the surgical unit where an IV line was started and blood transfusions were administered. The following narrative-style nurses' notes were recorded in her chart.

3/21/92

1300	The first unit of blood started to infuse into the right hand IV.—B. Smith, RN
1400	The right hand and fingernails became bluish in color. Radial pulse is palpable. Patient complains the hand feels numb and cold.—B. Smith, RN
1500	The right hand is purplish in color, but is not swollen.—B. Smith, RN
1600	Blood transfusion in progress infusing into right hand. The right hand is dark purple in color and swollen, the skin is cold and the hand is painful. Radial pulse is palpable. The IV was discontinued from the right hand and restarted in the left arm with an 18 gauge angiocath. The right hand was elevated on pillows and warm compresses were applied. Dr. Doyle was notified regarding the patient's hand. He states he will be in to see the patient as soon as possible.—J. Jones, RN

1800   Dr. Doyle in to examine patient's hand at 1630. See care plan for frequency of circulation checks and warm compresses. Continued to keep hand elevated on pillows. Medicated patient with 50 mg Demerol for pain, patient now states relief of pain. Hand remains swollen, purple in color, cool to touch with a palpable radial pulse.—J. Jones, RN

▶▶▶▶▶ Action Learning #62: Analyzing Documentation for Mrs. Hendricks

Examine the care B. Smith, RN (the first nurse) delivered to Mrs. Hendricks and answer this question: What components of the nursing process did B. Smith complete, beginning at 1400? It may be helpful to ask yourself: what did she assess, what did she plan, what did she do, and what did she evaluate?

Now, look at the notes written by J. Jones, RN beginning at 1600. Which components of the nursing process did she complete while caring for Mrs. Hendricks? Again, ask: what did she assess, what did she plan, what did she do, and what did she evaluate?

How were the approaches of the two nurses different?

DISCUSSION If you were a nurse–lawyer reading this record, what would you think of these nurses? How would you feel about defending their ability to use the nursing process?

Now, for the rest of the story. When B. Smith noticed that Mrs. Hendricks' right hand became blue, cold, and painful at 1400, those signs and symptoms should have indicated to the nurse the IV was no longer in the vein, but leaking into the subcutaneous tissues. The nurse should have been thinking about the relationship between pieces of data by using TOTAL RECALL of population norms for color, comfort level, and temperature of hands, along with signs and symptoms of IV infiltration. She should have used INQUIRY to ask herself if this situation was normal and what might be happening. When an IV leaks into subcutaneous tissue, it is necessary to discontinue the IV and restart it in another vein. However, Ms. Smith failed to do this. Instead, at 1500, the hand remained discolored; in fact, by then it was purple in color, and the IV blood transfusion continued into it.

At 1600, when J. Jones took over the care of Mrs. Hendricks, she assessed the hand, recognized the signs and symptoms as a problem, planned, and took action. She discontinued the IV, elevated the hand on a pillow, applied warm compresses to help reduce the swelling, and contacted the physician, who ordered pain medication. Ms. Jones treated Mrs. Hendricks' pain and the swelling and, at 1800, she reassessed and evaluated her previous care.

Because B. Smith did not discontinue the IV at 1400 (she did not plan and implement) when the first signs of infiltration occurred, and because it wasn't until 1600 (2 hours later) that the IV was finally discontinued, Mrs. Hendricks' hand became very swollen and gangrene eventually developed. Unfortunately, Mrs. Hendricks had to undergo surgery to amputate part of her index finger, as well as all of the other three fingers. She then had a second surgery to revise the stumps for possible placement of artificial fingers (prostheses). She had a third surgery to place the prostheses. To make matters worse, Mrs. Hendricks was right handed.

CASE STUDY #2: MS. ROSE

Ms. Rose was a 26-year-old admitted to the hospital for treatment of an abscess on the right side of her neck. She was treated with IV antibiotics and pain medications. Ms. Rose had a history of Raynaud's disease (poor circulation to the hands and feet). Her doctor, Dr. Bell, also diagnosed a clotting disorder. To treat the clotting problem, Dr. Bell prescribed a medication, Konyne, which contains clotting factors V, VII, and IX. These notes were recorded on the third day of Ms. Rose's hospitalization. Study this narrative documentation and look for evidence of the nurses' thinking during use of the nursing process.

2/22/93

1600   IV was restarted in the left thumb. Patient was given Tylenol grains X for complaint of left arm pain.——H. Hannon, RN

2000   Patient complains of tingling of left hand and fingers, IV is patent, no swelling is noted.——H. Hannon, RN

2200   Patient complains of pain in the left hand and arm, IV patent. Slight swelling of the entire arm is noted. It is cool to touch and firm, slightly discolored. Radial pulse is present.——H. Hannon, RN

2230   Dr. Bell was called regarding patient's left arm complaints. Ordered 3 inches of Nitropaste to be applied to the left arm. Paste was applied and the patient was given Percocet 5, two tablets, for pain. The IV was removed from the left thumb.——H. Hannon, RN

2/23/93

0045   Continued to complain of arm pain. Arm continues to be dusky in color. Lower arm and hand are swollen. IV was restarted in the right hand with 22 gauge angiocath.——T. Rizer, RN

0300   Percocet 5, two tablets were given for left arm pain.——T. Rizer, RN

0400   Left arm and hand continue to be swollen and painful, elevated on pillow.——T. Rizer, RN

0800   Left arm edematous, hand highly swollen. Finger joints highly swollen and spongelike. Skin cool, color dusky. Unable to palpate radial pulse due to edema.——D. Davis, RN

1000   Crying, complaining of much pain in left arm and hand. Demerol and Vistaril IM given.——D. Davis, RN

1130   Some relief noted, but pain not completely gone. ——D. Davis, RN

1200   Dr. Bell in to see patient. Ordered venous Doppler study and morphine for pain management.——D. Davis, RN

1400   Morphine 5 mg IV for complaints of severe pain.
Left arm is the same. Patient to Vascular Lab for
Doppler study.——D. Davis, RN

1600   Returned from Vascular Lab. Left arm, shoulder to
hand has major edema, firm, appears twice the size
of the right arm. From elbow to fingers, pale pur-
ple/blue in color, cool and very painful to touch.
——D. Davis, RN

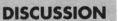

Action Learning #63: Part A. Analyzing Documentation for Ms. Rose

Study the documentation done by H. Hannon, RN from 1600 to 2230. Which
components of the nursing process did Mr. Hannon complete when caring for
Ms. Rose? Did he assess? Plan? Implement? Evaluate? Write the appropriate
component label next to each part of the documentation that it reflects.

DISCUSSION   You might have said, "There is documented evidence that
he identified all components as being done except evalua-
tion." The documentation reflects only assessing, planning, and implementing.
After Mr. Hannon described the condition of the hand and arm to Dr. Bell, the
physician thought Ms. Rose was having a Raynaud's disease attack (of poor
circulation, causing the discoloration and pain). The nurse applied Nitropaste
to the arm. Nitropaste is a vasodilator and, if this were a Raynaud's disease
attack, one would expect to see the circulation in the arm improve. This would
be evident by the arm returning to its natural pink color, the temperature becoming warm to the touch, and the patient having no further pain. Unfortunately, there is no documentation that anyone evaluated the results of
applying the Nitropaste to the arm. The documentation indicates that only partially processed nursing was given.

▶▶▶▶▶ **Action Learning #63: Part B. Further Analysis of Documentation for Ms. Rose**

Study the documentation done by T. Rizer, RN on the midnight shift. Which components of the nursing process did she document?

Was the patient still having problems with the hand and arm?

What could Ms. Rizer have done for Ms. Rose?

DISCUSSION Ms. Rizer's documentation shows that she assessed, planned, implemented, and evaluated her care. Unfortunately, her interventions were not effective. The patient's arm was getting worse; she required stronger pain medication, (Percocet is stronger than Tylenol), and the pain was not being controlled. As of 0400, the patient was still complaining of pain.

▶▶▶▶▶ **Action Learning #63: Part C. Further Analysis of Documentation for Ms. Rose**

Study the documentation of the day-shift nurse, Ms. Davis. Which components of the nursing process did Ms. Davis complete, as demonstrated by her documentation?

DISCUSSION Ms. Davis also assessed, planned, implemented, and evaluated, but was there still a problem? There certainly was! Look at her assessment of Ms. Rose's arm at 0800. The arm was getting worse instead of better. At 1000, she gave Ms. Rose a Demerol and Vistaril injection for pain (Demerol and Vistaril are stronger pain medications than Percocet).

The 1600 assessment showed the arm to be worse even after the patient was given more medication (morphine) for pain management. Obviously, there was something seriously wrong with this arm that was not being dealt with effectively by stronger and stronger pain medication.

CASE STUDY

At 1400, Ms. Rose had a venous Doppler study done that showed a large blood clot in the left subclavian vein. This clot was causing the poor circulation to the arm. The clot was caused by the Konyne (the medication with clotting factors) that Dr. Bell had prescribed. Dr. Bell had made an error in diagnosing the clotting problem from the beginning. Ms. Rose never should have received this medication and, in fact, it made her blood clot too much. (Dr. Bell was sued for misdiagnosing the clotting problem.) The patient was eventually transferred to another hospital, where many efforts were made to save her left arm. Unfortunately, the arm had to be amputated because it became gangrenous.

This scenario about Ms. Rose illustrates what can happen when all phases of the nursing process are not used well or are not documented. Continual evaluation of patient care is extremely important. If patients' conditions do not improve or if there is little progress toward goals and objectives, the nurse must reassess, replan, reimplement, and reevaluate. Nurses must communicate clearly all aspects of care with other health care providers. Without that communication, each nurse works without knowing what previous nurses assessed, planned, implemented, and evaluated. There is no continuity of care, patients suffer, and time is wasted.

Both written and verbal communication are needed to achieve continuity of care. In the preceding scenario, both written and verbal communication obviously were lacking. For example, if Mr. Hannon had said to Ms. Rizer: "I put some Nitropaste on Ms. Rose's arm and haven't had a chance to see if it did any good. Please be sure to check on that, and if it's not better, call Dr. Bell," the outcome may have been entirely different for this patient. Because Ms. Rizer's notes show no continuation of the work that Mr. Hannon started, one can assume that Mr. Hannon did not communicate his plan or his thinking processes to the next nurse.

▷ Clarity and Specificity of Documentation

In the preceding case studies, the nurses not only did not document safe nursing, they apparently did not provide it either. What about nurses who provide safe care but who still do not document that care? Unclear or missing documentation of care can cause as many problems as not doing the care. Notes must be clear and specific so that the care is fully communicated. It is not enough, however, merely to list what was done for a patient. The patient's response to care (evaluation) also must be noted so that patient progress can be tracked. Without that, the patient's condition may worsen without anyone noticing the change.

▶▶▶▶▶▶ **Action Learning #64: Charting Patient Responses and Nursing Care**

Compare the following two examples of nurses' notes on the same patient. Explain why the second one is better than the first.

Note #1: Assessment completed, AM care completed, medications given as ordered, tube feeding maintained and decubitus ulcer dressings changed per protocol.——I. Root, RN

Note #2: See Assessment Sheet and Care Flowsheet for details of assessment and routine care. Patient shows good response to morning dose of furosemide with 600 cc urine output and less edema present in his ankles. Tolerating tube feedings at 100 cc per hour, without evidence of aspiration; residuals are less than 5 cc. Decubitus ulcer dressings changed after the patient was premedicated with Demerol and Vistaril. Lesion on coccyx, 4 cm by 6 cm and 1/2 cm deep, has pink granulation tissue present, no drainage noted. The right heel ulcer, 2 cm by 2 cm, covered with black eschar. Travase ointment is beginning to debride the outer edge of lesion area. See nursing care plan for updated dressing protocol. Patient tolerated procedure with minimal discomfort.——B. Greenwald, RN

The second note is better because:

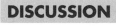 **DISCUSSION**   Does the first note tell you anything about the patient or how the patient is responding to treatments? The only thing you can deduce from this note is that the patient is receiving tube feedings and has a problem with pressure sores (decubitus ulcers).

It is expected that nurses assess their patients. If fact, in some institutions, there are requirements that there be a written assessment at specified

intervals, such as every 8 hours. It also is expected that patients receive proper attention to hygiene. Often this routine type of care is recorded on a flowsheet rather than in note format. Ms. Root's note is focused on those routine things that were done, rather than on the actual data found through assessment. Actually, the statement about the routine, "medications given as ordered," is worrisome. Would a nurse give medications as *not* ordered? That would be practicing medicine without a license! The statement as recorded is redundant.

In contrast to Ms. Root's note, Ms. Greenwald's note gives a clear picture of the patient's responses. For example, the medication furosemide is a diuretic, which causes the patient to remove excess fluid from his body by making more urine. The note clearly identifies how well this drug is working. The patient is also receiving tube feedings at 100 cc per hour. Problems that can occur with tube feedings include abdominal distention as the feeding sits in the stomach, diarrhea if too much is given, or aspiration of the feeding into the lungs if the patient vomits. The note tells how the patient is responding to the tube feeding so the reader would know that none of those potential problems had occurred.

There also is a clear description of the status of the decubitus ulcers. The nurse noted the size of the lesions and that granulation tissue was present. (Granulation is healthy tissue that fills in the wound. Eventually, skin will grow to cover the granulation tissue.) She also described a black eschar on one of the wounds. Eschar is dark, dead tissue, which must be removed (debrided) before the remainder of the wound will heal. These facts would let readers know exactly how the lesions looked on that day, so that nurses caring for this patient in the future would be able to judge how things have changed.

Also, note that the nurse in the second example did not simply repeat the nursing care plan; nor did she say that she had done this and that. By recording the results of what she did, others know she did these things. For example, there was no need to say, "Checked tube feeding residuals every shift." This appears on the care plan. But by recording, "Tube feeding residuals are less than 5 cc," one knows she executed her plan. Notes should be as brief as possible, because no one wants to read pages and pages of unnecessary information. By recording the results of one's actions, the reader knows the plan was executed and knows how the patient responded to the actions.

▼ THINKING-LEARNING CHECK

Pause here for a thinking-learning check. You should be able to elaborate on these ideas:

  - ▼ Nursing and documentation are both processes.
  - ▼ The nursing process and the process of documentation both follow a sequential pattern.

> ▼ Illustrations of what can happen when those patterns are not followed show how dangerous poor-quality nursing care can be.
>
> ▼ Clarity in documenting care is as important as the care itself.

▶ DOCUMENTATION AS PART OF QUALITY ASSURANCE

It is essential that patients have an assurance of high-quality health care. High-quality health care is not only cost effective in the long run ("Do it right the first time and you do not have to do it again," or "A stitch in time saves nine"), it is a matter of safety or even life and death.

▷ Who Assures Quality, and How?

High-quality care is the individual responsibility of each nurse, but there also are formal professional and institutional mechanisms to ensure that high-quality care is provided. High-quality nursing is defined and standards for that quality are set forth in such guidelines as State Nurse Practice Acts and Standards of Practice developed by the American Nurses' Association. Health care institutions also have formal programs for assuring high-quality care. Often there are representatives from all branches of health care delivery, including nursing, who serve on committees to oversee quality in the institution. There also are external agencies, such as the Joint Commission on Accreditation of Health Care Organizations, that send auditors to institutions to ensure that quality, as defined in specific criteria, is being maintained.

How nurses use and document the nursing process plays an important role in quality assurance. This role is played out in many ways, even in the specific parts of a documented plan of care. Look at the following example of a patient objective (outcome statement) found on a nursing care plan. "Patient will independently administer the correct dose of insulin subcutaneously using aseptic technique." If the nurse or an auditor were assessing for the quality of care related to this objective, that person would look for some documentation that the patient could or did achieve this outcome. One way to do that would be to see if the outcome was measurable and realistic for this patient, and, later, if the patient achieved this outcome.

The outcome statement is measurable, but because the patient is partially blind and has severe arthritis in his hands, it is not realistic. This patient would not be able to achieve this outcome. If the statement is revised, however, it can become realistic. A revised patient outcome statement for this particular patient might be as follows: "The patient's wife will independently administer the correct dose of insulin to the patient, subcutaneously using aseptic technique."

If the nurse had pursued the first outcome, the patient would never have achieved it. High-quality care would not be achieved. The nurse would have wasted valuable time and money while frustrating the patient and preventing him from receiving his insulin correctly once he was discharged home. With his insulin being given incorrectly, the patient's diabetes would be uncontrolled, and severe diabetic complications ultimately would develop that would necessitate future hospitalizations and diminish his quality of life.

By pursuing the second outcome statement (having the wife learn to give the injection), however, there is a much better chance of success. The second outcome statement is both measurable and realistic for this patient. With it, the nurse would not waste time and money; the patient, his wife, and the nurse would not become frustrated, and the patient's diabetes would be managed. Documentation of the second outcome statement reflects planning of high-quality care. Later, when the outcome is evaluated, documentation of that evaluation can reflect high-quality care as well.

▷ Quality Assurance Audits

Nursing documentation often is audited (reviewed and evaluated) through quality assurance programs. There are preset criteria that auditors use that are closely related to the policies of the institution. The records are reviewed to make sure everything that should be documented is indeed being documented. The person doing the auditing may be a staff nurse or a nurse specifically assigned to auditing duties. Here are some examples of policies that could serve as criteria for a medical record audit. The auditor would search records to ensure that these policies were being followed.

Nurses' notes:

1. Are written every 8 hours.
2. Reflect the patient's or family's response to nursing intervention.
3. Are signed with the appropriate nursing signature.

Nursing care plan interventions:

1. Reflect orders specific to each patient problem.
2. Are written in measurable, behavioral terms so staff know exactly what is to be done for the patient.
3. Are updated as the patient's condition changes.

▶▶▶▶▶ Action Learning #65: Mr. Smock's Missing Details

Assume you are a nurse quality assurance auditor. Read the following case study and documentation. Audit the notes by answering the questions, using the criteria provided.

CASE STUDY

Mr. Smock, 56 years old, was admitted for complaints of shortness of breath with any activity and a blood glucose level of 265 (normal is 60 to 120) on November 23rd at 8 AM. He has a history of congestive heart failure and insulin-dependent diabetes mellitus. He was placed on 2 L of oxygen. At home he took insulin, Lasix, and digoxin, but said the doctor told him his medications needed to be adjusted. The following admission note was found on his chart:

11/24/93

1600   56-year-old male admitted to bed 42B on 11/23/93 at 0800. Resting in bed with call light within reach, watching television.——BW, RN

Audit the above admission note using the following criteria:
Admission notes:

1. Address each patient problem within 12 hours of admission

2. Are accurately timed and dated

3. Are signed with the appropriate signature and title

Does the admission note meet criterion #1? Why or why not?

Does the admission note meet criterion #2? Why or why not?

Does the admission note meet criterion #3? Why or why not?

Practice writing a better admission note for Mr. Smock; then have a classmate audit your note to see if you meet the criteria.

| DISCUSSION | In the example given here, but hopefully not in your own, criterion #1 was not met because the nurse did not ad-dress Mr. Smock's problems. He had two medical problems—congestive heart failure and diabetes mellitus. The nurse did not record anything about those issues. Remember, monitoring medical problems is part of the interdependent function of nurses. The nurse did not record anything about independent nursing functions, so no one even knows what nursing diagnoses exist. Even with the limited information known, it was highly likely that the nursing diagnosis, "Activity Intolerance related to shortness of breath and congestive heart failure" should have been a conclusion.

Criterion #1 also was not met because the note was not written until 11/24 at 4 PM, 32 hours after the patient was admitted!

Assuming the date and time recorded were accurate, criterion #2 was met in this example.

Criterion #3 was not met. An appropriate signature is first initial, last name, and title. Initials and title do not constitute an appropriate signature. An appropriate signature would be "B. Walton, RN."

▶ DOCUMENTATION AND INCIDENT REPORTS

Even for great nurses, there are occasions when something happens to a patient that should not happen; the patient may be given the wrong medication or may fall out of bed. When something of this nature occurs, it is called an *incident*. It is important to document the incident because the patient may require follow-up medical and nursing care, and the health care institution needs to know the incident occurred to prevent the same type of incident from occurring again. For these two reasons, it is necessary to address the incident in the medical record as well as in an *incident report*. The note in the record will allow other care providers to follow up on any care, and the incident report allows the institution to monitor such risks. There are specific "Risk Management" committees or departments in most health care institutions that monitor incidents and plan actions to prevent them from reoccurring.

In documenting an incident, the following five basic guidelines should be followed:

1. The person who discovers the incident, even if he or she is not the person who was involved in the incident, should write the report.

2. In the medical record, nursing documentation should reflect the nursing process. In other words, what did the nurse assess, plan, do, and evaluate with regard to the patient relative to the incident?

3. The incident report form must be completed according to the institution's policy and procedure (these vary from institution to institution).

4. *Never* make reference to an incident report itself in the patient's medical record. The incident report is *not* part of the patient's medical record. The incident report belongs to the hospital and is used for internal tracking of incidents.

5. In the section of the incident report that calls for a description of the patient's condition and what the nurse assessed, simply copy the nurse's note from the medical record onto the incident report form.

▷▷▷▷▷▷ **Action Learning #66: Tracking an Incident: Mr. Katz's IV**

Read the case study and documentation. Then evaluate the documentation according to the guidelines for documenting an incident. You will be able to use numbers 1, 2, and 4 of the guidelines. For numbers 3 and 5, if possible, obtain a blank incident form from an agency where you practice and fill it out using the information in the case study and note.

CASE STUDY

The physician ordered an IV of 5% dextrose and water (D5W) at a rate of 20 cc per hour for Mr. Katz, who has a history of congestive heart failure. When Sally Tower, RN entered Mr. Katz's room on her initial rounds, she noticed Mr. Katz's IV was 0.9% saline infusing at a rate of 100 cc per hour. Sally slowed the IV rate, left the room, and obtained a bag of D5W. She returned to Mr. Katz's room, discontinued the 0.9% saline, and hung the bag of D5W. She double-checked the rate of infusion, making sure it was at 20 cc per hour, and auscultated Mr. Katz's lungs, noting that his lungs sounded clear. She also noted that Mr. Katz had no sacral or pedal edema, and asked him if he felt short of breath. She then called Mr. Katz's physician and informed him Mr. Katz had received approximately 700 cc of 0.9% saline and reported her other findings. Then Sally documented the following in Mr. Katz's chart:

11/30/93
1630   IV of 0.9% NS infusing at rate of 100 cc/hr. 0.9% NS discontinued. D5W at 20 cc/hr IV initiated. Patient's lung sounds are clear, no sacral or pedal edema noted. Patient has no complaints of dyspnea. Dr. Butler notified of patient's current status. Will continue to monitor patient for fluid overload.——Sally Tower, RN.

DISCUSSION Based on Sally's note, one can see that she assessed (wrong IV solution and rate), planned ("I need to correct this situation."), intervened (hung the correct solution, adjusted the infusion rate, and called the physician), and evaluated (the patient's lungs were clear, and he had no edema or difficulty breathing). After Sally documented the incident in the patient's medical record, she could copy her note directly from the record onto the separate incident report form for the hospital's use.

▶ **LEGAL RAMIFICATIONS OF DOCUMENTATION**

The medical record is the only legal record of the care the patient received as well as of the patient's response to that care. Documentation is a professional responsibility and is as important as delivering care. If a patient receives care, but no one documents it, there is no way other caregivers, auditors, or lawyers can know what was done and how the patient responded. How is the hospital to be reimbursed for the care provided to patients if there is no documented evidence of care? Documentation is a *must* (Marrelli, 1992).

If a patient decides to sue because of the care received or not received, one of the first documents the attorney representing the patient will request is the medical record. The attorney can request parts or all of a medical record as well as billing statements. Nurses' notes are part of the medical record and will be requested by the attorney.

If nurses' documentation reflects the nursing process and appropriate actions taken, chances are the documentation will stand up very well in a malpractice suit. In addition, the documentation will serve to remind nurses of the care they gave to that patient. By the time a suit is brought to court and nurses are questioned by attorneys about their practice, 2 or more years may have elapsed. It is possible, indeed likely, that the nurses would not remember this particular patient, let alone what they assessed and what they did for the patient. Documentation is what nurses have to rely on to refresh their memories. Documentation completed today that reflects the nursing process will be a welcome sight to the nurse who is facing a possible malpractice claim tomorrow.

▶ **CLOSING COMMENTS: THE IMPORTANCE OF THINKING AND DOCUMENTING**

The nursing process and the documentation process both require thinking. Thinking that occurs during the use of the nursing process allows the nurse effectively and efficiently to assess, plan, implement, and evaluate care. If thinking continues to be used in the documentation process, anyone reading the documentation will quickly recognize the quality of thinking and care provided. Thinking and great nursing care are most easily measured by great documentation of care and patient outcomes. The phrase, "If it's not documented, it didn't happen," is a useful reminder to both beginning and experienced nurses to dedicate time and energy to high-quality documentation.

▶▶▶ *THINKING LOG #11*

Think of a recent note you wrote in a patient's medical record. Recreate that note as accurately as possible. (*Remember* not to use the patient's name for the sake of confidentiality.) Describe how the note would help or hinder you if you had to defend your actions in court. Evaluate your note to see if it reflects the nursing process. Are all four components present? If not, what should be added to this note so that it does reflect the nursing process?

REFERENCE

Marrelli, T. M. (1992). *Nursing documentation handbook*. St. Louis: Mosby Year Book.

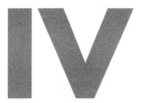

Thinking Through a Complex Patient Situation

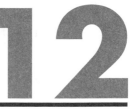

Assessing a Complex Patient Situation

After reading and doing the activities in this chapter you will be able to:

Track the thinking skills and content knowledge used to complete the assessment phase of the nursing process in a complex patient situation.

Set priorities for care in a complex patient situation.

This final section of this workbook, Chapters 12 through 15, is designed to pull all the pieces of thinking and doing back together into the "big picture" of great nursing. Looking at the big picture is an important theme that was introduced in Chapters 3 and 4, but the view from now on will be different. This time, the view will be enhanced because of the reader's growing sophistication in thinking about the nursing process and personal thinking abilities.

This section provides an opportunity to work with and think through a complex patient situation, from data collection and analysis (assessment) to determining the quality of care (evaluation.) Even though this is a more complex situation, the nurse uses the same thinking skills and the same nursing process that were used with simpler nursing situations. Those skills, however, are evolving with experience. The primary purpose of this section is to continue to acknowledge and nurture the reader's existing thinking skills as those skills grow toward achieving the goal of providing great nursing. A "Tracking Nursing Thinking" checklist is provided in Appendix B to aid this continuing learning process, and will be used throughout these last chapters.

This chapter briefly reviews the equation for great nursing that was introduced in Chapter 3, and then focuses on the case study of a woman named Betty. Her data base is presented on the Nursing Assessment Tool given in Display 12-1. The nurse's thinking, from the initial analysis to setting priorities for the assessment conclusions, is highlighted throughout this chapter.

Chapters 13 through 15 illustrate how care was designed and revised over time for Betty. Planning, implementing, and evaluating relative to each health concern are described.

To promote an appreciation of the qualitative differences in thinking during the nursing process, alternative care plans are presented in Chapters 13 and 14. Some of those plans are of poor to mediocre quality, and are critiqued and improved to illustrate the contrast in quality. The improved plans for actual problems and potential (high risk for . . .) problems illustrate not only increased quality but the differences in approaches for each of these types of problems. Planning for interdisciplinary problems, problems for referral, and wellness issues is discussed in Chapter 15.

As noted in the Introduction to this book, these final four chapters can be read and used at any point in the course of study. Some may find it helpful to examine this more complex "big picture" even before starting Chapter 1.

▶ RETURNING TO THE BIG PICTURE OF GREAT NURSING

The big picture, as described in Chapter 3, presented great nursing and its components. The components included the patient, the nurse (you), thinking skills, content knowledge, and the nursing process. A linear equation was presented to illustrate how all these components added up to great nursing:

$$\text{Patient} + \text{You} + \frac{\text{Thinking}}{\text{Skills}} + \frac{\text{Content}}{\text{Knowledge}} + \frac{\text{Nursing}}{\text{Process}} = \text{Great Nursing}$$

At that point, this equation was sufficient, but by now most readers should be questioning its simplicity. As you proceed through the next four chapters, give some serious thought to this equation. Reexamine the components and their relationships to each other in more depth. In Chapter 16, the final chapter of this text, the reader is asked to change this simple equation into something that better represents the dynamic qualities of the components.

▶ TRACKING THINKING

Even with of a deeper understanding of the concepts (components) contributing to great nursing and an increased awareness of individual thinking skills, it remains challenging for nurses to identify and track thinking because of its abstract nature. To assist the reader in systematically tracking the *thinking* and *doing* that occurred in the course of assessing, planning, implementing, and evaluating care for Betty, a simple checklist was developed. A checklist can never begin to measure the dynamic nature of thinking, but it can serve as a trigger to ensure the basics are addressed.

The checklist, called "Tracking Nursing Thinking" (TNT), is given in Appendix B. The TNT serves two major purposes. For chapters 12 through 15, it helps the reader track the *thinking* and *doing* of the nurse caring for Betty. But, more important, the TNT can serve as a guide for students as they use the nursing process. The TNT also may serve as a guide for self-evaluation and instructor evaluation. Student nurses using the prototype of the TNT found it to be dynamite!

▶ TRACKING THINKING THROUGH ASSESSMENT OF A COMPLEX PATIENT SITUATION

This section of the chapter examines a patient situation. Patient data are recorded on the Nursing Assessment Tool. The thinking that takes place from a point before data collection through to the major conclusions of assessment is studied. The final discussion of thinking focuses on working with the patient in prioritizing those conclusions.

The patient for this case study is Betty. Although Betty is not her real name, she is a real person with very real health concerns. High-level thinking is necessary to design individualized nursing care for her. Two years ago, Betty was told she had a progressive chronic disease affecting her motor neurons, amyotrophic lateral sclerosis (ALS). Betty is currently living at home in the northern part of the United States. The data were collected in late fall, as the first snows of winter were approaching.

▶ ENGAGING THINKING SKILLS AND CONTENT KNOWLEDGE

A certain amount of information (content knowledge) is helpful before the nurse begins collecting patient data. That knowledge helps the nurse collect the best data in the most efficient manner, and make sense of the data *during* collection.

▷ Basic Content Knowledge Needed Before Initial Data Collection

In all patient situations, the nurse must use content knowledge gained from TOTAL RECALL of information learned or from referring to some source to obtain that knowledge. For beginning students who are learning the content knowledge while they are simultaneously learning how to use that knowledge, there is that "cart before the horse" problem. It takes time to learn something and more time to learn how to apply that something in a patient situation. What expert nurses take for granted, novices must still learn. Novices must recognize that there are key areas of knowledge needed for each situation;

there are points in the process where the knowledge is needed and there are good, better, and best ways to use that knowledge.

Knowledge about the usual or "normal" provides standards for population norms. Knowledge of population norms allows the nurse to compare a patient's response to what is usually seen and make decisions about the significance of data. But knowledge of population norms alone does not help the nurse to develop individualized care; it only guides standardized care. To achieve individualized care, the nurse must know about the patient's individual norms and strengths, as well as about caring. Individual norms are discovered by asking the patient about them; caring leads the nurse to recognize the need to collect that individual data.

There are three general categories of knowledge that are helpful before major data collection takes place:

▼ Demographic data

▼ Major health issues affecting the patient

▼ Typical patient response patterns to the major health issues and corresponding nursing care issues

First, the demographic data include age (chronologic as well as developmental), gender, marital status, and the like. This basic information provides the nurse with a general starting point. With Betty, who is a 46-year-old, white, divorced woman with two sons, aged 16 and 20 years, knowing what is normal helps to identify relevant data (different from the norm) as they are collected later. The nurse must look up or RECALL the norms associated with these demographic data. For example, 46-year-old women are generally healthy, productive people who may be experiencing early signs of menopause.

Second, the major health issues affecting the patient include things like life stressors, situational or developmental crises, or medical diagnoses. In Betty's case these issues include a medical diagnosis of ALS and all the ramifications of having a chronic terminal disease. This knowledge guides the nurse's questions during data collection to focus on areas that typically are problems requiring nursing care.

Third, the typical patient response patterns to these major health issues and corresponding nursing care issues include how Betty is responding to her ALS disease in her eating patterns, sleeping patterns, elimination patterns, relationships with others, coping, and so forth. Understanding that all physiologic, psychological, social, cultural, and spiritual responses are affected by illness helps the nurse focus data collection on the "big picture." Applying this global understanding to assessment is key to grasping the holistic nature of nursing. Nurses must obtain a large amount of data to determine the full range of a patient's responses.

Although these content areas are very important to know for the nurse effectively to ask questions and make comparisons with the population norms, the nurse must be careful not to stereotype the patient by looking only for data that fit the classic cases (population norms). INQUIRY is critical here to keep an open mind and go beyond the standards to identify the patient's individual norms as well. For example, many patients with ALS become depressed and withdrawn as a way of coping with impending death. Data on Betty's emotional state do not indicate this typical coping response to ALS. Betty, therefore, does not fit into the population norm, but fits her own norm.

In most situations, the nurse will have this basic type of information either before working with the patient or at the very beginning of the interaction. For experienced nurses, with a great deal of stored content knowledge and experience, the timing of learning this basic information about the patient is not a big issue. The experienced nurse can process it all very quickly and draw on it as he or she collects and analyzes data from the very start of the encounter.

For the beginning nurse, however, having this knowledge before meeting with the patient allows for time to "look up" the necessary content knowledge. The beginning nurse can then plan ahead and know to assess for the most important information first, and not waste time on less relevant areas. For example, in Betty's situation, assessing her understanding of the safety precautions she can take to avoid respiratory infections is much more important than assessing her immunization status for DPT (diphtheria, pertussis, and tetanus) or her family history of breast cancer. A common problem for beginning nurses and students is to assume that a Nursing Assessment Tool needs to be filled out starting with the top of page one and ending with the bottom of the last page. If time permits, this is fine, but when time is limited, it is best to focus data collection and analysis on the critical areas first.

▷ Basic Content Knowledge Needed About Betty's Situation Before Data Collection

Typically, healthy, independent, 46-year-old divorced women with two sons experience the common concerns of "middle age," with children starting to leave home and prepare for their separate lives. In Betty's case, stages of growth and development have been accelerated from that typical of middle age (generativity versus stagnation, with creativity, productivity, and work) to one more typical of old age, integrity versus despair (Erikson, 1963). One son who had left home is returning to provide some care. Her younger son also is now responsible for some caretaking, which is more typical of an adult role. Betty's role has changed from one of extreme independence to a fairly dependent one.

Knowledge about the disease and its course (how it progresses) also is critical. Amyotrophic lateral sclerosis is a neurologic disease of unknown cause in which the motor neurons of the spinal cord, medulla, and cortex degenerate. The primary problems are muscle weakness and the multisystem changes that go along with the progressive weakness. The course of this illness is highly individual, with most people living 3 to 5 years, but some living 10 to 20 years; death is often the result of a respiratory infective process. There is no treatment for the disease itself, only for the symptoms of the disease. Betty was diagnosed exactly 2 years ago.

There are many risk factors associated with ALS that stem from the muscle weakness. As the disease progresses, patients become increasingly immobile; immobility is associated with numerous hazards in almost all body areas. Gastric motility decreases, with concurrent nausea, indigestion, and constipation. Circulation is decreased, which can cause kidney problems, decreased urine output, edema, and decreased healing ability.

The respiratory system is affected in several ways. The muscles of the diaphragm and the chest may be weakened from the disease itself, so respirations become more shallow; secretions are not moved effectively. This is the most life-threatening problem; ultimately, patients with ALS may need tracheostomies and mechanical ventilation because they do not have the muscle power to breathe, or they get respiratory infections that they cannot overcome. Risk to the respiratory system is increased by swallowing difficulties that occur as muscles in the mouth and throat weaken. These swallowing difficulties increase the chance of choking and aspirating food or liquid into the lungs, which leads to either sudden death or aspiration pneumonia. Betty has experienced swallowing problems, but has not had problems with severe choking or pneumonia.

Content knowledge regarding a chronic, terminal illness with its corresponding physiologic, psychological, social, cultural, and spiritual effects also is necessary preencounter information. The nurse must be knowledgeable and look for signs and symptoms of continually declining physical abilities to care for self and cope with the environment. How quickly patients experience the deterioration in functioning with chronic terminal illness is very individual, even for those with similar diseases. Nurses must be aware of the ranges of normal decline, and observe the degree and speed of change for each individual patient. Anticipating the patient's changing safety needs is particularly important with regard to declining functional abilities.

There also are several psychosocial concerns that accompany chronic terminal illnesses. Loss of independence and major role changes within the family and society are only two of the possible changes with which patients must cope. Some patients are anxious to know what to expect, and others prefer not to know. The nurse must assess the patient's readiness to learn about the illness and its ongoing impact on physical and psychosocial functioning. Grieving and impending death, which affect spiritual and cultural responses, are also paramount concerns that affect not only the individual but also the family and significant others.

►►►►►► **A**ction Learning #67: Identifying Possible Sources
for the Content Knowledge Needed to Prepare
for Data Collection With Betty

Make a list of at least three sources from which to gain the content knowledge
needed in Betty's situation. Follow the format below.

Area of Content Knowledge   *Sources of Information*

DISCUSSION   How much of the knowledge did you already have? The
more experienced you are, the more you will have already
stored in your memory for instant retrieval. How much time did it take to find
the proper sources? Most beginning students find the hunt for multiple
sources of information to be a very time-consuming activity that requires per-
severance. Did you identify the areas on the TNT checklist that fit with content
knowledge?

▷ **The Thinking Needed to Put All the Pieces
Together to Structure Data Collection Efficiently
and Effectively**

The following is a short example of the thinking used (combination of **TOTAL
RECALL** and **INQUIRY**) to begin one small but very important segment of effective, efficient data collection:

Betty has ALS.
ALS causes the muscles of swallowing to weaken.
Weakened swallowing muscles allow patients to aspirate food and liq-
uids.
Aspirated food and liquid can cause either immediate death or infec-
tions such as pneumonia.

Therefore, the following are key pieces of data needed from Betty:

How are her swallowing muscles right now?
If they are weakened, what types of problems occur with swallowing?
Certain types of foods or liquids? Saliva?

Has she ever choked? How did she handle it?
Does she know what to do for choking?
Do her significant others know what to do for choking?
What are her long-range plans for weakened swallowing muscles?
Does she understand the high risk she is at for aspiration?

This same process is used with all the available information about Betty. The more the nurse knows and *thinks* about before the initial encounter, the better prepared he or she is for focusing data collection and data analysis on the most important areas first.

▶ **COMBINING THINKING SKILLS, CONTENT KNOWLEDGE, THE NURSING PROCESS, THE PATIENT, AND YOU (THE NURSE)**

This section draws on what was learned in Chapters 7 and 8 regarding data collection (finding clues) and data analysis (making sense of the clues and clusters of clues). After the nurse prepared for the assessment by reviewing the areas of content knowledge that would be most needed, *thinking* about all the relationships possible, and identifying key questions to address, data were collected and initially analyzed using the Nursing Assessment Tool shown in Display 12-1.

Read through the data on the completed tool to obtain an overall picture of Betty's health status. Remember that the recorded data are "objective" (what the nurse can see, touch, hear, and so forth), "subjective" (what the patient or significant others say), and necessary inferences (objective data for which there is no precise means of measurement). Interaction was the primary method of collection, but observation and measurement were necessary as well. The use of D.E.T.A.I.L. (see Chapter 7) was helpful in collecting information about Betty's discomfort after her fall.

As data were collected, initial hunches were developed. Those hunches are noted by stars the nurse placed next to the nursing diagnoses (listed for each response area) that *could* be assessment conclusions about the data. As you read, think about the reasoning behind these initial hunches. Also, write down any additional ones you thought of that were not listed. Make a copy of the TNT checklist and keep it close by to track the thinking as it is described.

▷ **First Impressions**

As the data are collected (or read about), *thinking* also occurs—initial hunches and preliminary conclusions are formulated.

(text continues on p. 279)

Name _Betty_ **Age** _46_ **Sex** _F_ **Admit Date** _10/93_

Medical Diagnosis _ALS, Iron deficiency Anemia, Irritable bowel syndrome_

Allergies _None known_

Medications _Estrogen 0.625 mg QD, Baclofen 10 mg TID, Nortriptyline 75 mg Qhs. Metamucil 1pkt. prn.,_
Ferrous Sulfate 325 mg. QD

Persons/groups involved in care _Dep't. of Social Services, Methodist Church, County Hospice anticipated; Hannah Jones_
and Rhonda Smith (church friends)

COMMUNICATING: Sending messages
[Nsg. Dx.: Impaired Verbal Communication]

English (circle) (read,) (write,) (understand)

Other languages _Spanish (fluent)_

Speech impairments _Low, hoarse, monotone voice "its getting worse"_

Alternate form of communication _____

VALUING: Assigning relative worth
[Nsg. Dx.: Spiritual Distress]

Spiritual orientation _Methodist_

Important religious practices _None_

Cultural orientation _Mother is Greek, father from southern U.S._

Cultural practices _Likes southern cooking_

RELATING: Establishing bonds
Role
[Nsg. Dx.: Altered Role Performance, Altered Parenting, High Risk for Altered Parenting*, Sexual Dysfunction, Altered Family Processes, Caregiver Role Strain, High Risk For Caregiver Role Strain, Parental Role Conflict, Altered Sexuality Patterns]

Marital status or significant relationship _Divorced 15 years (mother in Ohio, father deceased)_

Age and health of significant other _N/A_

Number of children _2 sons_ Ages _20 & 16_

Role in home _16 yr. old son at home & in school; 20 yr. old son lives in same apt. complex_

Financial support _No income, but apt. rent & utilities paid by former employer; Appl. for SSI & Medicare completed_

Occupation _Retired (10/29/93) Apartment manager_

Job satisfaction/concerns _N/A_

Recent losses _job, independence, self care, ability to walk, some parenting activities_

Sexual habits _Celibate_

Relationships (satisfactory/unsatisfactory)

  Effects of illness on relationship _N/A_

  Sexual Concerns _N/A_

Socialization
[Nsg. Dx.: Impaired Social Interaction*, Social isolation]

Relationships with others _Close to Hannah & Rhonda "I have talked with ex-husband about caring for our son."_

 Patient's description _"My sons & friends are very helpful, I miss working."_

 Significant others' descriptions _per Hannah, pt's relationship with mother strained_

 Staff observations _Positive, open relationships_

KNOWING: Meaning associated with information
[Nsg. Dx.: Knowledge Deficit (Specify)*, Altered Thought Processes]

Perception of current health issues _"I've written my eulogy. I've come to accept the fact that I will die soon, probably this_
coming year. I have made plans for my funeral, talked with my minister, lawyer, ex-husband & sons about death."

Perception/knowledge of medications, treatments, procedures _Reported clearly what meds for. Said Nortriptyline for_
outbursts of laughing. Resists moving bed to first floor.

Previous illnesses/hospitalizations/surgeries _Perforated uterus during D&C (1974), Ruptured ovarian cyst (1978)_
Hysterectomy (1992) Several episodes of pneumonia & bronchitis (most recent 4 yrs. ago)

Display 12-1. Nursing assessment tool.

KNOWING (cont.)
History of the following:

	Patient	Family		Patient	Family
Anemia/Blood disorder	✓		Kidney Disease		
Cancer			Stroke		
Diabetes			Tuberculosis		
Heart Disease		_Father_	Alcohol/Substance Abuse		_Uncle_
Hypertension		_Father, Mother_	Smoking		_Parents_
Peripheral Vascular			Other		

Readiness to learn _Open, asks questions, listens attentively_
   Requests information about _Hospice, ALS_
   Education level _Business School Degree_
   Learning impediments _Fatigue & decreased vision ("difficult to read")_

Orientation
[Nsg. Dx.: High Risk for Injury]
Level of alertness _Alert_
Orientation: Person_____✓_____Place_____✓_____Time___✓___
Appropriate behavior/communication _Yes_

Memory
Memory intact: ⟨yes⟩/no Recent _____✓_____ Remote_____✓_____

Feeling: Subjective awareness of information
Physical Comfort
[Nsg. Dx.: Pain*, Chronic Pain]
Pain/discomfort: ⟨yes⟩/no If yes:
Date of onset/course _Yesterday, fell on kitchen floor, flat onto face_
Exact location _Teeth (broken front tooth), Lip (lacerated top lip), arm (left arm near elbow)_
Terms for quality and quantity _"My lip feels sore and puffy; my arm aches."_
Aggravating and alleviating factors _"Eating and chewing hot and cold liquids hurts my mouth, Tylenol helps dull the pain."_
Inter-system connections _Headache & nausea (Pt. went to Emergency Dep't. for this)_
Labeled by patient as: _"Frustrating," "Discouraging," "I should wear shoes more."_
Emotional Comfort
[Nsg. Dx.: Dysfunctional Grieving, Anticipatory Grieving, High Risk for Violence: Self directed or directed at others, High Risk for Self-Mutilation, Post-Trauma Response, Rape Trauma Syndrome, (Compound Reaction, Silent Reaction), Anxiety*, Fear*]
Recent stressful life events _Forced early retirement 2° ALS. Fall yesterday._
Many "hassles filling out forms for Social Security."
Verbalization of feelings of: _Frustration, anxiety about finances. "It's not death itself that I fear,_
but the interim time before I die."
Physical manifestations of emotions _None obvious_
Fears or concerns _" I've talked to my sons about how they will cope with my death and to my ex-husband about his caring for_
our youngest son." "I fear having to spend my final days with my mother."

MOVING: Activity
Activity
[Nsg. Dx.: Impaired Physical Mobility*, High Risk for Peripheral Neurovascular Dysfunction*, Activity* Intolerance, Fatigue*, High Risk for Activity Intolerance]
History of physical disability _ALS diagnosed 10/91_
Use of device _(cane, ⟨walker⟩ artificial limb) wheelchair ordered last week_
Limitations in daily activities _"I can walk short distances; it's hard to go up and down stairs, my son has to be behind me. I_
can't drive, cook, clean. My son does laundry and grocery shopping and drives me to my appointments."

Display 12-1. Continued.

MOVING (cont.)

Exercise habits _"I don't do any exercise at all"_

Physical symptoms with activity _Shortness of breath, fatigue, increased pulse, unsteadiness_

Rest

[Nsg. Dx.: Sleep Pattern Disturbance]

Hours slept/night _8-9_   Feels rested (yes)/no   Sleeps alone: (yes)/no

Position preference _Flat_ Naps during the day _None usually_

Sleep interruptions (number and type) _1-2 per night "I've always done this — just thinking"_

Sleep aids (pillows, meds, food) _"Just one pillow is fine"_

Difficulty falling/remaining asleep _None_

Recreation

[Nsg. Dx.: Diversional Activity Deficit]*

Usual leisure activities _"Shopping, going to movies and plays. I used to write poetry & read a lot."_

Usual social activities _Job had much social contact, lunch outings with Hannah and Rhonda_

Illness-related changes _Home alone; difficulty going to restaurants, ("smoke bothers me") "I get bored, I can go out only if_
someone takes me. I've worked all my life; I'm not used to so much free time."

Home Maintenance

[Nsg. Dx.: Impaired Home Maintenance Management]

Size & arrangement of home ((stairs)/bathroom) _2-floor apt; 2 bathrooms - full bath upstairs, & 1/2 bath downstairs, 2_
steps to enter apt, kitchen floor tiled & slippery, carpets in other rooms

Safety issues _Cluttered rooms, no safety bars in bathrooms. Safe neighborhood. Pt wearing socks._

Ability to maintain home _"I can't do housework." Sons & friends clean; sons do laundry and grocery shopping._

Health Maintenance

[Nsg. Dx.: Altered Health Maintenance]

Health insurance _HMO, Appl. for Medicare, SSI completed_

Schedule of health exams _MD seen monthly, Dentist every 6 months_

Access to health care _Friends, son must provide transportation_

Self exams (breast, testicular) _"I used to do self breast exams, but not as often as I should."_

Self Care

[Nsg. Dx.: Feeding Self Care Deficit*, Impaired Swallowing*, Ineffective Breastfeeding, Interrupted Breastfeeding, Effective Breastfeeding, Ineffective Infant Feeding Pattern, Bathing/Hygiene Self Care* Deficit, Dressing/Grooming Self Care Deficit*, Toileting Self Care Deficit]

Ability to perform ADLs (Indicate I for independent, D for dependent)

Feeding _I_, Infant feeding (as applicable) _N/A_, Bathing/Hygiene _D_, Dressing/(Grooming) _D_ Toileting _I_

Specific deficits _Feeding: Chew slowly, eat small amounts, swallowing difficulties; Bathing: can't sit in tub, uses chair, can_
shower when someone in the house; Grooming: "I can't shampoo my hair well, It's too much trouble to put my shoes on so I just
usually wear socks."

Types of assistance needed _Stand-by for bathing; minimal for grooming_

Growth and Development

[Nsg. Dx.: Altered Growth and Development*]

Developmental stage _Middle adulthood but (preparing for death)_

Ability to meet developmental responsibilities _Talks of death and funeral plans easily. "I had pictures taken while I still_
looked healthy (family & individual). Some parenting responsibilities can't be met."

Relocation

[Nsg. Dx.: Relocation Stress Syndrome]

Recent move: yes/(no) description_____

Adjustment to move_____

Display 12-1. Continued.

PERCEIVING: Reception of information

Self-Concept

[Nsg. Dx.: Body Image Disturbance, Self-Esteem Disturbance, Chronic Low Self-Esteem, Situational Low Self-Esteem, Personal Identity Disturbance]

Presenting appearance _Casually groomed, no make-up, no body odor_

Patient's description of self _"I've always been organized and logical. I liked to maintain control when I worked. I'm quiet around people I don't know. I like to be happy, I joke a lot."_

Effects of illness _"I can't do my hair well anymore. I'm surprised how many people have helped and brought food."_

Meaningfulness

[Nsg. Dx.: Hopelessness, Powerlessness]

Verbalization of hope/hopelessness _No specific comments_

Verbalization of control/loss of control _"I'm just frustrated with the system—all the red tape."_

Nonverbal cues about hope/control _None_

Sensory/Perception

[Nsg. Dx.: Sensory/Perception Alterations (Specify) (Visual*, auditory, kinesthetic, gustatory, tactile, olfactory), Unilateral Neglect]

History of restrictive environment _Confined to apt. due to weakness_

Vision deficits _I have trouble reading. I'm getting farsighted_ Glasses _None_

Hearing deficits _None_   Hearing Aid

Other Sensory/Perceptual changes _"I seem to have an exaggerated smell for things like perfumes and smoke."_

EXCHANGING: Mutual giving and receiving

Circulation

[Nsg. Dx.: Altered (Specify Type) Tissue Perfusion (Renal, cerebral, cardiopulmonary, gastrointestinal, peripheral), Fluid Volume Excess, Fluid Volume Deficit, High Risk for Fluid Volume Deficit, Decreased Cardiac Output]

Cerebral:

Neurological changes/symptoms _Dx ALS, weakness of arms & legs, esp. left side. Respiratory muscles and swallowing muscles weak_

Verbal response _Voice weak, hoarse, esp. in A.M._

Motor response _Unsteady gait, balance, weakness, weak grip, fine motor control (worse on left)_

Cardiac:

Heart rate and rhythm _86 Reg._ Blood pressure: R _118/78_ L _110/72_ Position _sitting_

Peripheral

Pulses _All palpable and equal bilaterally_   Skin temp. _Cool_

Color _Pale_ Moisture _Dry_ Capillary refill _Rapid_ Edema _L. & in ankles & feet_

Physical Integrity

[Nsg. Dx.: Altered Protection, Impaired Tissue Integrity, Altered Oral Mucous Membrane, Impaired Skin* Integrity, High Risk for Impaired Skin Integrity]

Tissue Integrity _Changes 2° fall yesterday_   Turgor _Adequate_   Rashes _None_

Lesions: _Lip: 1cm. cut with sutures_   Peteciae _None_   Bruises _L. arm — 8cm, circle above elbow_

Other (specify) _None_

Past history/treatment of skin breakdown _None_

Pressure sores (site/grade) _None_

Treatment _Keep lip clean, watch for infection. "I get stitches out in four days."_

Oxygenation

[Nsg. Dx.: Impaired Gas Exchange, Ineffective Airway Clearance, Ineffective Breathing Pattern*, Inability to Sustain Spontaneous Ventilation, Dysfunctional Ventilatory Weaning Response (DVWR)]

Complaints of Dyspnea _Yes_   Precipitated by _Activity, smoke, cold air, aerosol sprays_

History of pulmonary problems _Pneumonia & Bronchitis — last episode 4 yrs. ago_

Smoking: Y/(N) Pk Yrs._____ Respiratory rate _16_ Rhythm _Regular_ Depth _Shallow_

(Labored)/unlabored; use of accessory muscles _During activity_

Cough: (Productive/(nonproductive)) _"occasionally"_

Display 12-1. Continued.

EXCHANGING: Oxygenation (cont.)
Sputum: Color _N/A_ Amount _____ Consistency_____
Need for suction (frequency) _N/A_ Breath sounds _Decreased at bases_____
Oxygen percent and device _N/A_

Physical Regulation and Protection
[Nsg. Dx.: High Risk for Infection*, High Risk for Altered Body Temperature, Hypothermia, Hyperthermia, Ineffective Thermoregulation, Dysreflexia, High Risk for Injury*, High Risk for Suffocation, High risk for Poisoning, High Risk for Trauma, High Risk for Aspiration*, High Risk for Disuse Syndrome, Alt. Protection]
Temperature _98._ Route _Oral_____
Menstrual Period: Last _1992_ Frequency _N/A_ Duration _Hysterectomy, 1992_____
Immune Status _Not affected yet_____
White blood count _7200_ Differential _Not available_____
Clotting: PT _N/A_ PTT _N/A_ Platelets _Not available_____
Intermittent unusual sensations _None. "But I worry about choking. I don't know how to do the Heimlich maneuver,_
_neither do my sons."_____
Immunizations up-to-date _Yes (Flu shot & Tetanus October 1993)_____
Alcohol/caffeine/narcotic use _None except for occasional cola_____
Environmental/personal safety conditions _House cluttered, pt. rarely wears shoes. Kitchen floor slippery, showers alone_
_(someone in house, not in BR) No railings in BR, no use of transfer belt when walking upstairs_____

Nutrition
[Nsg. Dx.: Altered Nutrition: More than body requirements, *Altered Nutrition: Less than body requirements, Altered Nutrition: Potential for more than body requirements, Impaired Swallowing*, High Risk for Aspiration]*
Eating patterns:
Number of meals/day: Usual _2-3_ Current _2-3, plus snacks_____
Special diet _Soft—Dinners prepared and brought in by friends and neighbors 3-5 times per week_____
Food preferences/intolerances _Dislikes bananas & cottage cheese (too "sticky"), likes jello, mashed potatoes & pudding_
24-hour recall of food intake _Granola bar, applesauce, yogurt, meatloaf, potato, green beans, milk, 1 can pop_
Fluid intake/Type _water, pop_ Amount _1-2 glasses/day_ Preferences _Pop_____
Appetite changes _"I seem to eat less at each meal."_____
Swallowing difficulty _"Yes, I have to chew well & eat smaller portions; it takes longer to swallow."_____
History of ulcers _No_ Indigestion _No (but history of irritable bowel syndrome)_____
Anorexia/nausea/vomiting _Some nausea after fall yesterday, but OK now._____
Condition of mouth/throat/teeth _1 broken front tooth, mouth dry_____
Height _5'2"_ Weight _100 lbs._ Ideal Weight _110-130_____
Current diet therapies _None_____
Lab values (place * by abnormal values): (No recent values available)
Hemoglobin _11_ Hematocrit _32_ RBC _4.2_ Na_____ K_____ Cl_____
Glucose (fasting/not fasting) _____ Cholesterol _____ Triglycerides_____
Total protein _____ Albumin _____ Iron _____ Other_____

Elimination
[Nsg. Dx.: Constipation*, Perceived Constipation, Colonic Constipation, Diarrhea, Bowel Incontinence, Altered Urinary Elimination, Stress Incontinence, Reflex Incontinence, Urge Incontinence, Functional Incontinence, Total Incontinence, Urinary Retention]
Gastrointestinal/bowel:
Usual bowel habits _Every other day_ Changes from normal _"I get constipated easily"_____
Last BM _today_ Remedies used _Metamucil most days_____
Bowel sounds _Present 4 quds_ Abdominal examination _WNL_____
Stool Color _Brown_ Amount _Medium_ Consistency _Hard_____
Renal/Urinary:
Usual urinary patterns _2-3 times a day_ Changes from normal _"Perhaps a bit less"_____
Urine: Color _Amber_ Odor _No unusual_ Amount _Not measured_ per_____
Output for last 24 hours _Unknown_ Avg. hourly _____ Bladder distension: yes/no
Urinalysis _None available_ Urine C&S_____

Display 12-1. Continued.

CHOOSING: Selection of alternatives
Coping
[Nsg. Dx.: Ineffective Individual Coping, Impaired Adjustment, Defensive Coping, Ineffective Denial, Ineffective Family Coping Disabling, Ineffective Family Coping: Compromised, Family, Coping, Potential for Growth*]

Patient's usual problem-solving methods *"I try to be organized & logical."*

Family's usual problem-solving methods *"My son helps. We talk well."*

Patient's method of dealing with stress *"I talk to someone – often Hannah or Rhonda."*

Family's method of dealing with stress *"We talk"*

Patient's affect *Flat (probably related to muscle weakness of face 2° ALS)*

Physical manifestations of emotional state *None evident*

Support systems available *Church, friends, neighbors in apt. building. "My close friends from church help with negotiating the health care system to get services."*

Participation
[Nsg. Dx.: Ineffective Management of Therapeutic Regimen (Individuals), Noncompliance (Specify), Health Seeking Behaviors (Specify)]

Compliance with past/current health regimens *Usually, however stated, "I can't seem to decide to move my bed to the first floor."*

Willingness to comply with future health regimen *Yes*

Perceived barriers to compliance *"I feel bad about taking up so much of everyone's time. Every change seems to mean I'm more dependent on someone. For example, I need help to sort through things before the bed comes down, and this is such a busy time of year for my friends."*

Judgment
[Nsg. Dx.: Decisional Conflict* (Specify)]

Decision-making ability

Patient's perspective *"I make up my mind, but I change my mind often too. It's hard to accept all these changes."*

Others' perspectives *Betty has made realistic decisions about death, but she's prone to changing her mind about day to day decisions.*

PATIENT'S PRIORITIES FOR CARE

1. *Risks for aspiration, infection and injury*

2. *Self-care deficits*

3. *Constipation*

4. *"The decision about the bed"*

5.

6.

7.

8.

9.

10.

Tool adapted from: Guzzetta, C.E. Bunton, S.D., Prinkey, L.A., Sherer, A.P. & Seifert, P.C. (1989). Clinical assessment tools for use with nursing diagnosis. St. Louis, Mosby. (used with permission)

Display 12-1. Continued.

▶▶▶▶▶▶ **Action Learning #68: What Are Your First Impressions?**

Briefly list your first impressions after having read the data. What do you think about Betty as a person? What do you think are her greatest concerns? What do you think are her nursing needs?

DISCUSSION   One of your first impressions probably is "Wow, that's a lot of information; where do I even begin?" It can be overwhelming if you do not begin to see relationships among the data; there is too much information to remember as single pieces. How did the tool help you initially to cluster pieces to show relationships? When did your thinking move you beyond seeing the basic clusters of data in the tool to seeing more complex relationships among the data? How will your first impressions affect the rest of your data collection?

▷ 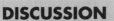 **Comparing Data With Norms and Standards to Identify Relevant Data**

Some of the information on the tool is either "normal" for the general population or "normal" for Betty. How do you tell the difference? The answer is by using your content knowledge for determining population norms, and asking the patient about her individual norms. Obviously, a medical diagnosis of ALS is not a population norm, and is relevant data. Examine the following pieces of data and judge whether or not they fit with population norms and Betty's individual norms.

▼ Retired at age 46
▼ Alert and oriented to person, place, and time
▼ Sleeps 8 to 9 hours a night
▼ Needs help with bathing and grooming activities
▼ Difficulty with chewing and swallowing
▼ Pulse = 86

This preliminary thinking—comparing data to norms and standards—is a major factor in accurately identifying the patient's health concerns. This phase of thinking is extremely dependent on content knowledge and experience, and thus presents a major challenge to beginning students. Beginners are expected to know that they don't know something and be able to look it up so they will know it. (Note the section on the first page of the TNT checklist, in which comparing data to norms is addressed.)

What is even more challenging is that looking something up does not complete the task. Even if the nurse has a "photographic memory" and can completely recall all the facts about ALS, that by itself is useless unless the T.H.I.N.K. modes are used to identify the relationships between those facts and this particular patient's responses to ALS.

▷ Developing Initial Hunches

The nurse's first set of hunches was based on the diagnostic labels (from the North American Nursing Diagnosis Association [NANDA] taxonomy) presented at the top of each pattern or subpattern on the tool. These initial hunches illustrate how the tool can provide logical "preclustering" of data. The nurse placed a star in the margin of each area that seemed to have relevant data during the data collection. The star was a reminder of the thinking that took place during data collection. Remember, collection (finding clues) and analysis (making sense out of clues) occur simultaneously. The star also served as a reminder to do more with the data.

There are many hunches that come to mind as the data are gathered. It is important to note them *and* keep an open mind to all possibilities. Many nurses jot down ideas in the margins or on separate paper as they use the assessment tool. Think about a system that works best for you to prevent you from narrowing your thinking too soon or forgetting some important hunch.

The initial hunches are the triggers to further thinking (mainly more TOTAL RECALL and INQUIRY) about what additional data are needed (data gaps). Directed data collection fills in data gaps to rule in or rule out hunches. Below is a list of initial hunches. Some of them overlap and may be considered as differential diagnoses for the same patient response. Read through the list and think about whether or not there is any foundation for these hunches.

Impaired Verbal Communication
Impaired Social Interaction
Knowledge Deficit about stair climbing problems
Fear of loss of independence and need to live with mother
Impaired Physical Mobility
Activity Intolerance
Fatigue
Diversional Activity Deficit
Impaired Home Maintenance Management
Self-Care Deficits: bathing and grooming
Altered Growth and Development
Pain
Anxiety about finances

High Risk for Peripheral Neurovascular Dysfunction
Ineffective Breathing Patterns
High Risk for Infection
High Risk for Injury
High Risk for Disuse Syndrome
High Risk for Altered Nutrition
Impaired Swallowing
High Risk for Aspiration
Constipation
Family Coping: Potential for Growth
Decisional Conflicts

▶▶▶▶▶▶ **Action Learning #69: Validating Hunches**

Pick three of the above hunches.

#1 _____

#2 _____

#3 _____

Ask yourself the following questions for each hunch (you will need a nursing diagnosis reference book or nursing theory text to help you answer the questions):

Are there data on the assessment tool to support these conclusions?

#1 _____   #2 _____   #3 _____

Do the formal label definitions in a diagnostic manual fit with this patient's situation?

#1 _____   #2 _____   #3 _____

Are there defining characteristics in the data base that fit with the defining characteristics in a diagnostic manual?

#1 _____   #2 _____   #3 _____

What additional data, if available, would help support the label?

#1 _____   #2 _____   #3 _____

Which differential diagnoses need to be considered?

#1 _____   #2 _____   #3 _____

| **DISCUSSION** | What was the most challenging part of this task? Did it get any easier by the third one? What shortcuts did you |

begin to develop to do this efficiently without sacrificing accuracy? What areas on the TNT checklist represent this activity of validating hunches?

▷ Overview of the Nurse's Thinking to Determine Conclusions of Assessment

Examine the nurse's thinking about the hunch "constipation." The Nursing Assessment Tool helped to identify basic clusters of single pieces of data. These clusters frequently led to the initial hunches. The following data cluster supporting the hunch "constipation" is found in the Nursing Assessment Tool.

▼ DATA CLUSTER

BM every other day
"I get constipated easily"
Metamucil most days
Drinks 1–2 glasses of water or pop/day
Walks only short distances
Medical Dx. of ALS
Takes iron, baclofen, and nortriptyline

Some basic content knowledge and thinking needed to determine that the data in this cluster are relevant to constipation are as follows:

Most adults have a bowel movement every day, but every other day is not that unusual.
Patients who say they are constipated usually are constipated, but some also have "perceived constipation," so this will need to be ruled out.
Metamucil increases bulk in the gastrointestinal (GI) tract and helps diminish problems with constipation.
Water intake of one to two glasses per day usually is not adequate fluid to maintain normal bowel movements.
Decreased physical activity (walking short distances) hinders GI motility and can lead to constipation.
A symptom of ALS is decreased GI motility, which can lead to constipation.
Iron, baclofen, and nortriptyline all have the side effect of constipation.

According to *NANDA Nursing Diagnoses: Definitions and Classification 1992* (NANDA, 1992, p. 16), the definition and defining characteristics for the diagnosis of constipation are as follows:

Definition: A state in which an individual experiences a change in normal bowel habits characterized by a decrease in frequency and/or passage of hard dry stools.

Defining characteristics: Decreased activity level; frequency less than usual pattern; hard formed stools; palpable mass; reported feeling of pressure in rectum; reported feeling of rectal fullness; straining at stool.

Other possible characteristics: Abdominal pain: appetite impairment; back pain; headache; interference with daily living; use of laxatives.

What other data in Betty's case, if added to the cluster, would better support the conclusion of constipation? There were data gaps in these areas:

▼ The patient's normal bowel movement pattern before ALS

▼ The effects of the Metamucil on her bowel patterns

▼ Other signs or symptoms of constipation identified under the defining characteristics or other possible characteristics

Another question the nurse had was, "What are the possible differential diagnoses to be considered?"

"Perceived constipation" and "colonic constipation" needed to be differentiated. The nurse examined the definitions and defining characteristics for these differential diagnoses in the same diagnostic manual. Because neither of these diagnoses fit this patient, the nurse made the decision to rule out these options and rule in her original hunch. This ruling-in process was the culmination of validating both the data and the diagnostic label. (Note the question on the TNT checklist about differential diagnoses.)

The nurse thought about all of the hunches in the same way. Most of the hunches were validated by definitions and defining characteristics. The next step was to consolidate the hunches into a manageable group for designing care. This required cluster analysis and a look at the big picture to determine what hunches were better dealt with as related factors to other problems. This task required that the nurse use INQUIRY and NEW IDEAS AND CREATIVITY to find the clusters best suited to become assessment conclusions. It also required that the nurse think ahead to planning by asking, "If I plan care for this problem, will it also cover that problem?" (Find the item on the TNT checklist that addresses this issue.)

This thinking is illustrated by the following example. Instead of writing three separate plans for Impaired Home Maintenance Management, Fatigue (weakness), and Impaired Physical Mobility (unsteady gait), the nurse recognized that all three issues could be handled in one diagnosis:

Impaired Home Maintenance Management related to weakness, unsteady gait, and living in a two-floor apartment

This is an example of how clustering hunches that are related to each other can streamline the design of care. This example also illustrates how two nurses caring for the same patient could label their conclusions somewhat differently while still being equally thorough in covering all concerns. Imagine the time it would take to write a plan for all of the original 24 hunches if they were all valid, or even if only half of them were valid. That would not be efficient use of valuable nursing time. Thinking ahead and finding the best clusters results in much better time management and coordinated patient care.

▶▶▶▶▶▶ **Action Learning #70: Finding the Best Clusters**

Reexamine the initial hunches. Look for the clusters that will allow the nurse to consolidate those hunches. In other words, what hunches are related to each other? Write out a nursing diagnosis that illustrates clustering of hunches. Don't hesitate to jot down ideas until you come up with the best cluster. Circle your final conclusion.

DISCUSSION   What was the most challenging aspect of this activity? What sources did you use to help guide your thinking as you were doing it? What will be the best way to validate your thinking and decisions?

▶ MAJOR CONCLUSIONS OF ASSESSMENT

The next area of focus during assessment is for the nurse to select the best labels for all the major conclusions of assessment, and then share those conclusions with the patient. Those conclusions include the patient's:

▼ Strengths

▼ Health concerns categorized as:

  Nursing diagnoses of actual problems, potential problems, and wellness issues

  Interdisciplinary problems

  Problems for referral

Although the nurse would have validated all conclusions with supporting data already, for the sake of this discussion the supporting data also are listed in Display 12-2.

(text continues on p. 288)

DISPLAY 12-2. Summary of the Major Conclusions of Assessment for Betty

STRENGTHS

High school graduate plus business college degree

Lives in a safe neighborhood with supportive neighbors who bring in meals three to five times a week

Twenty-year-old son lives in same apartment complex and provides transportation, shops for groceries, and does laundry

Close friends from church help in negotiating the health care system to get services she needs

Health and medical care coverage with HMO

Former employer (apartment management firm) is providing apartment and utilities at no cost to her now that she can no longer work for them

Making plans for her death with funeral home, minister, family, lawyer

Made arrangements with ex-husband to care for 16-year-old son after her death

Sixteen-year-old helps with laundry, meals, and getting up and down stairs to bedroom and full bathroom

Making arrangements with Department of Social Services for financial needs during extent of her illness

Sees MD regularly and dental checks every 6 months

Fairly well-balanced food intake

Bilingual

Alert and oriented ×3

Sleeps well

Likes to write poetry

Cares about personal appearance

Good sense of humor and good self-esteem

Vital signs stable

No smoking and no ETOH intake

Flu shot 10/93

Effective coping skills and problem-solving skills

HEALTH CONCERNS

Nursing Diagnoses

Actual Problems and Supporting Data

1. Constipation related to inadequate fluid intake, side effects of medications, decreased mobility, decreased intestinal motility 2° ALS

▼ DATA CLUSTER

Data supporting problem:	Data supporting related factors:
BM every other day	Drinks 1–2 glasses water or pop/day
Metamucil most days	Walks only short distances
"I get constipated easily."	Dx. of ALS
	Takes iron, baclofen, and nortriptyline (all of which can cause constipation)

Continued

2. Diversional Activity Deficit related to difficulty with reading, confinement to apartment, recently quitting job, limited energy 2° to ALS

▼ DATA CLUSTER

Data supporting problem:
"I get bored."
"I've worked all my life and I'm not used to all this free time."
"I don't do any exercise at all."
Home alone

Data supporting related factors:
"I'm becoming far-sighted; I have trouble reading."
Quit job 1 month ago
Can go out only if someone takes her out
Can walk short distances only
Uses walker

3. Bathing and Grooming Self-Care Deficits related to weakness, shortness of breath, and unstable movement 2° to ALS

▼ DATA CLUSTER

Data supporting problem:
Only takes shower when someone is there to help
"I can't shampoo my hair well anymore"

Data supporting related factors:
Unsteady gait
Weakness, esp. on left side
Can sit on chair, but not in tub itself
Gets short of breath and fatigued with activities
Dx. of ALS

4. Impaired Home Maintenance Management related to weakness, unsteady gait, and living in two-floor apartment

▼ DATA CLUSTER

Data supporting problem:
Home very cluttered
"I can't do housework."
"I can't drive, cook, or clean."

Data supporting related factors:
Unsteady gait
Weakness, esp. on left side
Uses walker for limited walking; wheelchair ordered
"It's hard to go up and down stairs"

5. Decisional Conflict about making changes in daily living activities and safety of home environment related to changes symbolizing decreased independence and reluctance to burden friends at holiday time.

▼ DATA CLUSTER

Data supporting problem:
"I can't seem to decide to move my bed to the first floor."
"I haven't started using the transfer belt."
"I'm still trying to manage the bath on my own."
"I make up my mind and then I change it."
Friends report patient is prone to changing her mind frequently about day-to-day decisions

Data supporting related factors:
"Every change seems to mean I am more dependent on someone."
"I need help to sort through things before the bed comes down, and this is such a busy time of year for my friends."
"I feel bad about taking up so much of everyone's time."

Continued

DISPLAY 12-2. *continued*

Wellness Nursing Diagnoses
Potential for enhanced effective preparation for death

▼ DATA CLUSTER

"I've talked to the minister and funeral home."

"I've come to accept the fact that I will die soon, probably this coming year."

"I had family and individual pictures taken while I still looked healthy."

"I've talked to my sons about how they will cope with my death."

"I talked to my ex-husband about caring for our youngest son."

"I wrote my eulogy."

"It's not death itself that I fear, but the interim time before I die."

"I've always been very organized and logical."

Potential (High Risk for . . .) Problems

1. **High Risk for Injury related to unsteady gait, weakness, living in two-floor apartment, spending much time alone, history of a fall, slippery kitchen floor, clutter on floors, and patient's usual pattern of wearing socks rather than shoes at home**

▼ DATA CLUSTER OF RISK FACTORS

Progressive weakness and unsteady gait 2° ALS

Weakness, esp. on left side

Bedroom and full bath on second floor of apartment

Lives with one son who is in school during the day

Son walks up stairs behind her but does not hold on to her or use a belt

Has not yet moved bed to first floor

No safety bars in bathroom

Kitchen floor tiled and slippery; carpeting in other rooms

"It's too much trouble to put shoes on so I usually just wear socks. I should wear shoes more."

Fell yesterday in kitchen and injured face

Clutter in many areas of apartment; patient unable to clean by herself

2. **High Risk for Infection (especially respiratory and urinary) related to weakness of muscles of respiratory system, decreased mobility, swallowing difficulty 2° ALS, insufficient fluid intake, environmental irritants during cold weather, and exposure to many people bringing in food**

▼ DATA CLUSTER OF RISK FACTORS

Shallow respirations 2° ALS

Increased chance of aspiration of food and fluids because muscles used for swallowing weakened

"Cold air, aerosols, and smoke make it hard to breathe."

Food prepared and brought to patient by several different people

Drinks 1–2 glasses of fluid per day

Continued

3. High risk for aspiration related to swallowing difficulties due to weakened muscles 2° ALS

▼ DATA CLUSTER OF RISK FACTORS

"It takes a long time for me to swallow; I have to chew a long time and eat small amounts."

"I don't know how to do a Heimlich maneuver; neither do my sons."

"I worry about choking."

Drinks thin liquids

Interdisciplinary Problem
   Altered Nutrition and Fluid Intake related to impaired swallowing and meal preparation by neighbors (Dietitian and Speech Therapist)

▼ DATA CLUSTER

5′ 2″, 100 lbs

Increased weakness/fatigue with activities, including eating

"I seem to eat less at each meal."

Drinks 1–2 glasses of water or pop each day

Dinners prepared and brought in by friends three to five times per week

"I have to chew well and eat smaller portions; it takes longer to swallow."

Uses walker; wheelchair ordered

Homebound alone, except for 16-year-old son who goes to school

Dx. of ALS

No income since retirement

Problem for Referral
   No income since retirement

The thinking behind these conclusions is discussed in more detail in the following chapters as the plans of care are examined. How did you rate the nurse's thinking when using the TNT checklist?

The final validation of the conclusions listed in Display 12-2 will not take place until the plan is evaluated after implementation. An important validation at this stage, however, is for the nurse to confer with Betty and see if she agrees with the nurse's decisions. A brief dialogue describing how this occurs, as well as how priorities are set, is presented in the next section.

▶ SETTING PRIORITIES WITH THE PATIENT

Guidelines for setting priorities were discussed in Chapter 9. Briefly, the guidelines suggested the following order of priorities:

1. Life-threatening issues
2. Safety issues
3. Patient priority health concerns
4. Nurse priority health concerns
   a. The overall picture of each health concern in relation to other concerns and the patient as a whole person
   b. Availability of time and resources

Keeping those guidelines in mind, the nurse proceeded with the validation of her conclusions and worked with Betty to determine the best use of their time and energy to plan care. The conversation with Betty went something like this:

> "Betty, I have asked you a lot of questions and found out a lot of information about you as a unique person with ALS. My job as a nurse is to determine what health care needs you have so we can decide what, if anything, you want to do about them."

> "Nursing has developed some standard labels for the different health care needs that people experience. We call these nursing diagnoses. I want to share with you my thinking about your health care needs and the resulting nursing diagnoses that I believe are appropriate to help us focus your care. There are also some conclusions about areas of need for which we can get help from others."

The list of conclusions was shared with Betty, and there was further discussion to explain and clarify any concerns she had. She agreed with all of the conclusions as stated above.

> "Now we need to decide which are the most important things to work on first, keeping in mind that we can work on several issues simultaneously. One system for deciding how to start is to use the following guidelines."

The guidelines are shared and explained to Betty.

> "Although you are not experiencing any immediately life-threatening issues, the high risks for infection, injury, and aspiration definitely qualify as safety issues. I believe it would be best for you if we address these areas first."

Betty agrees. If she didn't agree, however, the nurse would need to help her recognize the consequences of that decision. First, the nurse would attempt to increase Betty's understanding of the seriousness of these issues. Sometimes, additional information is all that is needed. Other times, the patient uses the defense mechanism of denial and has difficulty accepting the life changes that are occurring. This requires patience and support on the part of the nurse. Still other times, the patient just has a different set of values and is not willing to be concerned about safety issues. In this case, the nurse must focus on other areas of care, especially when the patient is not hospitalized and not in a health care-controlled environment.

With the life-threatening and safety parts of the guidelines addressed, the nurse then encourages Betty to identify which is the next area to work on. Betty says she is most concerned with the Self-Care Deficit and the Constipation. The nurse is concerned with the Decisional Conflict about making changes in daily living activities because this is strongly connected to the safety issues. Betty agrees that the safety issues are related, but really wants the other issues dealt with first. Both agree to work on all three areas simultaneously.

The remaining nursing diagnoses, interdisciplinary problems, and problems for referral also will be worked on. For example, the nurse can make the phone calls about the interdisciplinary problem with nutrition and the problem for referral to social services after her visit with Betty and before her next visit. Use the TNT checklist to rate the nurse's thinking while setting priorities.

▶ CLOSING COMMENTS

This chapter has provided an expanded view of how thinking skills, content knowledge, and the nursing process are combined, taking into account the patient and the nurse, to work toward great nursing. The *thinking* and *doing* in Betty's case study illustrate how the nurse moves from preencounter thinking to working with Betty in setting priorities for her care. The TNT checklist has provided some structure to follow the thinking as it occurs. The next chapters continue to track the nurse's thinking as plans of care are designed for the major conclusions of assessment.

▶▶▶ *THINKING LOG #12*

Part of being a caring nurse is thinking about how you would feel and what you would want if you were a patient. It is easy to distance oneself from patients and become impersonal. Put yourself in Betty's situation. What would you think about the nursing process being used with you? Write a short paragraph describing your thoughts and feelings.

REFERENCES

Erikson, E. (1963). *Childhood and society* (2nd ed.). New York: WW Norton.
North American Nursing Diagnosis Association. (1992). *NANDA nursing diagnoses: Definitions and classifications, 1992.* Philadelphia: Author.

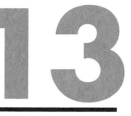

Designing, Doing, and Determining Quality of Care for Actual Problems With Multiple Related Factors

LEARNING OUTCOMES

After reading and doing the activities in this chapter you will be able to:

  Explain approaches to caring for a patient with nursing diagnoses categorized as actual problems.

  Discuss the importance of identifying all related factors for designing and doing care, and determining quality of care.

  Critique a poorly developed plan for selected actual problems with multiple related factors, and create a better plan.

It is now time to complete the phases of the nursing process for Betty. Assessment and the early stages of planning with Betty were covered in Chapter 12. To finish the process, designing, doing, and determining quality of care must be completed. As discussed in Chapter 9, "designing" refers to planning care *with* and *for* the patient. "Doing" refers to the implementation phase of care. "Determining quality" focuses on evaluation of the care. These three phases of the nursing process, which are constantly intertwined with assessment, must be accepted as tightly interwoven and approached as a collective set of activities.

This chapter explores care as it is planned, implemented, and evaluated for nursing diagnoses that are actual problems for Betty. Actual problems are those for which the defining characteristics (signs and symptoms) exist, and therefore the problem exists. Betty's potential problems (High Risk for . . .), wellness nursing diagnoses, interdisciplinary problems, and problems for referral are discussed in later chapters.

All five of Betty's actual problems have multiple related factors, each of which must be addressed in the overall plan for great nursing care to occur. The role of related factors is highlighted in this chapter to show how critical they are to individualized, thorough nursing care.

The number of factors contributing to problems varies from patient to patient. It often is easy to identify the most obvious related factor, stop at that point, and miss others. Because Betty's case has so many interrelated issues, her problems are complex, with many related factors. Studying her case provides a good example of the value of addressing *all* related factors.

For language clarification, remember that the terms "etiologies," "related factors," and "contributing factors" mean the same thing. Throughout this chapter, "related factors" is used most often.

Although all five of Betty's actual problems are discussed, only two are examined in detail. For those two, care plans of poor quality are presented for study. One of those plans is transformed to a better plan to illustrate the qualitative differences between poor and good plans.

There are two reasons for examining plans of poor and better quality. First, seeing what something should not be is a good way to learn what it should be. Think about that for a minute. Human nature seems to make it easier to critique something someone else did inadequately than to create something from scratch by oneself. Many people can offer suggestions or fix something that doesn't "look right" more easily than they can put words on a blank sheet of paper. Critiquing something that is done poorly is frequently less anxiety-producing than attempting to create a high-quality product from one's own resources.

The second reason involves trying to understand qualitative differences. One way to understand what something is is to describe what it is not. This works especially well for abstract ideas related to quality. Suppose, in planning to hire a nurse–manager, one tried to describe ideal characteristics. A first response might be, "We want someone who really works well with people." To clarify the abstract notion of working well with people, a common response would be to describe what is not wanted. "Someone who doesn't push her views over everyone else's" or "Someone who doesn't get upset easily" might be given as descriptions. Describing what one does not want is a common method of communicating what one does want. Therefore, studying some poorer-quality (but not unusual) care plans provides a safe, low-anxiety, learning opportunity that builds on human nature.

▶ REVIEW OF BETTY'S ACTUAL PROBLEMS

In Chapter 12, a list of the conclusions of assessment made from analyzing the data in Betty's situation was presented. Several nursing diagnoses were made, among which were five actual problems that fall within the domain of independent nursing practice:

Self-Care Deficits
Impaired Home Maintenance Management
Diversional Activity Deficit
Decisional Conflict
Constipation

Each of those problems has several factors contributing to it. The formal diagnostic statements included all the related factors. The next few pages explore those statements and the thinking involved in planning care for these problems. The first two diagnostic statements are:

Bathing and Grooming Self-Care Deficits related to weakness, shortness of breath, and unstable movement 2° amyotrophic lateral sclerosis (ALS) and no safety bars in bathroom

and

Impaired Home Maintenance Management related to weakness and unsteady gait 2° ALS and two-floor apartment living arrangement

Both are challenging problems. Because the related factors are similar, the thinking that goes into planning care for one of these problems can be applied to the other. The reason these are so challenging is that the related factors are brought on by the ALS, which will get progressively worse. Setting up objectives that focus on regaining function is unrealistic. If the weakness, shortness of breath, unstable movements, and unsteady gait cannot be reversed, one might well question if there is anything that can be done about these related factors.

A shift of thinking is needed away from regaining function to compensating for those deteriorating areas. Compensation calls for using the patient's strengths to overcome the deficits. Remember, Betty said she was logical and a good problem solver. A creative nurse will get her engaged in considering safe, energy-saving ways to manage some of her own care and decrease the clutter in her house.

The third diagnosis is

Diversional Activity Deficit related to difficulty reading, confinement to apartment, recently quitting job, and limited energy 2° ALS

This is a highly personal issue. Not everybody likes to watch TV, tie fishing flies, or play card games. Finding pleasurable diversional activities is important to emotional health. When usual activities are impossible, however, finding comparably rewarding ones calls for creativity and individualized interventions on the nurse's part.

The fourth diagnosis is

> Decisional Conflict about making changes in daily living activities and home environment to maintain safety related to changes being symbolic of decreased independence, reluctance to burden friends at holiday time, and limited finances to purchase support bars for bathroom

This is a complex problem. Because Betty is having trouble deciding to make changes, she is adding to her safety risks. A first impulse in planning care for this problem might be to say sternly to Betty, "You've just got to make these decisions because it is a matter of safety."

▶▶▶▶▶▶ Action Learning #71: Thoughts on Being Directive With Betty About Her Decisional Conflict

Think about the approach described in the preceding paragraph for dealing with Betty's decisional conflict, and answer these questions:

1. What are the advantages and disadvantages of this approach, the purpose of which is to promote patient safety?

2. Does this approach promote safety?

3. How does this approach reflect the nurse's knowledge and thinking about the intellectual and emotional components of behavior change?

4. How does this approach reflect planning *with* the patient?

5. What are some likely outcomes of this approach?

DISCUSSION   This approach might work; it could intimidate Betty into cooperation, which would result in safety being maintained, but at what cost? Decision making is an emotional and intellectual activity that is very personal. Simply knowing that something should be done is not enough. If you do not believe that, think about the health behaviors you know you should be practicing—exercising, dieting, quitting smoking, relaxing, and others. If you know you should exercise daily, why do you not just make up your mind and do it? Well, there are many reasons that are personal to you. Someone saying, "You've just got to exercise" is not going to make a big difference, is it? Remember this when you work *with* patients. This diagnosis is explored further, with poor and better care plans, later in this chapter.

The last nursing diagnosis concerns the actual problem of constipation. It also has multiple related factors.

Constipation related to inadequate fluid intake, side effects of medications, and decreased mobility 2° ALS

This diagnosis entails somewhat less complexity than the emotion-laden decisional conflict, but care for this problem must take into account other factors such as the patient's swallowing problems and the progressive nature of her mobility deficits. This diagnosis also is examined further, with a written care plan, later in this chapter.

Before moving to the written care plans, notice again that each of the actual problems has many related factors. The significance of related factors and their role in achieving great nursing care cannot be treated lightly.

▶ **THE ROLE OF RELATED FACTORS AND THEIR SIGNIFICANCE TO CARE**

Identifying all of the factors contributing to each actual problem is very likely one of the least well done parts of the nursing process. Yet it is one of the most valuable parts of designing individualized care. Find the item on the Tracking Nursing Thinking (TNT) checklist (Appendix B) that addresses related factors.

Often, nurses will identify the problem well, but then list only the medical diagnosis as the contributor to the problem. Betty's case illustrates how easily this can be done. Almost all of Betty's problems can be traced back to her ALS. It would be easy to say she has Constipation related to ALS, Self-Care Deficits related to ALS, Diversional Activity Deficits related to ALS, Impaired Home Maintenance Management related to ALS, and Decisional Conflict related to ALS. Except for Decisional Conflict, which seems to be pushing the issue a bit far, all of the problems are there because she has ALS. Any nurse recording nursing diagnoses in this short manner would be correct; however, such diagnoses would be hard to plan care for. Essentially, the ALS is a "done deal"— nothing can undo it—and the nurse therefore would have nothing to work with in planning care.

That is not to say that ALS is not a contributing factor to those problems. Indeed, it is important to know that ALS is a related factor. If Betty had self-care deficits because of a stroke, very different approaches could be taken. People who suffer strokes can regain some of their function; many return almost to prestroke function. Amyotrophic lateral sclerosis is, however, progressive; it gets worse instead of better. Care can focus only on compensating for the decreased function, not on regaining lost function.

The medical diagnosis may be listed as a related factor by itself or it may be linked to the functional changes brought on by it. In Betty's case, the term "secondary to" (2°) is added to make it clear which functional areas are linked to the medical problem.

By itself, however, the medical diagnosis as a related factor is limiting. It is much more helpful to stretch one's thinking to the next level and ask what functional issues are contributing to the problem. Those functional issues, although traceable to the medical problem, often are areas for which care can be planned. Knowing, for example, that Betty's difficulty with home maintenance is related to her living in a two-floor apartment, that she has trouble going up and down stairs, and has weakness and an unsteady gait secondary to ALS, allows the nurse to focus on helping Betty move her center of living to one floor and find ways to compensate for her weakness. ALS by itself would not provide that direction.

Delineating more specific related factors allows the nurse and patient to develop individualized objectives and corresponding nursing actions. In Betty's case, nursing actions might include, among other things, getting her a long-handled duster, putting a bin by the stairs where she could place things that needed to go upstairs, and getting devices to help her grip more easily.

Such nursing actions are much more individualized than they would be if the only identified related factor were the ALS. Individualization of care, therefore, depends almost completely on a well identified list of related factors that goes beyond the obvious one, which is usually the medical problem.

▷ Hindrances to Thinking Beyond the Medical Diagnosis as the Only Related Factor

Several obstacles limit the nurse in identifying all of the appropriate related factors. The primary cause is forgetting to engage all five thinking modes. Stopping the search for related factors once the medical diagnosis is listed is symptomatic of a nurse's use of just the HABIT mode; it can become a habit to link everything to the medical problem.

Second is the nurse's limited understanding of the domain of independent nursing practice. If only the medical diagnosis is listed as a related factor for a nursing diagnosis, it implies that the only reason nursing care is needed is to care for the complications of the medical diagnosis. A problem identified in this way actually becomes an interdisciplinary problem, and not a nursing diagnosis.

The third obstacle, one that takes a lot of time and energy to overcome, is limited experience and content knowledge. Limits in experience and content knowledge hinder the nurse from conducting more extensive data analysis, including:

▼ Looking for relationships among data and data clusters that point to related factors

▼ Accepting the fact that problems rarely have only one related factor

▼ Thinking ahead to planning

▼ Considering the big picture of the patient's situation as planning commences

The final obstacle that plagues even expert nurses is time. Thinking requires time. For beginning nurses, who may not be totally convinced they need to find all the related factors, the additional time it takes becomes a concern. Hopefully, the value of taking the time is becoming apparent.

▷ Recognizing When Related Factors Have Been Missed

Often it is not until a plan is being developed that less-obvious related factors are found. At other times, as a plan is implemented, additional factors become apparent; perhaps something is not working or something seems to be missing. An evaluation that reveals unmet goals also may be the point of realization. Suppose, for example, that while implementing Betty's care plan for Impaired Home Maintenance Management, the nurse found that Betty had always pampered and picked up after her son, who had a habit of leaving piles of stuff by the front door, rarely hung up his clothes, and left a trail of food wrappers and dirty dishes everywhere. A nurse might not see the behavior if the home visits occurred while the son was at school. Her son's behavior and Betty's past habits would be additional factors contributing to her inability to maintain her home. A plan that did not address these factors would fall short of the goal of a less cluttered, clean environment. Weeks might go by with Betty using her new techniques to no avail before that additional factor emerged.

Another clue that related factors have been missed is problems with planning care. The nurse looks at the problem and the related factors and feels stumped as to what can be done. The usual methods of linking the patient outcomes to the related factors just do not work, as might be the case when only the medical diagnosis is identified as a contributor. When that happens, and there seems to be no logical flow in "reversing" the related factor to find outcomes, the nurse should question the diagnostic statement. If the problem is one for which the nurse feels something can be done, but the outcomes are not being achieved, then there is a high probability that the related factors are not well defined. It is then time to look back to the existing data or collect more data to find all the factors contributing to the problem.

Still another clue to inadequate identification of related factors is when the nursing diagnosis for one patient looks just like that for other patients. Related factors are very individual. Although nursing diagnosis texts list many possible related factors for each nursing diagnosis, most patients will have specific factors not found in other patient situations or in books. In Betty's case, although the weakness and unsteadiness are common to many patients with ALS who have self-care deficits, the fact that she has no safety bars in her bathroom is unique to her living situation.

▷ Uniqueness of Related Factors to Patients

Very few, if any, patients have exactly the same response to anything, because everyone has unique resources and deficits. It is easy to lose sight of this while caring for several patients who do share many similarities. As an example, consider caring for several patients with Alzheimer's disease. Some nursing homes have units specially planned for these patients because they have many common problems. These patients lose part of their memory and often act in ways that are baffling to their families and care providers. There is no treatment for this disease, but these patients require extensive nursing care. Commonly, these patients wander, forget who they are and where they are, eat inedible things, get upset easily, and exhibit a host of other behavioral responses.

While planning care for these patients, it is easy to identify the related factor for most of their problems as the confusion secondary to Alzheimer's disease. However, there are unique factors that contribute to each person's responses as well. A man who was a soldier might get more confused around loud noises; a woman who was a piano teacher might be calmed when she hears music and more confused in a completely quiet environment. The challenge to nurses is to go beyond the obvious confusion factor to other, less obvious re-lated factors. Often, the less obvious factors are keys to effective interventions.

There is no magic number of related factors that one can expect to find for each problem. There may well be only one, but in most cases there are sev-eral. There also are cases in which the related factors are unknown. For exam-ple, "Anxiety related to unknown causes" might be a diagnosis for a person who has a vague feeling of dread, but who cannot figure out why that feeling is there. When the related factor is unknown, the nurse initially aims the care toward helping the patient identify the possible factors contributing to the problem. The goal of care would be for the patient to try to identify the causes of the anxiety. If that proved impossible, the next best plan would be to deal with the signs and symptoms of anxiety itself.

It also is possible that the nurse has a hunch about related factors, but does not feel a high degree of certainty about them. Rather than leave those less-certain factors out of the diagnostic statement, it is best for the nurse to add the word "possible" in front of those factors. An example of a nursing diag-nosis written in that format is "Functional Incontinence related to immobility and possible reluctance to ask for help." In a case like this, the nurse might suspect the patient is not asking for help, but may not know for certain that this is happening. Having that possible related factor is important for provid-ing thorough care; leaving it off until the nurse was certain of the factor would delay necessary interventions that focused on the patient asking for help. Including "possible" related factors is an excellent example of the nurse's thinking-in-process about the patient's problem. Find the item(s) on the TNT checklist that address, "Thinking toward planning . . . "

▶ DESIGNING CARE WITH BETTY FOR HER ACTUAL PROBLEMS

Each of Betty's actual problems was discussed briefly earlier. Now it is time to look at two of these in more detail. First, Decisional Conflict will be explored. Two plans of care are presented. The first is one done by Sue Swift, a fast-moving nurse whose major priority is efficiency. Her plans focus on the imme-diately recognized, usual interventions. Even though she has the benefit of a well worded, thorough diagnostic statement to start her plan, she develops a poor plan. Another nurse, Thelma Thoreau, expands that plan into a more in-dividualized, complete approach that addresses all the components of the problem and its related factors. Following the plan for Betty's Decisional Con-flict is a plan for Betty's Constipation, also done by Sue. You will be asked to take on Thelma's role and transform that plan into a better one.

▷ Sue's Care for Decisional Conflict

Look at Sue's Care Plan #1. Before reading Thelma's Care Plan, do Action Learning #72.

▼ Sue's Care Plan #1

Nursing Diagnosis:
  Decisional Conflict about making changes in daily living activities and home environment to maintain safety, related to changes being symbolic of decreased independence, reluctance to burden friends to help during holiday time, and limited financial resources to purchase support bars for bathroom.

Goal:
  By the end of 1 month, the patient will have made the right decision to make changes in her daily activities and home environment.

OBJECTIVES	NURSING ACTIONS	RATIONALE
Patient will:		
1. Identify three problem-solving techniques.	1a. Ask pt. what she knows about problem-solving techniques b. Teach her about problem solving c. Ask her to list three techniques	Determing what a pt. knows before teaching something new saves time
2. Select a technique she likes.	2. Explain which technique would be best in her situation and encourage her to use it	Helping pt. pick options increases chances of success
3. Learn how to use technique with decision conflict.	3a. Help her use technique with the changes she needs to make b. Correct errors in her use and support her	Correcting errors increases chances of success
4. Make good decisions.	4a. Talk to her friends and tell them she really needs them to help because she is having trouble asking b. Check out other community resources for financial assistance c. Monitor patient's follow-through on decisions	Using all available resources increases chances of success

▶▶▶▶▶▶ **A**ction Learning #72: Critique of Sue's Plan

Carefully analyze Sue's plan, write down what areas are poorly developed, and explain why you think they are less than ideal. Use the TNT checklist to help your critique.

DISCUSSION   Compare what you wrote with these observations:
Sue's care plan follows an appropriate format. It has a goal, objectives, and nursing actions. The goal is client centered and has a time frame. The goal comes close to flowing from the problem statement by addressing "decision making." The objectives and nursing actions and rationale are numbered sequentially.

This critique, however, exhausts the positive comments. Unfortunately, there are more problems with Sue's plan than there are positive aspects. First, the goal is quite value laden. The "right" decision implies there is only one "correct" choice. A month as a time frame is probably too long, considering the safety ramifications of this problem.

The objectives should flow from the goal and relate back to the related factors. In Sue's plan, the objectives are not focused on the related factors. There is no outcome that focuses directly on the symbolism of changes, reluctance to burden friends, or finding resources. Sue's objectives focus on teaching Betty problem-solving techniques, which are intellectual processes, but they are devoid of reference to the emotional issues in this conflict. The first two objectives are measurable and specific, but the last two are vague and not measurable. Objective Number 3 uses the verb, "learn" as a behavioral outcome. Although this term is often used, it is not measurable. Can one see learning? Not really; one can see the consequences of learning, such as passing a test, demonstrating something, or applying knowledge. If one is aiming for "learning" a technique as an outcome, then an objective such as applying the technique to the decision conflict would be measurable. The fourth objective has that vague, value-laden "good," which is like "right." What is "good?" The desired decision would need to be spelled out, such as, "will decide to ask for help."

On the whole, the objectives fall short because they are not individualized to Betty. The factors contributing to her conflict are not used as guides for the desired outcomes. They superimpose an intellectual fix onto an emotional conflict, which could seem to the patient to be a devaluation of her emotional concerns.

The nursing actions, on face value, fit with the objectives, but there is very little that is individual to Betty's situation. The actions are vague. "Teach her about problem solving" does not give much guidance or reflect much thought. Even if problem-solving teaching were what Betty needed, she would not get much with those general guidelines. How should those be taught?

Which techniques would be best in Betty's situation? Why teach her three techniques; why not two or four or one?

The nursing actions that accompany objective #2 do nothing to help Betty *select* a technique. The nurse is only advocating telling Betty which is best. If a nurse truly wants a patient to choose, then care should be directed to helping the patient make the choice, not to directing the choice.

Nursing actions for objective #3 are so vague, they are hardly worth writing down. "Help" is a catch-all word. The type of help needs to be specified. "Correcting errors" implies, again, that there is a right and wrong way to use a technique. It is a fluff-type of nursing action with very little depth to it.

The actions for the fourth objective simply do not fit with the objective. If the nurse wants the patient to make the decision, then why would the nurse make the decisions for her? That is what is recorded in 4a and b, under "Nursing Actions." These last actions could be seen as the nurse's true intent—to do this *for* the patient. It is akin to saying, "Here is what should be done; I'll just do it." It takes away the patient's participation in care.

▷ Thelma's Care Plan for Betty's Decisional Conflict

Thelma's plan of care shows thought that went back to the nursing diagnosis itself. There is a clear focus on the emotional aspects of this problem, and there are no attempts to devalue Betty or her dilemma.

The selection of Decisional Conflict as a valid nursing diagnosis was based on several factors. First, there is clear evidence that Betty is having a decisional conflict. The definition of Decisional Conflict fits with her situation, as do the defining characteristics and the related factors as found in a nursing diagnosis textbook.

Second, the decisional conflict is prohibiting her from restructuring her lifestyle and environment to maintain an acceptable level of safety. Without these changes, she is very likely to fall and experience unnecessary pain and discomfort from bruises or, worse, broken bones. This could increase her immobility, which would increase her chances for infection, especially respiratory infections. This could very likely accelerate her death.

In thinking through these issues, Thelma considered changing the nursing diagnosis instead of planning care for that specific problem. Looking at the big picture, it was obvious that one of Betty's major problems was " High Risk for Injury." Because this was already a diagnosis, Thelma thought, at first, that it would save time simply to add "Decisional Conflict" as an additional related factor to that conclusion. The resulting diagnosis would then read:

High Risk for Injury related to unsteady gait, weakness, living in a two-floor apartment, spending much time alone, history of falls, slippery kitchen floor, clutter on floors, patient's usual pattern of wearing socks rather than shoes at home, and **deci-**

▼ Thelma's Care Plan

Nursing Diagnosis: Decisional Conflict about making changes in daily living activities and home environment to maintain safety, related to changes being symbolic of decreased independence, reluctance to burden friends during holiday time, and limited finances to purchase safety bars.

Goal: By the end of 1 week, the patient will have made appropriate decisions to maintain safety in daily living activities and home environment.

OBJECTIVES	NURSING ACTIONS	RATIONALE
1. Share thoughts and feelings about changing her mind frequently, making changes that symbolize decreased independence, and her personal goals for dealing with her illness.	**1a.** Assist pt. to elaborate on her feelings about issues identified in objective #1 **b.** Actively listen, support, and comfort in decision making **c.** Discuss alternative ways to interpret change, eg, "change is reflection of strength and healthy problem solving"; encourage pt. to look at problem solving in different ways	**1.** Behavior change most successful if both cognitive and affective components are addressed Redefining the problem helps pt. explore new alternatives that may increase probability of change
2. List changes in daily living and home environment that will maintain safety.	**2a.** Help pt. identify most important changes to focus on first **b.** Explore with pt. current and new resources to help with changes, eg, other friends, church members, groups that assist the disabled	**2.** Clarification of pt.'s priorities helps nurse and pt. focus energy most effectively Use of outside resources increases probability of change
3. Describe consequences of making and not making changes regarding her goal/s for dealing with her illness.	**3.** Ask pt. to identify the pros and cons of making and not making changes, and impact on her goals	**3.** Helping pt. think ahead to outcomes of decisions helps pt. to select best decision
4. Agree to ask for help in 3 days for moving furniture, adding safety bars.	**4a.** Role-play with pt. to practice asking for help **b.** Contact alternative resources for moving and purchase of safety bars **c.** Assist pt. in setting date for taking action **d.** Monitor plan and modify as needed	**4.** Role-play, identifying additional resources and establishing set date increases probability of action occurring Ongoing evaluation increases probability of successful behavior change and maintaining patient safety

**sional conflict about making changes in daily living activities
and safety of home environment**

Although there is nothing wrong with this approach (it's one Sue would
be apt to take), Thelma did not believe it would be the best way to handle the
situation, for two reasons. First, it would make the care plan for "High Risk for
Injury . . . " very long and cumbersome. Second, that approach would not
highlight or recognize as clearly the strong emotional impact of these changes
for Betty.

By developing a separate plan, Thelma was able to channel more of Betty's energy into examining the underlying issues and how they relate to Betty's
goals for dealing with her illness. This could of course be done in the "High
Risk for Injury . . . " plan as well, but it was more likely to be slighted because
the plan had become so lengthy.

Once the thinking about the diagnosis itself was accomplished, Thelma
used the related factors to direct the expected outcomes for Betty's plan of
care. Because of the complexity of the related factors, there are several objectives that address each factor. With emotional issues, in particular, it often is
necessary to break down how each factor is addressed into measurable increments of change. Betty needs to process these changes; quick-fix outcomes as
seen in Sue's plan are unrealistic for an emotional issue with several related
factors.

The "how-tos" are clearly spelled out in the nursing actions. Specifics,
such as having Betty identify what is most important, give direct guidance to
any nurse who might need to follow through with this plan. There are many
references to helping Betty deal with her feelings. Ultimately, it is a plan that
helps Betty work through this problem, rather than one in which the nurse will
take care of the problem.

Now that Thelma's plan has been analyzed, check the TNT checklist
again, as you did for your analysis of Sue's plan. Look at how much better
Thelma's work is in comparison. For a second chance at analysis, consider another of Sue's plans.

▷ Sue's Plan for Constipation

Look at Sue's plan for Betty's constipation problem. Again, she has taken a
quick-fix approach. Unlike the decisional conflict problem, constipation may
seem like one that could be dealt with simply. There are few emotional issues
to take into account. However, other complex aspects of Betty's situation must
be kept in mind in dealing with this physiologic problem. Remember earlier
discussions of how no problem can be viewed in isolation from the other problems and the big picture of the patient's situation.

▼ Sue's Care Plan #2

Nursing Diagnosis:
  Constipation related to inadequate fluid intake, side effects of medications, and decreased mobility 2° ALS.

Goal: By the end of 1 week, the patient will have no constipation.

OBJECTIVES	NURSING ACTIONS	RATIONALE
Patient will: **1.** Increase fluid intake immediately.	**1a.** Teach patient about relationship between fluid intake and constipation **b.** Tell patient to drink things like coffee and prune juice that promote intestinal motility	**1a.** Fluid intake less than 1000 mL per day will lead to constipation **b.** Common sense
2. Change medications to ones without constipation side effects during next visit to MD.	**2a.** Tell patient to talk over medications with doctor and ask for changes to other medications	**2a.** Side effects of ferrous sulfate, baclofen, and nortriptyline = constipation
3. Continue to take Metamucil and Correctol daily.	**3a.** Let patient know that these may be necessary, considering the nature of her illness	**3a.** Limitations of activity will cause constipation

▶▶▶▶▶▶ **A**ction Learning #73: Becoming Thelma

Now it is your turn to try your hand at being Thelma. Analyze Sue's care plan and transform it into a plan that addresses the problem and all the related factors, taking into account the big picture of Betty's situation. Here is a hint: remember that Betty has trouble swallowing. Thin liquids are more apt to be aspirated into her lungs than are thick liquids. Remember, objectives should be measurable and specific. Nursing actions should be specific enough that another nurse could use the plan and continue interventions. Use the TNT checklist to help you check your work. Share your plan with a classmate. Note where your plans differ, and discuss how you each came to the conclusions you used in planning. So that you have plenty of room to write, think, revise, rewrite, you may want to do this exercise on a separate sheet of paper.

DISCUSSION	How did it go? Are you a better care planner than Sue? Was your plan similar to or different from that of your classmate?

How did the big picture guide your planning? What is the most useful thing you learned from this activity that will help you the next time you write a plan for a patient's constipation?

▶ DOING AND DETERMINING QUALITY OF CARE WITH BETTY

Most of the exploration of Betty's actual problems has focused on the designing of care, or care planning. As everyone knows, that is only part of the picture of the nursing process. Because this is a book, however, the implementation of care can only be discussed, not actually carried out. Because the care, as designed, cannot be implemented, it cannot be evaluated. Therefore, anything said about implementation and evaluation is conjecture only. Nevertheless, it is important to think about how Thelma's plans would be implemented and evaluated.

If the plan was developed *with* Betty, rather than *for* Betty, chances are that some of the implementing, or "doing" of the care, would have started as the plan was being developed. Betty would have started thinking about and sharing her ideas about the decisional conflict and, therefore, would already have started to meet some of the objectives. As the plan was implemented, the nurse and Betty would start to evaluate the outcomes by comparing Betty's progress to the preset objectives.

A most important thing to keep in mind is that implementing and evaluating must be considered during the planning phase. A well-designed plan of care will take into account the realities of doing the things on the plan. It will allow for ease of evaluation; the objectives will be specific and measurable, for example. Also, remember that implementing and evaluating may reveal new data that were not addressed in the original plan. In particular, additional factors contributing to the problems may emerge.

Thelma's plan for Betty's decisional conflict had a goal that was to be met in 1 week. If Thelma visited Betty daily, they might work on the decisional conflict plan a little bit each day. Thelma very likely would evaluate the plan as the week progressed and make changes as needed. Look at Thelma's SOAP note to see what may have occurred. (If you need to review the basics of the SOAP form of documentation, review Chapter 10.) Notice how the changes in the plan are based on the new data that were found when Thelma implemented the plan. The new data are documented in the "S" and "O" parts of the note. The "O" also includes the report of what the nurse did. Thelma specified which objectives had been met and which were not yet met in the "A" part. Remember, the "A" is the conclusion part of the SOAP note. The conclusions of evaluation focus on how the patient is progressing, as measured against the preset goals and objectives. In the "P" part of her note, Thelma referred to the plan's changes.

Here is Thelma's SOAP note:

12/20/93 3 PM Problem: Decisional Conflict

S: "It has been helpful to talk about this. I know I just need to get this done, but I really cannot ask anyone to help me until after the holidays. Could you check with the Independent Living Center (ILC) about putting in the safety bars in January?"

O: ILC offered as resource for installing bars without expense to patient. Lengthy discussions with patient about need to make decisions as soon as possible.

A: Goal partially met. Objectives 1, 2, and 3 met. Objective 4 unmet due to patient's insistence on waiting until after the holidays.

P: Time frame changed to 4 weeks for goal. Objective 4 time frame mid-January. Role playing will be done at that time. Will contact ILC in early January.—T. Thoreau, S.N.

Thelma's note documents what was done and how the patient is progressing toward the goal and objectives on the plan. The implementation and evaluation of care and Thelma's thinking are evident. Look at the TNT checklist and check which of the areas under "Conclusions of Evaluation" are completed well, as evidenced by Thelma's note.

▶ CLOSING COMMENTS

Betty's case illustrates the complexity of designing great nursing care. From Sue's care plans, one can see that quick-fix approaches compromise patient individuality and safety. Thelma's plan, although requiring more time to develop, reflects the type of individualized care that most people would want for themselves and their loved ones.

Taking the time and energy to discover all the possible related factors for each actual problem is worthwhile in terms of the guidance that related factors provide during care planning. Thinking through the complexities of each patient's unique situation and looking for the less-obvious relationships among data provide the nurse with a means to find those related factors.

Once the problems and all the related factors are identified, individualized care can be designed if the nurse is continually aware of the big picture of the patient's situation. Thinking about how each patient response affects others and thinking ahead to implementing and evaluating care gives the nurse the tools to design great nursing.

Implementation and evaluation complete the cycle of the nursing process. Evaluation "returns" to assessment as the nurse collects more information to see how the patient is progressing.

▶▶▶ *THINKING LOG #13*

Compare your thinking style to that of Sue and Thelma. Which nurse do you think you will be more like? Knowing how you think, what areas of designing care for actual problems will come easily to you? What areas will be most difficult? Hopefully, Thelma will be your ideal. Develop some memory aids for yourself so that you can think in the manner that Thelma does.

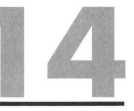

Designing, Doing, and Determining Quality of Care for Potential (High Risk) Problems

LEARNING OUTCOMES

After reading and doing the activities in this chapter you will be able to:

Explain approaches to caring for a patient with nursing diagnoses categorized as potential (high risk) problems.

Describe the differences in thinking, structure, and planning when working with actual problems and high risk problems.

Critique and improve a poorly developed plan for a selected high risk problem.

In this chapter, as in the last one, Betty's case is used to illustrate how great nursing is planned, implemented, and evaluated. Whereas the last chapter focused on actual problems, this chapter focuses on the problems for which Betty is at high risk. After some discussion of several important issues that differentiate actual problems from high risk problems, one of Sue's plans for a potential problem is presented. A critique of her plan and a revised plan illustrate differences in quality of planning. An additional plan of Sue's is presented for your critique and revision.

At several points in this chapter, the reader is reminded of other chapters in which particular concepts were first discussed or discussed in more depth. Use your KNOWING HOW YOU THINK mode to determine how you want to use these reminders. Some like to go back immediately and check the material. Others find that too disruptive to their continuity of thinking, and choose to ignore the cross-referencing for the time being. They would rather do the cross-referencing later, when they reread. Use whichever system works best for you.

▶ DEFINING POTENTIAL (HIGH RISK) PROBLEMS

▷ Terminology Clarification

As was mentioned in earlier chapters, two synonymous terms are used in the nursing literature to describe problems for which patients are at risk—"high risk problems" and "potential problems." The North American Nursing Diagnosis Association (NANDA) moved from using "potential" to "high risk" in 1992. Recently published nursing diagnosis books use the latter terminology; earlier books use the term "potential."

The change from "potential" to "high risk for" helps clear some of the confusion that can arise in distinguishing between the terms and among types of nursing diagnostic statements. For example, "possible" and "potential" are two terms that are sometimes confused. "Possible" problems are hunches, or problems that the nurse thinks exist but for which there is insufficient data to say for certain. With potential—or high risk—problems, the data exist, but they are risk factors for a problem that could occur, not data that support an existing problem.

Another clarification of terms is the distinction between risk factors for illness-related responses and risk factors for wellness responses, in which there is potential for change to a higher level of wellness. The terminology recommended by NANDA for wellness nursing diagnoses is "Potential for enhanced" —for example, "Potential for enhanced parenting."

A brief review of Chapters 6 and 8, which describe the conclusions nurses make after analyzing data, including conclusions about potential problems, might be helpful before continuing with this chapter.

▷ Differences Between Actual Problems and Potential (High Risk) Problems

Because actual problems exist, the focus of care is to diminish or remove them. Potential problems do not exist, so the focus of care is health promotion or illness prevention, which makes up a big part of a nurse's job. These activities are not simple, however. Identifying problems that are likely to occur and planning care to prevent those problems require a well-functioning thinking cap and a sound base of content knowledge.

Some of the differences between actual problems and high risk problems were discussed in Chapters 6 and 8. Three of those differences are reviewed and expanded on in this chapter: thinking differences, structural differences, and planning differences.

Thinking Differences

The biggest differences between diagnosing actual and potential problems lie in the thinking skills used and the amount of content knowledge and experience needed for the thinking. Actual problems are easier to diagnose because they are more easily supported by the patient data. Potential problems are a bit trickier. One has to "know" from books and from experience what conditions are likely to contribute to certain problems. The nurse must use INQUIRY to see that A + B + C, especially when D is present, will very likely lead to problem #1.

To illustrate this formula, consider a familiar nursing diagnosis, "High Risk for Impaired Skin Integrity," a potential problem that many patients have. In any given patient situation, the nurse needs to know, among other things, the following about skin:

Skin is the body's main defense against infection and needs to be maintained intact.

The skin does its job best when it is clean, dry, and has good circulation.

Breaks in the skin allow organisms to enter the body and disrupt normal functioning of the skin.

Organisms grow well in warm, wet, dark places.

Urine is irritating if left in contact with the skin for long periods of time (incontinent patients experience this).

Sitting for long periods of time cuts off circulation to parts of the body that are being sat on.

Skin that is overly dry and thin or fragile is more easily broken down than skin that is normally moist and healthy.

Good skin turgor means the skin will "bounce back" after it is moved or pressed.

Sitting for long periods of time in one place creates warm, moist, dark places on the perineum and the buttocks.

This list could be much longer, but the point is, a nurse must have at least this level of knowledge and experience to anticipate potential problems with skin integrity. Along with that knowledge, the nurse uses INQUIRY to see the relationships between these facts and the individual patient situation, and then comes to the conclusion that a patient is or is not at risk for impaired skin integrity.

▶▶▶▶▶ **Action Learning #74: What Is the Risk?**

Look at the following three situations and determine if the patient in each situation would be at risk, and if so, for what. Explain your thinking to a classmate and tell what knowledge was needed to make your decision.

1. Tommy has just started to crawl. His parents are collectors of blown glass art pieces and like to display them on floor-to-ceiling shelves

and the coffee table in the living room. The art work is also very colorful.
Is Tommy at risk?
If yes, for what?
Knowledge needed?

2. Mr. West has just read a new food fad book and is trying to convince you that nature's wonder food is bananas. He has decided to eat nothing but bananas for the next 2 weeks to cleanse his body of all the toxins it has built up over the years.
Is Mr. West at risk?
If yes, for what?
Knowledge needed?

3. Ms. North has just lost her husband. She is new to the city and has no close friends. She just started a new job and says she just wants to bury herself in her work and get on with life.
Is Ms. North at risk?
If yes, for what?
Knowledge needed?

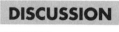 **DISCUSSION** How did you come to your conclusions? What pieces of your thinking fit with TOTAL RECALL? What fit with IN-QUIRY?

Structural Differences

Existence of the Problem

An actual problem exists when the patient data "paint a picture" of that problem. A potential problem exists when the problem is "likely to occur" if something isn't done; data that support the related factors are found, but the actual problem does not exist.

Terminology

For actual problems, the nurse simply states the nature of the problem (patient response). Examples of these are "Self-Care Deficit," "Impaired Gas Exchange," and "Parental Role Conflict." For potential problems, the problem label is preceded by the words, "High Risk for." Examples are, "High Risk for Self-Care Deficit," "High Risk for Impaired Gas Exchange," and "High Risk for Parental Role Conflict."

Existence of Defining Characteristics to Support the Problem

Defining characteristics *must* exist to support the problem if it is to be labeled as an *actual* problem. Defining characteristics *do not exist* for potential problems. If the defining characteristics existed, there wouldn't be a potential problem anymore; there would be an actual problem.

Data to Support the Related Factors

Data to support the related factors almost always exist for actual problems. Sometimes an actual problem can exist and the causes be "unknown," but there is no denying that the problem exists. A common example is, "Anxiety related to unknown causes." With a potential problem, however, there must always be data to support the related factors, or there wouldn't be a potential problem.

One might wonder how many related factors need to exist before the nurse diagnoses a potential problem. The answer comes with experience. In some cases, one factor is enough to alert the nurse; in other cases, several factors must exist before the nurse's antennae go up. This is another one of those probability issues. After nurses have taken care of several people with similar circumstances, they are able to make those judgments with a higher probability of accuracy. Think of this situation: An alien from another planet is driving a car. The car stops running when the gas gauge moved from "F" to "E." The first time it happened, the alien might not see the connection; however, when it happened a second or third time, she'd say, "Oh, when that little thing moves toward 'E,' the car is likely to stop; I'd better do something before that happens." She has learned from experience that there is a potential problem. She also could have read about this situation in a manual for operating a car to obtain some "content knowledge."

Planning Differences

Focus of the Patient Goal

When dealing with an actual problem, it obviously makes sense to try to remove or alleviate the problem. Basically, nursing is focused on *restoring* the patient to the optimum level of health, and that means diminishing or eliminating the problem. (An aside: It is important here to note that there are situations in which the patient has an actual problem but it is not feasible to restore health or eliminate the problem because the patient has a chronic or acute deteriorating condition. In these cases, maintenance and comfort are appropriate goals. Example: For a patient who has total incontinence because of irreversibly damaged nerves, a goal of continence is not realistic. A goal of comfort without constant wetness is the only option.)

The focus of the goal when dealing with a potential problem is different. Because the problem doesn't exist (yet), there are two basic approaches to planning care. One approach is to try to keep the patient at his existing level of health (*maintain*) and not let things get worse. Maintenance goals are often written in the negative form. The identified problem for which the patient is at risk will not occur; for example, "the patient will have no skin breakdown" if he is at risk for skin impairment. The other option is to help put the patient at even less risk (*promote* to a higher status of health). Here are two examples that show the difference between maintenance and promotion:

TABLE 14-1 Differences Between Actual and Potential Problems

TYPE OF PROBLEM	PROBLEM EXISTS	DEFINING CHARACTERISTICS SUPPORT PROBLEM	RELATED FACTORS EXIST	KNOWLEDGE, EXPERIENCE, THINKING SKILLS	FOCUS OF PLAN'S GOAL
Actual	Yes	Yes	Usually	Good to very good	Usually restore
Potential (High Risk for)	No	No	Yes	Very good to excellent	Maintain or promote

Maintaining status: A patient who has a stroke can easily get contractures (shortening of ligaments and tendons so that a part of the body stays in a permanently flexed position). A typical nursing diagnosis is "High risk for contractures related to paralysis and lack of active movement." The goal for this patient would be to **maintain** full range of motion. Stated another way, it could be, "The patient will not develop contractures."

Promoting higher status: A patient who has diabetes, but who does not follow his diet carefully and who does not take insulin as directed, can have many problems such as hypoglycemic or hyperglycemic reactions (too low or too high blood sugar levels), circulatory problems, infections, and many others. A typical nursing diagnosis is "High risk for hyperglycemic or hypoglycemic reactions related to nonadherence to diabetic diet and insulin schedule." The goal for this patient is to **promote** a higher level of care. Often the word "promote" is not actually used. Rather, the specific action that indicates health promotion is used; in this case that might be, "Patient will adhere to diet and insulin regimen."

Table 14.1 summarizes the differences between actual and potential problems.

▶ INTERFACE OF POTENTIAL PROBLEMS DIAGNOSED BY NURSES, MEDICAL PROBLEMS DIAGNOSED BY PHYSICIANS, AND PROBLEMS DIAGNOSED BY OTHER PROVIDERS

At times, diagnosing potential problems gets into the fuzzy realm of what is a nursing diagnosis, what is a medical diagnosis, and what is a diagnosis made by another health care provider. Recall earlier discussions of the conclusions nurses reach from analyzing data—patients' strengths and health concerns—

with the health concerns being nursing diagnoses, interdisciplinary problems, and problems for referral.

Usually, the distinctions among the three different types of health concerns in the domain of nursing are easy to see. If a patient has severe chest pain, obviously a nurse would refer that person to a physician. It is fairly easy to see that a person who has hypertension and who needs counseling on diet and lifestyle changes, has interdisciplinary problems. If a patient who has trouble getting to the bathroom because of mobility deficits is incontinent, a clear nursing diagnosis conclusion can be made (Functional Incontinence related to mobility deficits). Or if the family is adjusting well to the new baby and wants to continue, the wellness diagnosis is Potential for enhanced family growth. Other times, however, the distinction is not so clear. Subtle differences must be distinguished.

In the realm of nursing diagnoses, nurses focus on patients' response patterns, not on diseases. The actual problems that nurses are licensed for and capable of treating independently are human responses. When it comes to diagnosing and treating areas of risk, however, nurses go beyond the confines of responses to include risks for diseases as well. Diagnosing *actual* pathologic conditions (illness or disease) is the domain of physicians. But diagnosing the *risk* for a disease is within the realm of nursing because nurses can intervene to prevent a disease from occurring.

For an illustration of the difference between diagnosing an actual disease and diagnosing the risk for a disease, look at these examples:

Mrs. Grey has an indwelling urinary catheter and she does not drink very much. Mr. Brown, the nurse, knows that most people who have indwelling catheters get urinary tract infections, especially those who do not drink lots of fluids. Although the nurse would not diagnose an actual urinary tract infection, the nurse would diagnose the patient's high risk for urinary tract infection and work with Mrs. Grey to increase her fluid intake to prevent the infection from occurring. If Mr. Brown suspected the patient had a medical problem, because of blood in the urine and an elevated temperature, he would refer the patient to a physician to diagnose that problem.

Ms. French, the school nurse, talks with a group of adolescents about their sexual practices. She finds that very few of the sexually active youths use condoms. She concludes that they are at high risk for pregnancy, contracting AIDS or other sexually transmitted diseases. She diagnoses the high risk, although she would not diagnose the diseases themselves. Her interventions include helping the adolescents change their behaviors to decrease their risk.

This review and enhancement of previous information on potential problems is presented to help the reader see how the nurse came to the conclusions about Betty's high risk problems and how care was planned, implemented, and evaluated for those risk areas.

▶ DESIGNING CARE WITH BETTY FOR HER POTENTIAL PROBLEMS

In Chapter 12, these three nursing diagnoses of potential problems were made based on the data in Betty's case:

High Risk for Injury related to unsteady gait, weakness, living in two-floor apartment, spending much time alone, history of a fall, slippery kitchen floor, clutter on floors, and patient's usual pattern of wearing socks at home.

High Risk for Infection (especially respiratory and urinary) related to weakness of muscles of respiratory system, decreased mobility, swallowing difficulty 2° amyotrophic lateral sclerosis (ALS), insufficient fluid intake, environmental irritants during cold weather, and exposure to many people bringing in food.

High Risk for Aspiration related to swallowing difficulties due to weakened muscles 2° ALS.

At first glance, these diagnoses seem very long-winded. That is often the nature of "high risk" nursing diagnoses for patients who have many factors contributing to one area of risk. Betty, like many patients with chronic illnesses, has many risk factors with which to deal. Some nurses shorten the diagnostic statement by indicating the risk factors just once (such as on the care plan), and then recording only the area of risk (injury, infection, aspiration) for future documentation (such as SOAP notes). That would seem logical in the first two diagnoses here.

▷ How the "High Risk" Nursing Diagnoses fit Into the Big Picture of Betty's Care: The Nurse's Thinking

One could ask why the nurse decided on these three areas of risk. Here is some of the nurse's thinking that took place as the areas of risk were considered relative to the big picture of Betty's care:

Is there a need to address the risk of infection and the risk for aspiration separately? Yes, the two are closely related because aspiration ultimately can lead to pneumonia, which is an infection, but aspiration can also be immediately life threatening because Betty could completely occlude her trachea and not be able to breathe. If the aspiration risk is addressed only in terms of the infection, a plan of action for an aspiration emergency might not be addressed.

Are these potential problems more of a priority than the actual problems? Yes, although they are not life threatening yet, they are potentially more life threatening than the Constipation, Self-Care Deficit, Diversional Activity Deficit, and Impaired Home Maintenance Management, which have been identified as actual problems. The Decisional Conflict actual problem is closely related to the High Risk for Injury, so it is of equal priority to the potential problems. The injury, infection, and aspiration could each result in early death; therefore, it is a high priority to intervene to prevent those things from occurring.

How do these "high risk" diagnoses overlap with the other health concerns? High Risk for Injury is closely related to Betty's decisional conflict. If she can make decisions to move her bed downstairs, she will eliminate some risks for injury. The plan of care for the decisional conflict should be referred to in the plan for decreasing the risks for injury. The high risks for aspiration and infection are related to the interdisciplinary nutrition problem. Interventions by the dietitian and speech therapist could decrease Betty's risk for aspiration and therefore decrease her risk for infection. As plans are developed for the aspiration and infection risks, the interdisciplinary plan should be addressed simultaneously.

How well did the nurse do in achieving the items on the Tracking Nursing Thinking (TNT; see Appendix B) checklist, under the category "Consider the 'big picture' when finalizing all conclusions of assessment?"

▷ Sue's Plan for Betty's High Risk for Aspiration

Once again, Sue's nursing care plan provides food for thought. With her usual speed she developed a plan for Betty's "High Risk for Aspiration" nursing diagnosis. Read Sue's Care Plan #1 and think about how it could be better.

Sue's goal is that the patient will have no episodes of aspiration. This is the easy way out—to say the problem for which Betty is at risk will not occur. In Betty's case, however, this goal, although ideal, is not realistic. In spite of all that Betty or her nurse might do, Betty still could have an episode of aspiration. Sue should be focusing on decreasing the risks for aspiration. In other words, she should be promoting a higher level of functioning (decreasing the risk) rather than just maintaining present functioning.

Sue then merely repeats the goal as an objective. There is very little that can be measured in terms of patient's outcomes based on that objective. This objective only offers two options, either there is *no* aspiration or there is aspi-

▼ **Sue's Care Plan** #1

Nursing Diagnosis: High Risk for Aspiration related to swallowing difficulties due to weakened muscles 2° ALS

Goal: Patient will have no episodes of aspiration

OBJECTIVES	NURSING ACTIONS	RATIONALE
1. No aspiration.	a. Make sure patient knows about dangers of aspiration	Aspiration can occur when muscles in mouth and throat are weakened
	b. Teach patient and son the Heimlich maneuver	Everyone should know this emergency procedure
	c. Make sure patient sits upright when eating	Gravity helps food and liquids go down
	d. Tell patient not to drink thin liquids	Thin liquids can be aspirated more easily when muscles of swallowing are weakened

ration. There is no in-between option for the reality of Betty's situation. The related factor of the nursing diagnosis is not addressed in the objective. The swallowing difficulties are what put Betty at risk. Outcomes that provide criteria to measure the status of the swallowing difficulties are needed; otherwise there is no way to determine if any change in the risk factors has occurred.

The nursing actions, in Sue's usual form, are very short and provide very little detail for any other nurse who might need to follow this plan with Betty. The first action (a) is important, but if implemented as stated, it could scare the patient into not eating. Betty is already nutritionally compromised, so it would not be clinically sound to act in any way that would make one problem worse while trying to correct another problem.

The second action (b) is a good idea, but there is not enough detail as to how the teaching would best be done. Considering the age of Betty's son and the fact that Betty could be alone when she aspirated food or fluid, individualized approaches to teaching should be spelled out in more detail, especially considering Betty's decreased mobility.

The third action (c) is not realistic for the nurse to do. Sue could not "make sure patient sits upright when eating" because Betty lives at home and does not have a nurse present at all times. The nursing action must focus on how the patient can manage at home. Betty needs to understand how sitting upright is relevant to decreasing her risk of aspiration, so she can adapt her life at home to doing just that. The nursing actions do not suggest ways for nurses to help her do that.

The fourth action (d) is dangerous because of Betty's existing low level of fluid intake. Merely telling Betty not to drink thin liquids will make the fluid intake problem worse, and would be counterproductive to the plans to alleviate Betty's risk for infection and her constipation problem (see Chapter 13).

Each rationale in Sue's plan is related to its corresponding nursing action. The list of rationales, however, is incomplete because Sue's planned nursing actions are incomplete. If she studied any references on care of patients who are at risk for aspiration, she would have found that there are much better rationales for much better nursing actions.

▷ Thelma's Plan for Betty's High Risk for Aspiration

Thelma's plan is much more comprehensive and reflects much more study of the principles of care for patients at risk for aspiration. She clearly had the big picture of Betty's case in mind as she developed this individualized, clinically sound plan. As you examine Thelma's plan, compare her work with the items on the TNT checklist.

The goal of Thelma's plan is realistic. It does not indicate that Betty will not aspirate, as Sue's plan did. Considering the nature of Betty's illness, it would be impossible to ensure that Betty never had an episode of aspiration. Thelma focused on decreasing Betty's risk by promoting a higher level of functioning. She also focused on Betty's need to have an emergency plan for an aspiration episode.

The objectives on Thelma's plan are specific and measurable. When the time comes for evaluation, Thelma has clear outcomes developed to compare with Betty's future behaviors to determine change. The objectives also focus on controlling the factors contributing to the risk (the swallowing difficulties). By aiming for control of the related factors, Betty's risk will be decreased, which is the goal. In acknowledging that full control is impossible, Thelma's objective of Betty having an emergency plan is realistic.

Thelma's planned nursing actions are specific enough that any nurse could continue the plan in Thelma's absence. Rather than just making comments like "teach the patient . . . ," Thelma records teaching strategies. She advocates using pictures and how to make a dummy for Heimlich maneuver practice.

Thelma's actions are individualized for Betty. There are actions that focus on assessing Betty's usual patterns so that necessary changes can be incorporated into the patient's individualized habits and tastes. There is a clear orientation of the actions to a home care situation. Whereas Sue wrote "make sure patient sits upright while eating," Thelma addressed her actions to an adaptation of Betty's usual position for eating, and helping Betty come to the conclusion that sitting upright was best. Thelma's individualized plan also addressed Betty's strengths. Betty already knew that she needed to chew longer and eat slowly. By reinforcing that behavior, Thelma was acknowledging the strength and using it to overcome a potential problem.

All nursing actions are clinically sound. There are no actions that would be harmful to other areas of Betty's health. Clearly, Thelma kept the big picture of Betty's situation in mind and did some research on swallowing problems

▼ Thelma's Care Plan

Nursing Diagnosis: High Risk for Aspiration related to swallowing difficulties due to weakened muscles 2° ALS.

Goal: Within 2 weeks, patient will decrease risk of aspiration and have plan for dealing with aspiration emergency, as evidenced by:

OBJECTIVES	NURSING ACTIONS	RATIONALE
1. Describing the mechanisms of swallowing and how her muscle weakness puts her at risk (week 1).	1a. Explain to Betty how swallowing muscles work to prevent food from going into trachea b. Use pictures to show her the anatomic landmarks that are relevant to swallowing c. Reinforce Betty's present understanding of need to chew longer and eat slowly	1a. An increased level of knowledge will allow patient to understand the risks b. Multisensory learning will enhance understanding of abstract information c. Building on present knowledge and strengths will enhance learning
2. Agreeing to eat and drink only while sitting upright with head tilted slightly forward (week 1).	2a. Determine Betty's usual position for eating b. Using pictures, show Betty how the position of the body and head helps food move into the esophagus, not the airway	2a. Eating is often associated with other behaviors that are unique to each person b. The upright position keeps the tongue forward and allows food to be better formed into a bolus; tilting the head back opens the airway
3. Describing the best foods and fluid consistency to prevent aspiration (week 1).	3a. Assess Betty's food likes and dislikes and help her plan how to adapt these to a mechanical soft consistency b. Help Betty plan for moving to pureed foods as muscles weaken further c. Reinforce need to eat foods that are not too hot d. Encourage Betty to maintain a fluid intake of at least 2000 mL per day e. Suggest drinks that are of nectar consistency by adding thickening agent (eg, gelatin) to favorite juices and eating foods high in fluids, such as custards, creamed cereals, creamed soups, and milk shakes	3a. Adapting patient's favorite foods to therapeutic diet will increase compliance with dietary changes b. Pureed foods are less apt to be aspirated c. Hot foods can cause a gasp reaction, which could trigger aspiration d. Fluid intake is vital to maintaining circulation and kidney function, and to preventing infection. e. Thin liquids may be aspirated more easily than thick liquids; thick liquids allow patient more time to swallow, giving weakened muscles a better chance to work fully

Continued

▼ **Thelma's Care Plan** *continued*

OBJECTIVES	NURSING ACTIONS	RATIONALE
	f. Incorporate all diet changes into written list for neighbors who bring food	**f.** People who prepare foods need guidelines; otherwise patient has to adapt foods
	g. Coordinate actions with interdisciplinary plan with dietitian and speech therapist	
4. Developing a plan for managing an aspiration emergency (week 2).	**4a.** Teach Betty and her son how the Heimlich maneuver is done, using a stuffed shirt and pants "dummy" for practice Help Betty find furniture of correct height to use to push against if she should choke while alone	**4a.** Actual practice with the technique will allow for better learning and will allow nurse to correct imperfections in technique
	b. Provide a written set of directions to post in the house as reminders	**b.** Written reminders will allow others to be prepared for an emergency and will reinforce teaching
	c. Encourage Betty to eat alone as little as possible; suggest that she eat high-risk favorite foods only when someone is present	**c.** It is much more likely that effective removal of aspirated food can be accomplished by others than by patient herself

For more details on swallowing disorders, see Emick-Herring, B., & Wood, P. (1990). A team approach to neurologically based swallowing disorders. *Rehabilitation Nursing, 15*(3), 126–132.

and risks of aspiration. She adapted what she found to Betty's individual situation without compromising the soundness of the proposed actions.

The rationales listed give additional testimony to Thelma's focus on clinically sound nursing actions. Each rationale is clearly linked to a nursing action, and no action (except for the self-explanatory note about coordinating this plan with another plan) is left without a rationale to explain it. Thelma even added a note about a good reference on the subject of swallowing difficulties. Other nurses could check that reference if they wanted more details on this clinical problem.

Did Thelma miss any of the items on the TNT checklist?

▷ Sue's Plan for Betty's High Risk for Infection

Are you ready to critique Sue's second plan? She approached Betty's risk for infection in much the same way she approached the aspiration risk. Again, you get to critique the plan and make it better. It is time to readjust your thinking cap and take on Thelma's role.

▼ Sue's Care Plan #2

Nursing Diagnosis: High Risk for Infection (especially respiratory and urinary) related to weakness of muscles of respiratory system, decreased mobility, swallowing difficulty 2° ALS, insufficient fluid intake, environmental irritants during cold weather, and exposure to many people bringing in food.

Goal: Patient will have no infections, as evidenced by:

OBJECTIVES	NURSING ACTIONS	RATIONALE
1. Having a regular exercise program.	1a. Teach patient how she can get regular exercise b. Explain the value of exercise to prevention of infection	Increased mobility decreases risk of infection by improving circulation and respiratory function
2. Following recommendations of dietitian and speech therapist for swallowing problems.	2. Coordinate plan with other providers	
3. Increasing her fluid intake.	3a. Let patient know she should have about 2000 mL of fluid each day b. Remind patient to avoid too many thin liquids	2000 mL per day recommended for optimal fluid intake Thin liquids increase swallowing risks
4. Avoiding contact with too many people.	4a. Explain to patient how increased contact increases her exposure to germs	The more people, the more chances of infection

▶▶▶▶▶▶ Action Learning #75: Becoming Thelma Again

In the last chapter, you had an opportunity to try your hand at improving Sue's plan for Betty's constipation problem. Now you can do the same for Betty's high risk for infection. Examine Sue's plan; find some books that address risks for infection, think about the big picture of Betty's case, and develop a plan as you think Thelma would. Use the planning part of the TNT checklist to check your work. Share your plan with a classmate and compare your approaches. As you did with Action Learning #73 in Chapter 13, you may want to use a larger sheet of paper so you can "think" on paper as you develop your plan.

DISCUSSION   How has your thinking evolved? Did this exercise go faster than the one in the last chapter when you first took on Thelma's role? Chances are, it still took you a long time to develop the great plan. Planning great nursing care takes time, especially for beginners, but each plan you develop gets easier. Through practice, you start to home in on the important issues more quickly.

▶ DOING AND DETERMINING QUALITY OF CARE WITH BETTY FOR HER RISKS

Consider now how Thelma would implement and evaluate care for Betty. (Continue to track her activities on the TNT checklist.) Thelma's plan for the aspiration risk will be discussed to show how this is done. Although only one plan is discussed in this section, remember that Thelma would be implementing and evaluating all parts of Betty's care, including care for the actual problems discussed in Chapter 13 and the wellness, interdisciplinary, and referred concerns discussed in Chapter 15. She would use the same process for each of those parts of the plan.

To implement the plan for the aspiration risk, Thelma would set up a visit with Betty. First, because she probably wrote much of the plan after her last visit to Betty, she would share all elements of the plan and ask Betty what she would like added to the it. Thelma would want to find out from Betty the best times to focus on the aspiration issues. At the specified time, Thelma would begin the implementation with data collection. There are several places on the plan where actions indicate a need to assess Betty's usual patterns—positions for eating and Betty's food likes and dislikes. Getting Betty's personal perspective early on would allow Thelma to incorporate more personalized information into the other actions.

Because much of the plan involved teaching, Thelma would stop periodically to see if Betty was clear about what was discussed. She would ask Betty to explain what she had learned. Doing this would allow Thelma and Betty to evaluate the care because Betty's answers would indicate if the objectives were being met.

Thelma and Betty had set a 2-week time frame for meeting the goal of this plan. The first three objectives had 1-week time frames. Thelma and Betty, therefore, would aim to meet the first three objectives during the first visit and would set up a second visit to focus on the fourth objective. Such a time frame and plan would make sense, considering that Betty is being seen at home and that her son needed to be involved in the last part of the plan, which focused on objective number four.

Thelma therefore would have come to the first visit with her teaching materials for objectives one through three. If Betty didn't have any other pressing needs, Thelma would have implemented all the actions for the first three objectives and adapted those actions to whatever came up during the session with Betty.

At the end of the first visit, Betty and Thelma could evaluate the first three objectives. Using a SOAP note format (review Chapter 10 for discussion of SOAP note), here is what an evaluation of the care at the end of week 1 might be:

12/14/93 3 PM Problem: High Risk for Aspiration

S: "It really helps to see the pictures of my muscles involved in swallowing. I know how easy it is to choke now. I will definitely sit up whenever I eat. I've already started to see how much easier it is to swallow thicker liquids, but I never thought about using gelatin to thicken things like juice. My son should be here in the evening next Tuesday so we can practice the Heimlich maneuver. I will remember all of this much better if I can have everything in writing."

O: Patient participated actively in all parts of interventions and picked up information quickly.

A: Objectives 1–3 met. Interventions effective. Goal of decreased risk being met.

P: Next visit Tuesday, 12/21/93. Focus on objective #4; son will be present. Bring written information to leave with patient. Review areas covered this week and reinforce with written materials.—T. Thoreau, S.N.

This note shows how Thelma reviewed the patient's response to the interventions by recording selected quotations from Thelma as subjective data. Thelma also recorded objective data—her observations of Betty's response. Under the "A," Thelma recorded her conclusion, which related to how the objectives and goals were being met. Under the "P" section, Thelma recorded any plans for the future. She could have written the additional information on the plan itself and stated, "See changes in plan."

This example of evaluation shows the nursing process cycle and how nursing care is constantly adapted according to the patient's changing responses. It also shows that the nurse is thinking about the patient's progress in this area of risk.

How effective was Thelma's care according to the TNT checklist? Did you see any areas for improvement?

▶ **CLOSING COMMENTS**

This chapter has reviewed some of the issues surrounding nursing diagnoses of patients' health concerns that are areas of risk. Applying that knowledge to a complex patient situation, one can appreciate the importance of defining the conclusion (nursing diagnosis) well, viewing that conclusion as part of the big picture of the patient's situation, and planning sound care for the patient. The cycle of the nursing process continues as the nurse evaluates and revises care after it is implemented.

Although Betty's case is more complex than the case studies presented earlier in this book, the same nurse thinking processes apply as did earlier. As patient complexity increases, there are more pieces of information to add to the thinking, but the thinking itself is not new.

▶▶▶ *THINKING LOG #14*

> Continue your role-playing of Thelma and develop a plan for the nursing diagnosis "High Risk for Injury . . . ." As you develop the plan, track your thinking according to the T.H.I.N.K. modes (**T**otal Recall, **H**abits, **I**nquiry, **N**ew Ideas and Creativity, and **K**nowing How You Think). If you do not have time to develop a new plan, go back to the plan you created in Action Learning #75 for the "High Risk for Infection" diagnosis, and track your thinking through that process.

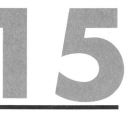

Designing, Doing, and Determining Quality of Care for Wellness Diagnoses, Interdisciplinary Problems, and Problems for Referral

After reading and doing the activities in this chapter you will be able to:

Explain approaches to care for wellness diagnoses, interdisciplinary problems, problems for referral.

Examine the differences, similarities, and overlap among all the major conclusions of assessment: strengths, actual problems/wellness diagnoses, potential problems, interdisciplinary problems, problems for referral.

Wellness diagnoses, interdisciplinary problems, and problems for referral are the topic of this final discussion on the conclusions of assessment. That these are discussed last in no way implies they are of less importance. Great nursing means that nurses have identified all relevant conclusions of assessment and have acted on all aspects of patient's health care needs.

This chapter focuses on brief descriptions of wellness diagnoses, interdisciplinary problems, and problems for referral as well as the thinking behind planning, implementing, and evaluating these conclusions in Betty's case. By this time it should be self-evident that all five modes of thinking are needed to address all conclusions of assessment.

▶ WELLNESS DIAGNOSES

Wellness diagnoses have been the focus of much debate within the nursing profession over the last decade. One point of view is that wellness issues are simply strengths. People taking this stand note that the word "diagnosis" implies a problem; wellness issues, therefore, do not really fit well within the existing taxonomy. It appears that most nurses on that side of the fence work primarily in acute care settings.

Another point of view is that wellness diagnoses are very appropriate nursing diagnoses because the basic foundation of nursing is health promotion and illness prevention. Many proponents of the wellness diagnoses work in community health, maternal–child, or well child nursing settings.

The debate has been addressed in several of the North American Nursing Diagnosis Association (NANDA) conferences. Ongoing debate has focused on the taxonomy itself. Some nurse scholars propose a companion wellness taxonomy to parallel the current taxonomy. Another proposed approach is to consider one taxonomy with different axes to incorporate the wellness diagnoses as options for any area of care.

This debate will probably continue, but meanwhile, NANDA has added wellness diagnoses to the existing taxonomy. In the proceedings of the ninth NANDA conference (Carroll-Johnson, 1991), the following guidelines for review of wellness nursing diagnoses were established:

> A wellness nursing diagnosis is a clinical judgement about an individual, family or community in transitions from a specific level of wellness to a higher level of wellness.

> 1. Label: The term "Potential for Enhanced" will be the designated qualifier. Enhanced is defined as made greater, to increase in quality, or more desired. Wellness diagnoses will be one-part statements.

> 2. Definition: The definition of the label provides a clear, precise description. The definition delineates its meaning and helps differentiate this diagnosis from all others.

> 3. Literature/Clinical Validation: A narrative review of literature is required to support the rationale for the diagnosis. A sample one-part wellness nursing diagnostic statement with related outcome criteria and nursing-prescribed interventions must accompany the submission. (pp. 375–376)

▷ Designing Care With Betty for Her Wellness Diagnosis

Although Betty has several areas that might be considered wellness diagnoses, there was one area that particularly lent itself to a wellness diagnosis—her acceptance of and planning for her death. A search of the NANDA taxonomy did not reveal an appropriate diagnostic label for Betty's situation. Therefore, the nurse and Betty created a diagnosis to fit the situation, "Potential for Enhanced Effective Preparation for Death."

If the nurse finds this to be a useful diagnosis, and it can be supported with literature and clinical validation, he or she might submit it to NANDA to review for inclusion in the taxonomy at a future date. Right now, however, the nurse's primary concern is helping Betty to continue to prepare effectively for her death. The accompanying care plan was developed.

The goal of this plan is to maintain the healthy attitudes and behaviors that Betty is already demonstrating. The objectives (outcome behaviors) also reflect continuance of specific attitudes and behaviors. The nursing orders in-

▼ Care Plan for Betty's Wellness Diagnosis

Nursing Diagnosis: Potential for Enhanced Effective Preparation for Death

Goal: Betty will maintain attitudes and behaviors that promote effective preparation for death

OBJECTIVES	NURSING ORDERS	RATIONALE
1. Continue to share thoughts and feelings with nurse and significant others.	1a. Maintain therapeutic relationship by active listening and support b. Monitor for any decrease in her sharing	1. Maintaining and monitoring nurse–pt. relationship increases opportunities for caring
2. Continue to follow through on decisions regarding legal, financial, and child care issues.	2a. Discuss status of decisions, what is finalized, what is in progress b. Provide assistance in further problem solving and decision making as needed	2. Support and assistance increases effective problem solving
3. Continue to meet with pastor on weekly basis.	3. Monitor frequency of contact with pastor and pt.'s responses to those meetings; suggest increase or decrease as needed	3. Monitoring effectiveness of resources promotes effective use
4. Continue to modify living arrangements to maintain safety and minimal stress.	4. Monitor impact of declining functions and modification of lifestyle on effective coping with impending death	4. Because increase stressors can diminish coping skills, additional help may be needed soon
5. Identify changing needs as death approaches.	5. Assess for changing needs and add additional resources to plan of care when required, eg, hospice care, increased frequency of home care, respiratory equipment, and the like	5. As functioning declines additional resources can support coping skills

clude monitoring and adjusting as needed, especially as Betty's physical condition worsens. The emotional stress of declining functional abilities can decrease energy for dealing with the emotional aspects of impending death.

▷ Doing and Determining Quality of Care With Betty for Her Wellness Diagnosis

As of this point in Betty's care, this plan is working very well. The nurse includes time to address Betty's preparation for death during each visit. A SOAP note after one visit might look like this:

12/14/93 3 PM Diagnosis: Potential for Enhanced Effective Preparation for Death

- S: "I really enjoy the visits from the pastor, he is a very caring person. I know he is busy but I wouldn't mind seeing him more often, I'm just afraid to bother him."
- O: Patient's voice tone and body language relaxed and peaceful when discussing conversations with pastor. Receptive to gentle encouragement to ask pastor for additional visits.
- A: Objective #3 met, interventions effective, goal of maintaining effective preparation for death being met.
- P: Next visit 12/21/93. Follow up to see if pastor was asked and if he can increase his visits. Continue to monitor her need and family's need in this area. Continue to monitor Objectives 1, 2, 4, and 5.

The note shows how the nurse documented implementation and evaluation of care. Betty's progress is tracked clearly by using the plan's objectives as the standards for desired outcomes.

▶ INTERDISCIPLINARY PROBLEMS

Before examining interdisciplinary problems specifically, it is helpful to review briefly the concept of collaboration. Collaboration is best described as cooperation and working together. It does not mean one person supervises, directs, or manages other people. Those activities are called supervising, directing/delegating, or managing.

Collaboration means that people with different areas of expertise are working as equals to define issues, design solutions, and achieve high-quality outcomes. In a sense, all conclusions made about a patient's situation are collaborative because the nurse collaborates with the patient; however, collaboration with patients is a given in great nursing care. The term "interdisciplinary problem" is applied to issues that require collaboration between nurses and other health care disciplines.

In health care, as in other arenas, collaboration among professionals occurs along a continuum. The continuum refers to the back-and-forth flow of accountability and responsibility for different aspects of the patient's care. All health care providers are considered equal partners in the team providing care, but there are times when one partner's expertise has a predominant influence on the design of specific aspects of care. For example, Mr. Jidou, age 83 years, is experiencing severe pain in his knees from degenerative joint disease. He is being seen in a primary care clinic on an outpatient basis. His health care team includes the physician, the home care nurse, and the physical therapist. Both the physician and the nurse know that the Mr. Jidou needs exercises, but the physical therapist is the primary designer of the details for this aspect of care. The physical therapist will design the type and frequency of exercises needed for achieving the physician's order of "Nonweight-bearing exercises to the lower extremities," and the nurse will work with the patient and family to find the best ways for the patient to do the exercises at home.

A nursing conclusion in Mr. Jidou's case, categorized as an interdisciplinary problem, would be written as, "Pain in both knees related to chronic degenerative joint disease." With a more complete data base there would likely be additional related factors that would help to individualize care better. Additional data might include information such as Mr. Jidou's inability to tolerate most over-the-counter medications for reducing pain, or a chronic respiratory condition that limits his activity tolerance for nonweight-bearing strengthening exercises.

Another way of writing interdisciplinary problems is in the format of "high risk for . . . ." Consider an example of a patient who is admitted to an alcohol rehabilitation unit. The first priorities for care include life-threatening and safety issues, and are matters of collaboration between nurse and physician. The major life-threatening and safety issues in alcohol rehabilitation are related to the signs and symptoms of withdrawal of the toxic chemical, ethyl alcohol, from all body systems, especially the cardiovascular system. A typical interdisciplinary problem at this point of treatment is, "High risk for complications of alcohol withdrawal." The related factors will vary depending on the patient. An example of a related factor for this diagnosis might be, "related to detoxification after 20 years of daily alcohol intake averaging 1 pint/day."

There is a relationship among the type of health care setting, the nature of the patient's health concerns, and the number of interdisciplinary problems that are identified as nursing conclusions. In most cases, in the inpatient settings where patients experience more acute levels of health problems, there are more nursing conclusions in the realm of interdependent practice (interdisciplinary problems). In outpatient settings, home care, or wellness care settings, there usually are more nursing conclusions in the realm of independent nursing care (nursing diagnoses). These generalities are by no means always the case, however.

▷ Designing Care With Betty for Her Interdisciplinary Problem

Five nursing conclusions made in Betty's case were classified as actual problems, the care of which could be provided in the independent realm of nursing. Another nursing conclusion is in the realm of interdependent nursing practice. This conclusion required collaboration with other health care providers: "Altered Nutrition and Fluid Intake related to impaired swallowing and meal preparation by neighbors." To design effective care in this area, the nurse enlists the expertise of a dietitian and a speech therapist to define the issues accurately, design treatment plans, and evaluate outcomes.

This interdisciplinary problem is closely related to the High Risk for Aspiration diagnosis addressed in Chapter 14. Because the risk for aspiration pointed to a need for immediate action, the nurse will have started the interventions on that plan already. One of the actions on that plan was to coordinate those actions with recommendations on this interdisciplinary plan.

Because collaboration can take more time when the patient is at home, the nurse could not wait and address the risk for aspiration and the nutrition and fluid intake problem together as one issue. If Betty had been hospitalized, the nurse would have had quick access to the speech therapist and the dietitian and, therefore, could have combined the high risk diagnosis and the interdisciplinary problems into one plan. Further along in Betty's care, those two plans would very likely become one interdisciplinary plan.

The first part of the *preliminary* care plan for "Altered Nutrition . . . " is presented in the Preliminary Care Plan for Betty's Interdisciplinary Problem. This plan illustrates the first steps in incorporating the collaboration aspect. The actual interdisciplinary plan cannot be completed until after the collaboration occurs with the other health care professionals.

Notice that the goal of this plan is focused on improving a condition that is not currently acute but probably will be if left untreated. The time frame of 1 month probably is realistic, depending on how quickly the nutritionist and speech therapist can make recommendations.

The objectives are patient centered, measurable, and flow from the related factors. They focus on the patient, describing her understanding of the seriousness of the problem, her willingness to participate in the evaluations, and her compliance with the recommendations. The last objective brings the focus back to the need to share information with the neighbors who prepare her meals, by addressing the second related factor for this interdisciplinary problem.

The nursing actions are nurse centered, realistic, and clearly flow from their respective patient objectives. The actions (as well as the objectives and rationales) specifically related to collaboration with other health care providers are in **boldface**. The speech therapist will assess and diagnose the degree of swallowing difficulty, and make suggestions for swallowing techniques and the types of foods and liquids that are least likely to stimulate choking. The

▼ Preliminary Care Plan for Betty's Interdisciplinary Problem

INTERDISCIPLINARY PROBLEM:

Altered Nutrition and Fluid Intake related to impaired swallowing and meal preparation by neighbors

Goal: Within 1 month, Betty will have attained adequate nutrition and hydration

OBJECTIVES	NURSING ORDERS	RATIONALE
1. Describe significance of impaired swallowing to maintain adequate food and fluid intake.	1a. Ask Betty to describe her understanding of the problem and assess her awareness of the importance of dealing with it b. Explain as needed the purpose of collaboration with speech therapist and dietitian	1. Patients who understand the reason for change are more cooperative in seeking change
2. Participate in evaluation of swallow status and nutritional and fluid intake.	2. Collaborate with MD, speech therapist, and dietitian, and help Betty set up appointments for evaluation	2. Effective referrals include getting patient to proper providers
3. Follow up on recommendations of speech therapist and dietitian.	3a. Discuss recommendations with Betty and ask her to explain them and share how she feels about them b. Assess how well she can follow recommendations at home c. Consult with dietitian and speech therapist to modify plans as needed to fit best her individual needs	3. Effective referrals include evaluation of the results.
4. Share needs for specific food requirements with neighbors.	4a. Discuss how she will share needs with neighbors, role-play as needed b. Develop a written list that can be given to neighbors for reference	4. Helping patients adapt recommendations to their specific needs improves quality of care

nutritionist will assess and diagnose the current nutritional state, and make suggestions on how to maintain adequate intake of food and fluids without increasing the risk of aspiration. If all works well, the dietitian and the speech therapist will collaborate in their final recommendations and a revised care plan will be designed. An interdisciplinary care plan has many of the same characteristics of a nursing care plan but includes the special recommendations of all the collaborators, including the patient.

▷ Doing and Determining Quality of Care With Betty for Her Interdisciplinary Problem

One of the recommendations of the dietitian was the following objective, "Increase fluid intake to eight glasses of thickened fluid a day." This recommendation did not work well for Betty. It increased her need to urinate to the point of diminishing any activities outside the home. Diminished ability to be far from a toilet created increased problems related to Diversional Activity Deficit. This recommendation also caused nausea and occasional gagging. The nausea was unpleasant, but the gagging was dangerous for Betty.

After the nurse begins to implement this objective, a SOAP note might look like this.

12/17/93 10 AM Interdisciplinary Problem: Altered Nutrition and Fluid Intake

S: "The nutritionist and the speech therapist both said to add the thickening agent to fluid and drink eight glasses a day. I have been trying, but I have to go to the bathroom so much I can't leave the house, and I added the thickener to water and it made me sick to my stomach. I'm gagging at times."

O: Dietitian contacted by nurse and recommendations changed to drinking three glasses of thickened apple juice and three glasses of apricot nectar. Betty agreed to try this change.

A: Objective #3 partially met. Modifications above made. Goal of attaining adequate nutrition being achieved.

P: Call Betty tomorrow and assess for decreased frequency of urination and decrease or absence of nausea. Follow up on Betty's interaction with neighbors, Objective #4.—G. Rubenfeld, R.N.

Both the speech therapist and the nutritionist will continue to see Betty for modifications as her chronic terminal illness progresses. It is important for the nurse to maintain contact with all health care providers involved in the patient's care. This task is somewhat easier in an acute care setting, where all the providers usually are in the same organization. But, in other settings, such as clinics and homes, it becomes particularly important for the nurse to assume the role of case manager—coordinator. This role provides for increased continuity and completeness of care.

▶ PROBLEMS FOR REFERRAL

The nurse's skill in effectively identifying and referring problems depends directly on three factors: accepting that nursing cannot be all things to all people, the nurse's content knowledge about the domains of other health care disciplines, and the nurse's degree of experience. Beginning nursing students generally make fewer referrals than do experienced nurses, but this is not always the case.

▷ Accepting the Limitations of the Nursing Profession and Oneself

The first factor that influences the nurse's skill in identifying problems for referral and making effective referrals requires some additional thinking. From the beginning of nursing school, nurses are taught how to assess, plan, implement, and evaluate care for nursing problems. At some point, nurses also must learn about the limitations of their profession. Nurses cannot do everything for everybody. There are situations in which patients' problems and concerns do not fit at all within the domain of nursing. It is the responsibility of the nurse to recognize this and properly refer the patient to providers who can meet those needs. This is part of the nurse's professional responsibility.

Nurses may make referrals to other nurses as well as to nonnurse providers. For example, it is perfectly appropriate for a nurse who has worked for 20 years in obstetrics to say that he or she is not qualified or comfortable caring for gerontologic patients. It is, however, that nurse's responsibility to assist the patient or family in finding the proper resource to deal with the problems related to gerontologic concerns. Those other resources very likely may be gerontologic nurses or other specialists in gerontology.

Accepting one's own limitations goes beyond accepting a lack of knowledge and experience in another area of care. Sometimes a nurse's values and beliefs are in conflict with an area of patient need. Deciding when one's values and beliefs are hindrances to care is not an easy judgment. There are professional and ethical issues to consider as well. Nurses, for example, cannot simply refuse to care for people they do not like; however, if nurses honestly feel that their values and beliefs could interfere with the quality of their care in any given situation, they should refer patients to other providers, whether they be nurses or other health care workers.

▷▷▷▷▷▷ **Action Learning #76: Identifying Problems for Referral**

As a beginning nurse, examine the following situations and think about your knowledge and experience, values and beliefs. Which would you consider as problems for referral and which you would deal with yourself or collaboratively? Why? Share your reasoning with a classmate.

Peter is experiencing all the signs and symptoms of diabetes—frequent urination, excessive thirst and hunger. He has a strong family history of diabetes. He asks you for help.

Alicia is 13 years old and tells you she needs an abortion and wants you to help her in finding out how to get one.

Fred is complaining of bad stomachaches after 2 weeks of eating only chili dogs and French fries. He is asking for help getting rid of the stomach aches.

Bill has been gaining weight and is asking you for help in finding a weight management program that he can live with. He is feeling very stressed because his companion, John, just moved out and John did all the cooking.

DISCUSSION   What criteria did you use to determine if you could deal with the patient's requests, or if you needed to make a referral? How did your values and beliefs about each situation influence your decisions? Except for the first situation with Peter, all of the situations could appropriately be handled by experienced nurses. It would not, however, be inappropriate for even experienced nurses to make referrals if they believed their values and beliefs about abortion or homosexuality would interfere with the objectivity of their thinking or their judgments about care.

▷ **Content Knowledge**

Content knowledge about the domains of other health care disciplines is initially obtained through nursing education programs, reading, attending conferences, and so forth. The more the nurse knows about the other health professions, the more likely patient problems for referral will be recognized and appropriately referred. Most nursing programs include a large amount of information in the biomedical field. This knowledge, plus the close collaboration between nurses and physicians, makes referrals to the physician fairly easy to identify. It takes more effort on the part of the nurse to learn about the kinds of care other health care professionals can provide, and to learn how to make referrals.

▶▶▶▶▶▶ **Action Learning #77: Increasing Your Content Knowledge for Referring Problems**

Select a health care profession other than nursing or medicine. Find someone who works in that profession and ask that person the following questions. Share your findings with a classmate. (This Action Learning exercise will be helpful for interdisciplinary problems as well.)

1. What is your primary responsibility in patient care?

2. What kinds of things should I be looking for in patient behaviors, signs or symptoms, and the like, to make appropriate referrals to you?

3. What is the most effective way to make sure you and the patient get connected?

DISCUSSION What was your most interesting finding? What is the best way for you to store this information in your long-term memory for future use?

▷ Experience

Experience is also a great teacher. The more the nurse works directly with other providers, the clearer the understanding of their roles and responsibilities. Probably one of the best role models for knowledge and experience about health care services, patient resources, and how to make referrals is a community health nurse. A major responsibility of all community health nurses is to know who in the community can do what for whom, and how to get patients effectively connected with the resources they need.

Display 15-1 lists some basic guidelines for making effective referrals. These guidelines are broad enough to be used in many settings. Additional specific guidelines usually are found in the policy and procedure manuals of each health care setting.

DISPLAY 15-1. Basic Guidelines for Making Referrals

GUIDELINES	QUESTIONS TO BE ANSWERED
Collaborate with patient	What specifically is needed? How soon is it needed? How does the patient think the need could best be met?
Identify available resources	Which providers/resources focus specifically on this patient's needs? What is the cost? Does the patient go to them or will they come to the patient? Does the patient meet the criteria for obtaining help from this resource?
Assist patient in making contact	How is contact made: by phone, letter of referral, in person? Can the patient complete forms? Does patient have transportation, baby sitting, and so forth, to keep appointment?
Determine quality of results	Did patient get connected? Was need met? How does patient feel about the resource? Are modifications in plan needed?

▷ Designing, Doing, and Determining Quality With Betty for Her Problem for Referral

The area of finances frequently presents problems that require a referral. Even community health nurses, who directly assist patients with examining the impact of finances on their overall health and living situation, usually make referrals to other organizations to work on the details. Such organizations include the Department of Social Services, Credit Counseling Services, emergency rent payment groups, and the like.

The nurse worked with Betty to define the issues with regard to finances. This frequently is a very difficult subject for the patient and the nurse to discuss. Many people are taught from a very early age that it is inappropriate to discuss one's financial status with anyone but a personal banker. Discussion of a person's financial situation is sometimes more difficult than talking about elimination or sexuality. The nurse approached this delicate topic by saying,

> "Betty, many people have a lot of difficulty sharing information about their financial situation. These are very private matters. It is important, however, for us to discuss this because it significantly affects your and your sons' future lifestyle. I am not an expert in financial matters but I can begin to help you find resources as they are needed.
> "The other reason to discuss this is to make you aware of resources that you are entitled to and eligible for as a hardworking taxpayer of many years.
> "Tell me how you feel about talking about your financial situation and what I can do to make it easier. I should remind you at this point that all of this information, as is all the information about you and your family, is strictly confidential."

Once the discussion began, it became clear that Betty had had no income since her retirement, which had been necessary for medical reasons. The nurse knew from experience that Betty was probably eligible for disability income through Social Security and contacted the Social Security Office. Because of Betty's difficulty in talking for any length of time on the phone, the nurse contacted the agency directly. In other circumstances, the nurse would have helped the patient to make the contact and learn how to negotiate the system. Negotiating the health care delivery system to obtain the needed resources is a skill that is invaluable to all patients.

The appointment was set up, transportation was arranged, and Betty kept the appointment. She was, however, disappointed. Because she has a small Certificate of Deposit in a local bank, she was not eligible to receive her disability benefits at that time. A plan was developed for her to use up the funds, after which she would be eligible to reapply in 3 months. In the meantime, the nurse worked with other agencies to be sure Betty received home care services and additional food until she could receive her benefits. Luckily, she did not have to worry about paying rent and utilities because her former employer was providing that.

▶ **CONCLUDING COMMENTS ON DESIGNING, DOING, AND DETERMINING QUALITY OF CARE FOR WELLNESS DIAGNOSES, INTERDISCIPLINARY PROBLEMS, AND PROBLEMS FOR REFERRAL**

Providing care for these last three conclusions of assessment require the use of all five modes of thinking just as much as they were needed to address actual and potential problems. Wellness diagnoses require more NEW IDEAS AND CREATIVITY, simply because there are currently fewer options in this area on the NANDA taxonomy. Interdisciplinary problems and problems for referral also require extra content knowledge to be identified effectively. Skill in identifying these last three conclusions of assessment significantly enhances the delivery of comprehensive, great nursing care.

▶ **SUMMARY OF CHAPTERS 12 THROUGH 15**

The last four chapters were meant to show how thinking and the nursing process are applied in a complex patient situation. Although no written description can ever capture the full scope of any real-life situation, we hope the reader has been able to appreciate how the nurse's thinking was used to coordinate the many aspects of care.

Betty's case required that the nurse collect and analyze a large amount of data and make many conclusions. There also were many conclusions about Betty's strengths that were addressed in care plans as a means to help her deal with her health concerns. The conclusions about Betty's health concerns touched on all categories—nursing diagnoses of wellness issues, actual problems, and potential problems; interdisciplinary problems; and problems for referral.

While these examples in Betty's case are fresh in the reader's mind, it may be helpful to review the differences and similarities among all the major conclusions of assessment. As was pointed out in early chapters, nursing is like life in general: Things don't always fit into nice, neat boxes or categories. There are always gray areas and fuzzy edges. Keeping the gray areas and fuzzy edges in mind, examine Table 15-1, which gives the characteristics of each of the major conclusions of assessment. Remember, there are always exceptions to any rules, but these distinctions work for most situations.

TABLE 15-1 Overview of the Differences and Similarities Among the Major Conclusions of Assessment

QUESTIONS TO ASK	WELLNESS NURSING DIAGNOSIS	ACTUAL PROBLEM NURSING DIAGNOSIS	POTENTIAL PROBLEM NURSING DIAGNOSIS	INTERDISCIPLINARY PROBLEM	PROBLEM FOR REFERRAL
Who identifies the concern?	Nurse	Nurse	Nurse	Nurse or other provider	Nurse or other provider
Who deals with the concern?	Nurse (independent practice)	Nurse (independent practice)	Nurse (independent practice)	Nurse (interdependent practice)	Other provider
What content knowledge is needed?	Nursing science Sciences Basic studies	Nursing science Sciences Basic studies	Nursing science Sciences Basic studies	Nursing science Sciences Basic studies Domain of other providers	Nursing science Sciences Basic studies Domain of other providers
What minimum work experience is needed?	Average	Average	Better than average	Average	Average
What modes of thinking are needed?	All five modes	All five modes	All five modes	All five modes	All five modes
What does first part of conclusion statement look like?	"Potential for Enhanced . . ."	Taxonomy label or other descriptive label	Usually taxonomy label of "High Risk for . . ."	Taxonomy label or other descriptive label	N/A
Are related factors included?	NO—N/A	Yes, unless unknown	Yes (mandatory)	Sometimes	N/A
What might complete statement look like?	Potential for Enhanced Family Coping; Growth	Self-Esteem Disturbance r/t knowledge deficit, ineffective coping as new mother, and loss of job	High Risk for Impaired Skin Integrity r/t immobility, incontinence and fragile skin	High risk for complications of kidney transplant	Unsafe housing

▶▶▶▶▶ **Action Learning #78: Distinguishing the Category of the Conclusion of Assessment**

Examine the conclusions listed below. Select the most likely conclusion category from Table 15-1 that would fit with the conclusion. Explain your reasoning to a classmate.

Conclusion Label	*Conclusion Category*
1. Unsafe sanitation in day care center	
2. High risk for complications of open heart surgery	
3. Altered Cardiac Output related to . . .	
4. High Risk for Injury to toddler related to unsecured kitchen cabinets containing cleaning fluids	
5. Potential for Enhanced individual coping	

DISCUSSION   How well did you do? Did you consider #1 as a problem for referral? For most beginning nurses it might be, but for an experienced community health nurse it could also be considered a community-focused interdisciplinary problem. This wasn't meant as a trick question, but to show you how the "rules" are not rigid; there are always exceptions.

▶▶▶ *THINKING LOG #15*

The best way to internalize everything you have been reading and thinking about over the last four chapters is to continue to put your learning to work. Select a patient you have previously care for, or one you are currently caring for. Using the Tracking Nursing Thinking checklist (Appendix B) as a guide, plan care for all the major conclusions of assessment. Share your plan with a classmate and explain why you did what you did.

If you haven't begun to collect your care plans already, start now. Create your own Care Plan Portfolio, and include this one in it. You will find your portfolio to be a valuable resource for many years to come.

REFERENCE

Carroll-Johnson, R. M. (Ed.). (1991). *Classification of nursing diagnoses: Proceedings of the ninth conference.* Philadelphia: JB Lippincott.

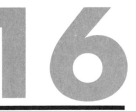

Thinking Into the Future: From Linear Equation to a Paradigm of Great Nursing

LEARNING OUTCOMES

After reading and doing the activities in this chapter you will be able to:

Discuss learning and thinking as it has evolved from the beginning chapters through the last chapter.

Design and explain a visual illustration of the relationships among all the components of great nursing.

Embrace the future of *your* professional nursing practice.

This final chapter is an overview of where you started, where you are, and where you are going as you continue your journey in nursing. The journey has just begun.

▶ WHERE YOU STARTED

The first three chapters of this text introduced the basic concepts of *thinking*, *doing*, and *the nursing process*. The second and third sections of the text, Chapters 4 through 11, explored the details of the nursing process and the importance of effective verbal and written communication. The fourth section, Chapters 12 through 15, examined thinking, doing, and the nursing process in the context of a more complex patient situation. You have come a long way.

Knowing the five modes of thinking is the foundation for critical thinking and sound clinical judgment. Clearly understanding the multiple roles of direct and indirect care activities helps define the domain of what nurses do, and appreciating the intertwining of thinking and doing with the multiple pro-

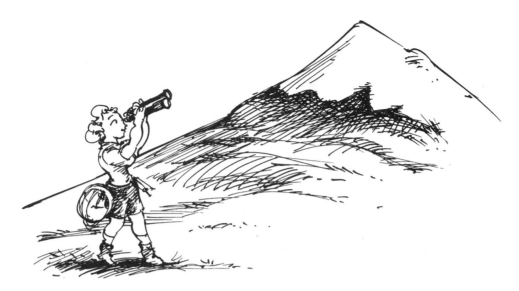

Figure 16-1. Thinking into the future.

cesses within the nursing process is necessary to move beyond the role of be-ginner.

In Chapter 3, a linear equation for great nursing was examined. It looked like this:

$$\text{Patient} + \text{You} + \frac{\text{Thinking}}{\text{Skills}} + \frac{\text{Content}}{\text{Knowledge}} + \frac{\text{Nursing}}{\text{Process}} = \text{Great Nursing}$$

At that point in time, this basic equation was sufficient, but by now, read-ers who have expanded their thinking are questioning its simplicity. It is time to examine where your thinking is now, after reading, rereading, and doing the many Action Learning exercises and Thinking Logs throughout all the chap-ters. It is time to reexamine the equation with your ever-growing thinking skills.

▶ WHERE YOU ARE

The basic components of the equation are still appropriate; however, their defi-nitions need expanding. The simple addition of each component to the others does not do justice to the dynamic relationship among the components and the resulting great nursing.

Appreciating the phrase, "The whole is greater than the sum of the parts," is critical to this discussion. Consider as an example the now famous cake that has served to illustrate several issues. The ingredients of the cake are the parts of the whole. The cake itself, the finished product, is the whole. How different are the separate parts from the whole? The cake is a tasty result of the appropriate amounts of each ingredient, blended in the proper sequence, and then baked at the appropriate temperature for the optimum length of time. The cake is a new and unique whole that cannot simply be separated back into its original parts.

Likewise, the simple equation of the five components, added to each other to achieve great nursing, does not fully represent the whole of great nursing. To illustrate how your thinking has moved beyond this early understanding, review the components and complete the last of the Action Learning exercises.

▷ Thinking Skills

By now you have gained new insight into your thinking skills as well as how to nurture and develop their growth. Reflect back, using your KNOWING HOW YOU THINK mode, to appreciate fully some of the changes in your thinking. You have every reason to be proud of you accomplishments thus far.

▶▶▶▶▶▶ **Action Learning #79: Thinking Skills**

List the changes that have occurred in your thinking since you started this activity book. Share your findings with a classmate.

DISCUSSION What have you learned about thinking in general and your thinking in particular? Could you recognize differences in quality as well as quantity? What is (are) the biggest change(s) in your thinking now, and what is (are) the area(s) you want to work on the most?

It is the growing level of comfort and ease in using all five modes of thinking skills that is of particular importance at this point. The key modes of thinking that were introduced in Chapter 1 (TOTAL RECALL, HABITS, INQUIRY, NEW IDEAS AND CREATIVITY, and KNOWING HOW YOU THINK) have been identified consistently throughout this text.

Now, to broaden your perspective on thinking, consider these thinking skills as more than separate entities. Picture these five modes as working in harmony with each other all at the same time. Compare the modes of thinking to the strings on a guitar. Each mode, like each string, has its own special purpose, but when all the strings are used together to play a piece of music, the result is much nicer than if just one or two strings were played alone. The same idea applies to the use of the thinking modes. The more they are used in harmony with each other, the better the result.

Also consider the fact that the five modes of thinking are integral parts of the patient as well as the nurse. Thinking skills are developed over time and can be enhanced for both nurse and patient. One of the major roles of nursing is to help patients learn how to help themselves. Guiding and enhancing patients' understanding of their own thinking and problem-solving skills is one of the major goals of all nursing care.

KNOWING HOW YOU THINK is the key mode for nurturing the growth of all thinking modes for both the nurse and the patient. Some refer to this mode as "reflective thinking." Reflective thinking has been studied for over a decade. Even the popular literature considers reflective thinking to be the common denominator among the world's great thinkers (Begley, 1993).

▷ Content Knowledge

There is never an end to the learning of content knowledge. What is learned today may be different tomorrow, or maybe even in a few minutes. Great nursing is impossible if nurses stop learning content knowledge.

Content knowledge was first discussed in Chapter 2, when the *doing* part of nursing was explored. If nurses do not understand the many direct and indirect aspects of nursing care, great nursing is impossible.

Nurses also must know about the activities of other health professionals to effectively identify, collaborate on, and refer health concerns. The major content knowledge required of nurses, besides nursing knowledge, is in the biomedical field. Although many expert nurses are sophisticated enough in their content knowledge to determine medical diagnoses, it *is* **not** *within the legal realm of nursing practice to make medical diagnoses*.

The purpose of having strong content knowledge in the biomedical field is not to make medical diagnoses but to supplement nursing practice. For example, a patient with all the signs and symptoms of diabetes can be identified by the nurse and referred to the physician for the official diagnosis. The nurse then diagnoses the many possible and probable nursing needs of the patient, who must manage the activities of daily living affected by the disease. The nurse determines how the diabetes is affecting sleep patterns, activity patterns, eating patterns, skin care, and so forth. All of those effects of the disease become the human responses for which nurses are responsible as they diagnose and design care.

The sources of content knowledge are ever-expanding. Lectures, workshops, books, journals, computer searches, other health professionals, patients, significant others, and experience are only some of the many sources of information.

The strong connections between content knowledge and thinking become obvious as the nurse looks for the many possible and probable relationships among the multiple content areas: the patient's individual responses to the situation at hand; the patient's strengths and resources; what the nurse knows or needs to look up about health and illness; the domain of nursing; and the domain of other health care professionals.

Action Learning #80: The Relationship Between Thinking Skills and Content Knowledge

Think about the dynamic relationship between thinking skills and content knowledge and draw a simple diagram to illustrate the relationship. Share your creation with a classmate and explain it. If needed, revise your diagram to make the visual image clearer.

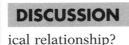 **DISCUSSION** How challenging was it for you to represent this relationship? How will this drawing help you remember this critical relationship?

▷ The Nursing Process

Several chapters have addressed the details of the components of the nursing process—assessing, planning, implementing, and evaluating—as well as the big picture of the nursing process components working together. The components of the process each require thinking skills (all five modes) and content knowledge to be completed effectively. Each of the components also has many subcomponents or subprocesses within the overall process. The components also interact and interrelate constantly, like guitar strings, if they are working well. Thus, the nursing process is a dynamic entity consisting of multiple processes within a larger process, all working in harmony to achieve great nursing care.

A brief review of Chapters 3 through 9 will refresh the reader's perspective on the details as well as the whole of the nursing process.

▶▶▶▶▶▶ **Action Learning #81: The Relationship Between the Nursing Process, Thinking Skills, and Content Knowledge**

Use your TOTAL RECALL to remember how assessing, planning, implementing, and evaluating work together, and then draw a diagram to illustrate how they fit with thinking skills and content knowledge. Incorporate your diagram from Action Learning #80 if it will work here. Share your work with a classmate and ask that person to critique your work for clarity in representing the concepts. Ask the classmate to make suggestions as needed, but you make the final decision as to what best represents your understanding of the relationship among the concepts.

DISCUSSION   How does this diagram add to your understanding of the interrelationships among the concepts?

▷ **The Patient**

This activity book consistently has considered the "patient" as an individual. It is important to remember, however, that families, groups, and communities also are patients, and have their own unique nursing needs and interventions. After you become skilled in applying the nursing process to individuals, you will need to expand your skills to work with families, groups, and communities.

It also is important to remember that patients have thinking skills, content knowledge, and feelings just as nurses have. Patients are unique individuals with unique needs. On top of that, the patient has automatic ownership of the health situation. Great nursing cannot exist if the patient is depersonalized and not recognized as the ultimate controller of his or her health situation.

All of these factors make patients special individuals who deserve thinking nurses—nurses who do not simply dole out standardized, cookbook care.

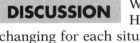

Action Learning #82: Adding the Patient to the Diagram

Create a symbol or character to represent the patient. Add this symbol to the your evolving diagram in a way that shows the interconnectedness and the relationships among the components of the equations discussed so far—thinking skills, content knowledge, the nursing process, and the patient.

DISCUSSION   Why is the patient such a critical part of your diagram? How can you represent the patient as being different and changing for each situation, to avoid cookbook care?

▷ You—The Nurse

The next component of this equation to diagram is you. You, and every other nurse, are a unique blend of thinking skills, content knowledge (including knowledge of the nursing process), and, the most vital part of all, a unique personality. It is your personality that provides the values, the feelings, and the caring. It is your personality that makes your nursing practice unique to you. Without you and your caring, "great nursing" is simply a nice-sounding phrase with a very hollow ring.

Action Learning #83: Incorporating the Unique You Into the Diagram

Create a symbol or picture of yourself to add to the diagram. Create this symbol carefully, because it will always be you and no one else. It will not represent just any nurse or nursing in general; it is you alone. This symbol or picture will change over time as you grow and change, but it will always stand for you and your special blend of thinking, doing, and caring.

DISCUSSION How challenging was it to create a symbol to represent yourself? How does it feel to be recognized as one of a kind and so important to the development of great nursing care?

▷ Great Nursing

This brings us to the last part of the original equation, great nursing. It continues to be a concept that is not easy to describe precisely and clearly. Great nursing usually is easy to recognize when it is found, but it is elusive to pin down with words. Consider the following comparison of adequate nursing to great nursing to help make the distinction clearer.

> *Adequate nursing care:* Safe care because all parts of the the nursing process are used. (Unsafe, poor nursing care is the result of skipping one or more of the parts.) The nurse who provides adequate care mechanically plods through all the components of the nursing process in a series of separate steps that simply follow each other in a linear fashion. The primary thinking modes used are TOTAL RECALL and HABITS.
>
> *Great nursing care:* Safe, efficient, and effective care that results from using the nursing process as the dynamic tool it was designed to be. Assessing, planning, implementing, and evaluating are done by nurses using all modes of thinking. The nursing process becomes embedded into the nurse's thinking process. The nursing process is no longer a separate entity that requires retrieval from a textbook or even from conscious memory, during each patient encounter. Care is focused on the patient as a unique individual. When nursing is great, it is a caring art as well as a sophisticated science.

Great nursing is not an elusive ideal that can only be written about by nursing scholars. Great nursing is practiced hourly, by nurses in all health care settings: homes, long-term care facilities, schools, clinics, intensive care units, urgent care clinics, and hospitals, to name only a few. Great nursing will be practiced by *you* as you incorporate the components of the equation into your practice.

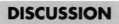**ction Learning #84: From Linear Equation to Paradigm**

A paradigm is a model that represents two or more concepts and their relationships and outcomes. You have been creating a paradigm over the last few pages as you recreated your perceptions of the components and relationships in the original linear equation for great nursing. Now it is time to complete your paradigm. Continue to use your thinking cap and put all the pieces together into one paradigm—thinking skills, content knowledge, nursing process, patient, you, and great nursing. Share your paradigm with a classmate. Save your paradigm and reexamine it when you graduate.

DISCUSSION What do you think of your creation? How is it similar to and different from those created by classmates? What parts do you think will change the most by graduation? Are you willing to make the changes at that time and continue to grow toward great nursing? In particular, remember that this is *your* paradigm; it will be similar to others, but no others will have "you" as a critical component.

The preceding review and paradigm development were designed for two reasons. First, they demonstrate how you have grown in your thinking and your ability to see relationships among the components of great nursing. Identifying relationships and examining their values are extremely valuable abilities. Seeing relationships permits you to see the "big picture" of the patient's needs.

The second, and equally important, reason for designing your own paradigm is to help you internalize the concepts of the original equation. To "internalize" means to absorb new information into your existing understanding so you can use the new information automatically. It is the process of developing HABITS, very useful HABITS. The better you incorporate the concepts into your repertoire of thinking and doing, the more likely you are to use the concepts effectively and efficiently in nursing practice. Concepts that are not internalized can be "parroted" back on an examination, but can rarely be applied to real-world nursing care.

One of the best ways to internalize information is to feel a sense of ownership of the information. The diagram you have created is yours and yours alone; you own it. It took your thinking, your personality, and your energy to create it. You are more likely to value, remember, and use what is your private property, than you are likely to use someone else's diagram memorized from a textbook. Therefore, you were encouraged to create a personal paradigm, in the hope that it would mark your entry into a new level of thinking and doing in your journey toward great nursing.

▶ WHERE YOU ARE GOING

Now that you have identified where you are, what about where you are going? The future holds many challenges for nursing and nurses. For example, technology threatens to depersonalize both the patient and the nurse while it leads nursing into the new age. Cost-containment measures are eliminating many nursing positions, while, at the same time, they force the use of NEW IDEAS AND CREATIVITY to find better ways to deliver great care. Proposals for new national health care policies are seen as threats by some and blessings by others. One predicted consequence of national policy change is a significant increase in the need for nurses to be primary providers of service to many populations.

To coin a cliché, there are no crystal balls to help predict where you or health care are going. Change, however, is guaranteed, and the best you can do is be prepared for it as you continue your journey into the future. As you prepare, consider incorporating these three basic principles to navigate successfully the troughs and waves (maybe even tidal waves) as they come:

▼ Nurture and value your thinking in all five modes: TOTAL RECALL, HABITS, INQUIRY, NEW IDEAS AND CREATIVITY, and especially KNOWING HOW YOU THINK.

▼ Acknowledge the patient as a unique individual with strengths and health concerns *and* as the person who has the final word in determining his or her own health care.

▼ Know that great nursing is an achievable goal if you believe in and internalize your own paradigm.

The future of the nursing profession and patient care is in your hands, your heart, and your head. Great wishes, great health, and GREAT THINKING.

REFERENCE

Begley, S. (1993, June 28). The puzzle of genius: Where do great minds come from? And why are there no Einsteins, Freuds or Picassos today? *Newsweek*, pp. 46–50.

NANDA APPROVED NURSING DIAGNOSES

Pattern 1: Exchanging

1.1.2.1	Altered Nutrition: More than body requirements
1.1.2.2	Altered Nutrition: Less than body requirements
1.1.2.3	Altered Nutrition: Potential for more than body requirements
1.2.1.1	High Risk for Infection
1.2.2.1	High Risk for Altered Body Temperature
1.2.2.2	Hypothermia
1.2.2.3	Hyperthermia
1.2.2.4	Ineffective Thermoregulation
1.2.3.1	Dysreflexia
1.3.1.1	Constipation
1.3.1.1.1	Perceived Constipation
1.3.1.1.2	Colonic Constipation
1.3.1.2	Diarrhea
1.3.1.3	Bowel Incontinence
1.3.2	Altered Urinary Elimination
1.3.2.1.1	Stress Incontinence
1.3.2.1.2	Reflex Incontinence
1.3.2.1.3	Urge Incontinence
1.3.2.1.4	Functional Incontinence
1.3.2.1.5	Total Incontinence
1.3.2.2	Urinary Retention
1.4.1.1	Altered (Specify Type) Tissue Perfusion (Renal, cerebral, cardiopulmonary, gastrointestinal, peripheral)
1.4.1.2.1	Fluid Volume Excess
1.4.1.2.2.1	Fluid Volume Deficit
1.4.1.2.2.2	High Risk for Fluid Volume Deficit
1.4.2.1	Decreased Cardiac Output
1.5.1.1	Impaired Gas Exchange
1.5.1.2	Ineffective Airway Clearance
1.5.1.3	Ineffective Breathing Pattern
1.5.1.3.1	Inability to Sustain Spontaneous Ventilation
1.5.1.3.2	Dysfunctional Ventilatory Weaning Response (DVWR)
1.6.1	High Risk for Injury
1.6.1.1	High Risk for Suffocation
1.6.1.2	High Risk for Poisoning
1.6.1.3	High Risk for Trauma
1.6.1.4	High Risk for Aspiration
1.6.1.5	High Risk for Disuse Syndrome
1.6.2	Altered Protection
1.6.2.1	Impaired Tissue Integrity
1.6.2.1.1	Altered Oral Mucous Membrane
1.6.2.1.2.1	Impaired Skin Integrity
1.6.2.1.2.2	High Risk for Impaired Skin Integrity

Pattern 2: Communicating

2.1.1.1	Impaired Verbal Communication

Pattern 3: Relating

3.1.1	Impaired Social Interaction
3.1.2	Social Isolation
3.2.1	Altered Role Performance
3.2.1.1.1	Altered Parenting
3.2.1.1.2	High Risk for Altered Parenting
3.2.1.2.1	Sexual Dysfunction
3.2.2	Altered Family Processes
3.2.2.1	Caregiver Role Strain
3.2.2.2	High Risk for Caregiver Role Strain
3.2.3.1	Parental Role Conflict
3.3	Altered Sexuality Patterns

Pattern 4: Valuing

4.1.1	Spiritual Distress (distress of the human spirit)

Pattern 5: Choosing

5.1.1.1	Ineffective Individual Coping
5.1.1.1.1	Impaired Adjustment
5.1.1.1.2	Defensive Coping
5.1.1.1.3	Ineffective Denial
5.1.2.1.1	Ineffective Family Coping: Disabling
5.1.2.1.2	Ineffective Family Coping: Compromised
5.1.2.2	Family Coping: Potential for Growth
5.2.1	Ineffective Management of Therapeutic Regimen (Individuals)
5.2.1.1	Noncompliance (Specify)
5.3.1.1	Decisional Conflict (Specify)
5.4	Health Seeking Behaviors (Specify)

Pattern 6: Moving

6.1.1.1	Impaired Physical Mobility
6.1.1.1.1	High Risk for Peripheral Neurovascular Dysfunction
6.1.1.2	Activity Intolerance
6.1.1.2.1	Fatigue
6.1.1.3	High Risk for Activity Intolerance
6.2.1	Sleep Pattern Disturbance
6.3.1.1	Diversional Activity Deficit
6.4.1.1	Impaired Home Maintenance Management
6.4.2	Altered Health Maintenance
6.5.1	Feeding Self Care Deficit
6.5.1.1	Impaired Swallowing
6.5.1.2	Ineffective Breastfeeding
6.5.1.2.1	Interrupted Breastfeeding
6.5.1.3	Effective Breastfeeding
6.5.1.4	Ineffective Infant Feeding Pattern
6.5.2	Bathing/Hygiene Self Care Deficit
6.5.3	Dressing/Grooming Self Care Deficit
6.5.4	Toileting Self Care Deficit
6.6	Altered Growth and Development
6.7	Relocation Stress Syndrome

Pattern 7: Perceiving

7.1.1	Body Image Disturbance
7.1.2.	Self Esteem Disturbance
7.1.2.1	Chronic Low Self Esteem
7.1.2.2	Situational Low Self Esteem
7.1.3	Personal Identity Disturbance
7.2	Sensory/Perceptual Alterations (Specify) (Visual, auditory, kinesthetic, gustatory, tactile, olfactory)
7.2.1.1	Unilateral Neglect
7.3.1	Hopelessness
7.3.2	Powerlessness

Pattern 8: Knowing

8.1.1	Knowledge Deficit (Specify)
8.3	Altered Thought Processes

Pattern 9: Feelings

9.1.1	Pain
9.1.1.1	Chronic Pain
9.2.1.1	Dysfunctional Grieving
9.2.1.2	Anticipatory Grieving
9.2.2	High Risk for Violence: Self-directed or directed at others
9.2.2.1	High Risk for Self-Mutilation
9.2.3	Post-Trauma Response
9.2.3.1	Rape-Trauma Syndrome
9.2.3.1.1	Rape-Trauma Syndrome: Compound Reaction
9.2.3.1.2	Rape-Trauma Syndrome: Silent Reaction
9.3.1	Anxiety
9.3.2	Fear

Purposes of the Tool

1. Guidance while preparing a student care plan to make sure all aspects of thinking and doing are included.
2. Self-evaluation to determine if one's care plan has included all the key elements.
3. Peer or instructor evaluation of plans to provide either initial evaluation or validation of the care planner's self-evaluation.

How to Use

1. Make a photocopy of the tool for each plan to be evaluated.
2. Compare the items listed on the far left with any evidence on the written care plan that indicates the item has occurred.
3. Use the "self ranking" scale at the top of each page to judge how well each item was achieved. If there is no evidence indicate a "0" or "N/A" for "not applicable."
4. Add any additional supporting comments or ideas for improvement in the column on the far right.
5. At the end of each of the three sections, in the areas provided, briefly discuss the care planner's overall ability in thinking and doing.
6. Write a summary of additional comments or suggestions for growth in the final section.

Optional Uses for Tracking Nursing Thinking

1. Assign numerical value to each of the items and tally the scores for each. Some items can have more weight than others, for example, "are [objectives] client centered" might be weighted at 1 point, and "Provide rationale for all nursing actions" might be weighted at 2 points. The number of points would then be multiplied by the self-ranking number for a total score for that particular item.
2. Develop a grading scale based on the scores.
3. Keep a notebook of all the checklists completed over the semester or course to document and acknowledge growth and improvement.

TRACKING NURSING THINKING CHECKLIST		
Student _____	**Patient Initials** _____	**Date** _____
What is the concern? **(Conclusions of Assessment)**	**Self** **Ranking**	**Supporting Comments/Plans For** **Improvement**
Did I ...	0...No 1...Good 2...Better 3...Best	
Develop a therapeutic relationship		
Collect objective, subjective data and necessary inferences?		
Know population norms for comparison? (content knowledge)		
Compare data to population norms?		
Compare data to individual norms?		
Use branching questions?		
Use D.E.T.A.I.L. questions?		
Develop hunches?		
Identify data gaps?		
Use directed data collection to fill gaps?		
Cluster data effectively?		
Select the best clusters?		
Select the best labels for the clusters?		
Identify all conclusions of assessment (strengths, nursing diagnoses, interdisciplinary problems and problems for referral)?		
Develop conclusions that reflect strong content knowledge?		
Consider alternative conclusions, differential diagnoses?		
Use proper nursing diagnosis format?		
Support all conclusions with data?		
Support all related factors with data?		
Identify all related factors for all nursing diagnoses?		
Think toward planning when finalizing all conclusions?		
Place self in patient's shoes?		
Consider the "big picture" when finalizing all conclusions of assessment?		
Clearly document all data and conclusions of assessment?		

MY OVERALL ABILITY IN THINKING AND DOING DURING ASSESSMENT IS:

TRACKING NURSING THINKING Checklist p. 2 Student_____Date_____		
How can the concern be altered by nursing care? (Conclusions of Planning and Implementation)	Self Ranking	Supporting Comments/Plans for Improvement
Did I...	0=No 1=Good 2=Better 3=Best	
Make the patient a partner in planning?		
Use the patient's strengths in planning?		
Use the best resources to design care?		
Set priorities based on the guidelines, and the "big picture"?		
Considered life threatening issues?		
Considered safety issues?		
Considered the patient's priorities?		
Considered the nurse's priorities?		
Establish goals that:		
Match with the conclusions?		
Are client-centered?		
Have a realistic time frame?		
Are indicators of direction to move?		
Establish objectives that:		
Fit with their respective goals?		
Are client-centered?		
Are measurable?		
Include specific criteria?		
Address all behaviors, cognitive, affective, psychomotor, and changes in patient conditions beyond the patient's control?		
Develop nursing orders that:		
Fit with each objective?		
Are nurse-centered?		
Give clear directions?		
Are realistic?		
Are clinically supported by sound rationale?		
Provide rationale for all nursing orders?		
Identify sources of rationale?		
Design care for all nursing diagnoses, interdisciplinary problems and problems for referral?		
Design care that used effective time and resource management?		
Use standardized care plans as a trigger to thinking and individualized care?		
Clearly document the nursing care plan?		
Implement care safely?		
Implement care efficiently?		
MY OVERALL ABILITY IN THINKING AND DOING DURING PLANNING AND IMPLEMENTATION IS:		

TRACKING NURSING THINKING Checklist p. 3 Student_____Date_____		
Did the plan work? **(Conclusions of Evaluation)**	**Self Ranking**	**Supporting Comments/Plans for Improvement**
Did I...	0=No 1=Good 2=Better 3=Best	
Establish appropriate outcome criteria (objectives) during the planning?		
Ask patient to assist in the evaluation process?		
Determine patient's progress toward objectives and goals?		
Clearly document patient's progress toward objectives and goals?		
Determine degree of patient's achievement of all goals and objectives?		
Clearly document patient's achievements toward all goals and objectives?		
Determine if the patient's concerns/problems were resolved?		
Clearly document the status of concerns/problems?		
Modify the plan of care periodically to adapt to the patient's changing needs?		
Clearly document modifications in plan?		
Backtrack through the nursing process to find areas of breakdown in thinking if there were any?		

MY OVERALL ABILITY IN THINKING AND DOING DURING EVALUATION IS:

ADDITIONAL COMMENTS/SUGGESTIONS FOR GROWTH:

Bibliography

Allen, D.G., Bowers, B. & Diekelmann, N. (1989). Writing to learn: A reconceptualiztion of thinking and writing in the nursing curriculum. *Journal of Nursing Education, 28*(1), 6–11.

American Nurses' Association. (1980). *Nursing: A social policy statement*. Kansas City: ANA.

Bandman, E. L. & Bandman, B. (1988). *Critical thinking in nursing*. East Norwalk, CT: Appleton & Lange.

Becker, H. A. & MacCabe, N. (1994). Indicators of critical thinking, communication, and therapeutic intervention among first-line nursing supervisors. *Nurse Educator, 19*(2), 15–19.

Belenky, M. F., Clinchy, B. M., Goldberger, N. R., & Tarule, J. M. (1986). *Women's ways of knowing: The development of self, voice, and the mind*. New York: Basic Books.

Bell, E. A. (1991). Debate: a strategy for teaching critical thinking. *Nurse Educator, 16*(2), 6–7.

Benner, P. (1984). *From novice to expert: Power and excellence in nursing practice*. Menlo Park, CA: Addison-Wesley.

Benner, P. & Tanner, C. (1987). Clinical judgement: How expert nurses use intuition. *American Journal of Nursing, 87*, 23–31.

Bevis, E. O. (1993). All in all, it was a pretty good funeral. *Journal of Nursing Education, 32*, 101–105.

Bowers, B. & McCarthy, D. (1993). Developing analytic thinking skills in early undergraduate education. *Journal of Nursing Education, 32*(3), 107–114.

Brookfield, S. (1993). On impostorship, cultural suicide, and other dangers: how nurses learn critical thinking. *Journal of Continuing Education in Nursing, 24*(5), 197–205.

Brookfield, S. D. (1987). *Developing critical thinkers*. San Francisco: Jossey-Bass.

Brown, H. N. & Sorrell, J. M. (1993). Use of clinical journals to enhance critical thinking. *Nurse Educator, 18*(5), 16–19.

Brykczynski, K. A. (1989). An interpretive study describing the clinical judgment of nurse practitioners. *Scholarly Inquiry for Nursing Practice: An International Journal, 3*(2), 75–112.

Burnard, P. (1989). Developing critical ability in nurse education. *Nurse Education Today, 9*, 271–275.

Cameron, J. (1992). *The artist's way: A spiritual path to higher creativity*. Los Angeles: Tarcher/Perigee.

Carnevali, D. L. & Thomas, M. D. (1993). *Diagnostic reasoning and treatment decision making in nursing*. Philadelphia: J.B. Lippincott.

Carpenito, L. J. (1993). *Nursing diagnosis application to clinical practice* (5th ed.). Philadelphia: J.B. Lippincott.

Chaffee, J. (1990). *Thinking critically*. Boston: Houghton Mifflin.

Chinn, P. L. (1989). Nursing patterns of knowing and feminist thought. *Nursing & Health Care, 10*, 71–75.

Cholowski, K. M. & Chan, L. K. S. (1992). Diagnostic reasoning among second-year nursing students. *Journal of Advanced Nursing, 17*, 1171–1181.

Costa, A. L., Hanson, R., Silver, H. F., & Strong, R. W. (1985). Building a repertoire of strategies. In A. L. Costa (Ed.), *Developing minds: A resource book for teaching thinking* (pp. 141–143). Alexandria, VA: Association for Supervision and Curriculum Development.

Diekelmann, N. L. (1992). Learning-as-testing: A heideggerian hermeneutical analysis of the lived experiences of students and teachers in nursing. *Advances in Nursing Science, 14*(3), 72–83.

Dreyfus, H. L. & Dreyfus, S. E. (1986). *Mind over machine.* New York: The Free Press.

Eyres, S. J., Loustau, A., & Ersek, M. (1992). Ways of knowing among beginning students in nursing. *Journal of Nursing Education, 31*(4), 175–180.

Facione, P.A., Sanchez, C.A. & Facione, N.C. (1994). *Are students disposed to think?* Millbrae, CA: The California Academic Press.

Facione, P.A. (1992). *Critical thinking: What it is and why it counts. A resource paper for students.* Millbrae, CA: The California Academic press.

Facione, P.A. (1991). *Using the California critical thinking skills test in research, evaluation, & assessment.* Millbrae, CA: The California Academic Press (ERIC Doc. No: ED 337 498).

Farrel, P. & Bramadat, I. J. (1990). Paradigm case analysis and stimulated recall: strategies for developing clinical reasoning skills. *Clinical Nurse Specialist, 4*(3), 153–157.

Gehrke, P. (1994). Finding voices through writing. *Nurse Educator, 19*(2), 28–30.

Gordon M. (1994). *Nursing diagnosis process and application* (3rd ed.). St. Louis: Mosby.

Harbison, J. (1991). Clinical decision making in nursing. *Journal of Advanced Nursing, 16*, 404–407.

Hart, L. A. (1983). *Human brain and human learning.* New York: Longman.

Heinrich, K. T. (1992). The intimate dialogue: journal writing by students. *Nurse Educator, 17* (6), 17–21.

Jones, E. A. & Ratcliff, G. (1993). *Critical thinking skills for college students.* University Park, PA: National Center on Postsecondary Teaching, Learning, and Assessment.

Jones, S. A. & Brown, L. N. (1991). Critical thinking: impact on nursing education. *Journal of Advanced Nursing, 16*, 529–533.

Kintgen-Andrews, J. (1991). Critical thinking and nursing education: perplexities and insights. *Journal of Nursing Education, 30*(4), 152–157.

Klaassens, E. (1992). Strategies to enhance problem solving. *Nurse Educator, 17*(3), 28–30.

Lipman, M. (1991). *Thinking in education.* New York: Cambridge University Press.

Marrelli, T. M. (1992). *Nursing documentation handbook.* St. Louis: Mosby.

McCloskey, J. C. & Bulechek, G. M. (Eds.). (1992). *Nursing interventions classification (NIC).* St. Louis: Mosby.

McFarland, G. K. & McFarlane, E. A. (1993). *Nursing diagnosis & intervention* (2nd ed.). St. Louis: Mosby.

McKeachie, W. J. (1986). *Teaching tips: A guidebook for the beginning college teacher* (8th ed.). Lexington, MA: D.C. Heath.

McPeck, J. E. (1990) *Teaching critical thinking.* New York: Routledge.

Miller, M. A. (1992). Outcomes evaluation: measuring critical thinking. *Journal of Advanced Nursing, 17*, 1401–1407.

Miller, M. A. & Malcolm, N. S. (1990). Critical thinking in the nursing curriculum. *Nursing & Health Care, 11*(2), 67–73.

Myers, C. (1986). *Teaching students to think critically.* San Francisco: Jossey-Bass.

Norris, S. (Ed.). (1992). *The generalizability of critical thinking: multiple perspectives on an educational ideal*. New York: Teachers College Press.

North American Nursing Diagnosis Association. (1992). *NANDA nursing diagnoses: Definitions and classification 1992*. Philadelphia: NANDA.

Nosich, G. M. (1994). Where to begin? How to design classes to teach for thinking. *Educational Vision The Magazine for Critical Thinking*. 2(2), 20–21.

Pascarella, E. & Terenzini, P. (1991). *How college affects students*. San Francisco: Jossey-Bass.

Paul, R. (1992). *Critical thinking: What every person needs to survive in a rapidly changing world* (rev. 2nd ed.). Santa Rosa, CA: The Foundation for Critical Thinking.

Perkins, D., Jay, E., & Tishman, S. (1993). *Assessing thinking: A framework for measuring critical thinking and problem solving skills at the college level*. Paper prepared for the National Center for Education Statistics.

Perry, W. G. (1970). *Forms of intellectual and ethical development in the college years*. New York: Holt, Rinehart and Winston.

Pesut, D. J. & Herman, J. (1992). Metacognitive skills in diagnostic reasoning: Making the implicit explicit. *Nursing Diagnosis*, 3, 148–154.

Polin, L. (1993). Three ways writing is thinking. *Writing-Notebook: Visions for Learning*, 10(4), 31–33.

Pond, E.F., Bradshaw, M. J., & Turner, S. L. (1991). Teaching strategies for critical thinking. *Nurse Educator*, 16(6), 18–22.

Reinsmith, W. A. (1993). Ten fundamental truths about learning. *The National Teaching & Learning Forum*, 2(4), 7–8.

Saarmann, L., Freitas, L., Rapps, J., & Riegel, B. (1992). The relationship of education to critical thinking ability and values among nurses: Socialization into professional nursing. *Journal of Professional Nursing*, 8(1), 26–34.

Sarosi, G. M. & Taylor, J. J. (1994). Strategies for teaching nursing research. *Western Journal of Nursing Research*, 16, 221–25.

Schank, M. J. (1990) Wanted: nurses with critical thinking skills. *Journal of Continuing Education in Nursing*, 21(2), 86–89.

Swartz, R. J. & Perkins, D. N. (1990) *Teaching thinking: Issues and approaches*. Pacific Grove, CA: Midwest Publications.

Tanner, C. A., Padrick, K. P., Westfall, U. E., & Putzier, D. J. (1987). Diagnostic reasoning strategies of nurses and nursing students. *Nursing Research*, 36, 358–363.

Villas, P. (1993). Thinking and writing. *Journal of Health Education*, 24 (1), 57.

White, N. E., Beardslee, N. Q., Peters, D., & Supples, J. M. (1990). Promoting critical thinking skills. *Nurse Educator*, 15 (5), 16–19.

Worrell, P. J. (1990). Metacognition: implications for instruction in nursing education. *Journal of Nursing Education*, 29 (4), 170–175.

Yura, H. & Walsh, M. B. (1988). *The nursing process: Assessing, planning, implementing, evaluating* (5th ed.). East Norwalk, CT: Appleton & Lange.

The letter *f* following a page number indicates a figure;
the letter *t* indicates a table; and *d* indicates a display.

Rubenfeld G./Scheffer B.: Critical Thinking in Nursing: An Interactive Approach. © 1995 J.B. Lippincott Company